Carbon-Based Nanocarriers for Drug Delivery

Mihir Kumar Purkait,
Ankush D. Sontakke, and Anweshan

CRC Press
Taylor & Francis Group
Boca Raton London New York

CRC Press is an imprint of the
Taylor & Francis Group, an **informa** business

First edition published 2024
by CRC Press
2385 Executive Center Drive, Suite 320, Boca Raton, FL 33431–2742

and by CRC Press
4 Park Square, Milton Park, Abingdon, Oxon, OX14 4RN

CRC Press is an imprint of Taylor & Francis Group, LLC

© 2024 Mihir Kumar Purkait, Ankush D. Sontakke, and Anweshan

Library of Congress Cataloging-in-Publication Data
Names: Purkait, Mihir Kumar, author. | Sontakke, Ankush D., author. |
   Anweshan. (Anweshan), author.
Title: Carbon-based nanocarriers for drug delivery / Mihir Kumar Purkait,
   Ankush D. Sontakke, Anweshan.
Description: First edition. | Boca Raton, FL : CRC Press, 2024. | Includes bibliographical
   references and index.
Identifiers: LCCN 2023020515 (print) | LCCN 2023020516 (ebook) | ISBN 9781032414447
   (hardback) | ISBN 9781032414478 (paperback) | ISBN 9781003358114 (ebook)
Subjects: MESH: Nanoparticle Drug Delivery System | Carbon | Nanostructures
Classification: LCC RS201.N35 (print) | LCC RS201.N35 (ebook) | NLM QV 785 |
   DDC 615.1/9—dc23/eng/20230727
LC record available at https://lccn.loc.gov/2023020515
LC ebook record available at https://lccn.loc.gov/2023020516

ISBN: 978-1-032-41444-7 (hbk)
ISBN: 978-1-032-41447-8 (pbk)
ISBN: 978-1-003-35811-4 (ebk)

DOI: 10.1201/9781003358114

Typeset in Times
by Apex CoVantage, LLC

*This book is dedicated to our families and friends,
for their endless support and motivation.*

Contents

Preface

It is well known that "Health is wealth" for every individual living on the earth. The rapid industrialization, pollution, and current living style of humans have created numerous threats to their health by several death-causing diseases. Meanwhile, these diseases can be cured by modern medical practices such as allopathic drugs. Still, these drugs could cause numerous side effects and suffer from a lack of efficacy due to several factors. It was observed that drugs would react with the substrates of targeted sites such as cancer cells for employing the therapeutic tasks and may interact with the normal tissues and result in side effects. However, the application of suitably designed targeted drug delivery systems (DDSs) via novel drug carriers can surmount all such obstacles and limitations of drugs. Recent advances in nanotechnology have investigated a variety of nanomaterials with improved surface characteristics for their application in targeted DDSs. Carbon as a parent material and its nano-derivatives, such as fullerene, graphene, graphene oxide (GO), and carbon nanotubes (CNTs), have provided great adaptability for targeted DDSs with numerous therapeutics.

This book is designed to give a practical approach to the use of carbon-based nanomaterials (CBNs) as nanocarriers in targeted DDSs for the treatment of cancer, neurodegenerative diseases, gene and peptide delivery, and other major therapeutics. This book deals with the fundamentals and principles of CBNs with their sources, attributes, classification, and real-world applications. It elucidates the significance of DDSs, their historical aspects and classification, followed by the efficacy of CBNs as drug carriers. The extensive chapters in this book further represent the recent developments in the synthesis, functionalization, and application of CBNs such as graphene, GO, graphene quantum dots (GQDs), fullerene, CNT, and their nanohybrids in major therapeutics. In addition, smart carbon-based nanocarriers and toxicological aspects related to the use of these CBNs in DDSs are explored with their remediation strategies. Subsequently, this book explores various case studies related to the delivery of Doxil® and Docetaxel-PNP. The chapters will provide a detailed description of various CBNs, their surface characteristics, synthesis, functionalization methods, and application in targeted DDSs.

The content of the book was designed based on the belief that the recent developments, knowledge gaps related to new research areas, their implications, and future prospects must be addressed continuously for vigorous research outputs. It will widen the scope for a better and fundamental understanding of the topic as well as provide potential future research opportunities in DDS to the reader. Apart from undergraduate and postgraduate students, this book is strongly recommended for people concerned with the chemical, biomedical, material science, biotechnology, and pharmaceutical fields of research. We are also grateful to all the owners of copyright who have kindly allowed us to reproduce diagrams and tables from their publications (reference in the text).

Finally, we continue to acknowledge our families, who provided patience, understanding, and encouragement throughout. We believe that this book is the right blend of both experimental and theoretical studies providing tremendous potential for knowledge and helping researchers and academicians to contribute toward a sustainable solution on health.

Prof. Mihir Kumar Purkait
Ankush D. Sontakke
Anweshan

About the Authors

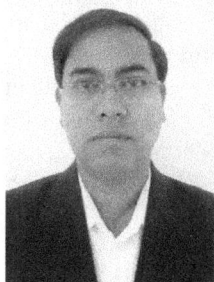

Dr. Mihir Kumar Purkait is a professor in the Department of Chemical Engineering at Indian Institute of Technology Guwahati (IITG). Presently, he is Chair Professor of National Jal Jeevan Mission (NJJM), Ministry of JalShakti (Government of India). He is energetically involved in frontier areas of chemical engineering with his major research interest in the field of advanced separation processes and material science.

Prof. Purkait has made outstanding contributions in translational and applied research. The quality and quantity of his research are reflected in the large number of publications, patents, technology transfers, start-ups, projects, consultancies, and involvement with various national and international scientific committees. His work has remarkable relevance in societal as well as industrial sectors.

He has more than 20 years of experience in research and academics. He has published more than 300 papers in different reputable international journals with h-index of 69, has 12 granted patents, and made three technology transfers. He has authored 15 books and completed 42 sponsored projects/consultancies from various funding agencies. Prof. Purkait has supervised 22 PhD students on fundamental and applied research.

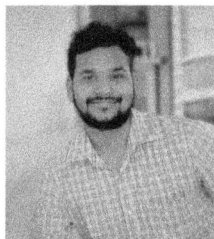

Ankush D. Sontakke is pursuing his PhD in the Department of Chemical Engineering from the Indian Institute of Technology Guwahati (IITG). He received his master's degree (2016) in chemical engineering from Sant Longowal Institute of Engineering and Technology, Longowal, Punjab and B. Tech degree (2013) from Jawaharlal Darda Institute of Engineering and Technology, Yavatmal, Maharashtra. He worked at Multi Organics Private Limited, Chandrapur, Maharashtra, for one year (2013–2014). Also, he served as an assistant professor in the Department of Chemical Engineering at Chandigarh University, Gharuan, Mohali, Punjab, during 2016–2017. His research activities are focused on graphene and related materials such as graphene oxide (GO), graphene oxide nanoscrolls (GONS), graphene quantum dots (GQDs), and their application in drug delivery systems (DDSs). He is working on the advancement in DDS using various structural, morphological, and functional modifications of carbon-based nanocarriers to improve their surface characteristics, biocompatibility, toxicity toward cancer cells, loading, and release behavior. He has been closely working in the area of carbon-based nanocarriers and nanohybrids for their sustainable synthesis as well as application in anticancer drug delivery and stimuli-responsive carriers for the controlled release of drugs. He is also exploring strategies for therapeutic targeting and controlled drug delivery. He has published many peer-reviewed articles in reputable international journals and published several book chapters.

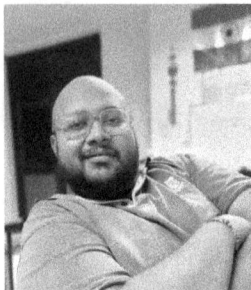

Anweshan received his B. Tech degree (2012) in chemical engineering and technology from the National Institute of Technology Durgapur, West Bengal, India. After completing his B. Tech, he joined the Tinplate Company of India Limited (manufacturing sector) and continued his services there as a senior engineer for three years (2012–2016). He then explored the start-up ecosystem growing in India and joined the Grow Green India Foundation as a junior research associate and then transferred to RD Grow Green India Pvt. Ltd., an enterprise of the foundation, as a research associate (2016–2018). He is pursuing his doctorate in chemical engineering from the Indian Institute of Technology Guwahati, Assam, India. His research work is dedicated to the detection of contaminants in water and wastewater using low-cost green synthesized nanoparticles and their subsequent treatment through electrocoagulation. He is working on the fabrication of metallic oxide nanomaterials via green pathways for sensing trace organic compounds and pathogens in water. He is also working on synthesizing carbon-based nanohybrids focused on metal-impregnated nanohybrids and hydrogels for their applications as absorbents to remove pathogens. Further, his works involve the design of stand-alone electrocoagulation reactors and integrated systems for the remediation of arsenic, fluoride, and iron-infested groundwater. He has several patents and published many peer-reviewed articles in reputable international journals.

1 Fundamentals of Carbon-Based Nanomaterials

1.1 INTRODUCTION TO CARBON-BASED NANOMATERIALS (CBNS)

Carbon is among the most adaptable element in the periodic table, primarily due to its enormous, diverse array of types and degrees of bonds that may establish together with it or with numerous other elements [1,2]. Furthermore, the possibility of a diversity of allotropes is enabled by the potential of carbon orbitals to hybridize in the sp, sp^2, and sp^3 orientations. Up until this point, the three naturally prevalent allotropes of carbon, namely, graphite, diamond, and amorphous carbon, have been supplemented by those produced artificially, like graphene and its derivatives, fullerenes, carbon nanotubes (CNTs), quantum dots (QDs), and nanodiamonds (NDs) [2,3]; contemporary attention on carbon-based nanomaterials (CBNs) has expanded significantly over the past several decades, beginning with the advent of fullerenes (1985) and subsequently with those of CNTs (1991) and graphene (2004). Due to their unique characteristics, these CBNs are employed extensively in a diverse array of sectors, including material science [4], energy generation and storage [5], environmental studies [6], biological [7,8], and biomedical [9,10].

Graphene and CNTs, two of the myriad carbon nanomaterials, are perhaps the best-known examples and have been the subject of in-depth research because of their exceptional mechanical robustness, thermal and electrical conductivity, and optical characteristics. Graphene and CNTs have superior Young's modulus and tensile strengths, which may approach 1–1.2 TPa and 120–150 GPa, respectively [9,11]. In comparison to copper, which has a thermal conductivity of 401 W/mK, graphene has a thermal conductivity of ~5000 W/mK. With a conductance of 10^6 S/m and an impedance of 31 Ω/sq, graphene's electrons may move with ultra-high mobility of (2×10^5 cm^2/V. s), which itself is 140 times greater than silicon's. The sp^2 hybridization, whereby it provides an additional electron to the π bond and results in strong conductivity at ambient temperature, is the cause of this exceptionally high mobility [12]. CNTs exhibit thermal conductivities of around 2000–3500 W/mK, and the current density in their metallic form was several times greater than that of metals like copper [13]. Single-layer graphene has a maximum light absorption ratio of 2.5% [14]. Utilizing these features for a variety of applications, such as photovoltaic and energy storage, membrane processes, ultra-light composites, and biomedical engineering, constituted a significant share of scientific research [15,16]. Graphene and CNTs are excellent electrical conductors by nature, and it is possible to regulate their biocompatibility [17].

DOI: 10.1201/9781003358114-1

The potential of CBNs to transport therapeutic drug molecules and enable the imaging of cells and tissues essential for diagnosing and treating unhealthy and destroyed tissues had a significant influence on the biomedical domain in recent years. The potential biological uses of CBNs include drug and gene delivery, photothermal and photodynamic treatment, as well as bioimaging, biosensing, fluorescent labeling of cells, and regenerative medicine [10,18]. Since CBNs have inherent fluorescence, a limited emission spectrum that can be tuned, and excellent photostability, they may be used to sequence and diagnose cells and tissues. Additionally, their surfaces can be altered with a variety of functional groups to improve their attributes. CBNs are among the most preferred and competent alternatives for drug delivery applications due to their high surface areas and superior opto-electronic and electromechanical features [19].

One of the most important concerns for the real-world applications of CBNs is their toxicity or biological safety, which is associated with their aqueous stability and interactions with tissues and cells [20]. The potential applications of CBNs in cancer and inflammation therapies have been sparked by certain recent investigations. For instance, when CBN is ingested by cancer cells, it stimulates the generation of reactive oxygen species (ROS), which causes lipid and DNA destruction as well as induces cell apoptosis [21]. Additionally, the enzymatic activity of monocytes is impacted by graphene nanomaterials, which raise ROS levels and damage the mitochondrial membrane, leading to apoptosis, the cell death mechanism [22,23]. Contrarily, biofunctionalized CBN enhances delivery effectiveness by reducing clearance and promoting retention throughout the body.

As stated, CBNs comprise graphene and related materials, CNTs, fullerene, QDs, etc. Excluding the capped ends of CNTs, wherein carbon atoms form pentagons, or active functional groups, each of the previously mentioned nanomaterials contains a substantial portion of sp^2-bonded carbon atoms; however, each of them has various forms based on the way the hexagonal lattice is configured. The fact that these various forms bestow distinctive and differentiating characteristics despite being made up of identical atoms is a significant attribute that must be explored. The physicochemical properties of CBNs are the deciding parameters for their relevant applications. Therefore, it is necessary to investigate and understand the structure, morphology, and other surface characteristics, such as electrical conductance, mechanical strength, aqueous stability, and biocompatibility of these nanomaterials through advanced characterization and biological assay techniques.

In line with this, the present chapter describes the fundamentals of CBNs, including their structural attributes, physicochemical properties, and related application in the practical world. It also elucidates the classification of CBNs such as fullerene, QDs, CNTs, graphene nanosheets, nanoribbons, nanoscrolls, and graphene oxide (GO) based on their dimensionalities along with their surface characteristics and scope of applications. Numerous characterization techniques generally employed to investigate the surface morphology and other properties of CBNs are described in brief. Furthermore, the recent advances in the applications of CBNs in therapeutic, sensing, environmental remediation, and catalysis are highlighted. It is believed that the fundamental understanding and recent developments in the applications of CBNs will provide substantial information to the scientific community working in material science, nanotechnology, biomedical, and pharmaceutical sectors to further explore the potential of these nanomaterials in real-world applications.

1.2 CLASSIFICATIONS AND ATTRIBUTES OF CBNS

The CBNs are classified into four categories based on their dimensions higher than the nanoscale (100 nm), namely, zero-dimensional (0-D), one-dimensional (1-D), two-dimensional (2-D), and three-dimensional (3-D) nanomaterials. In the case of 0-D nanomaterials, all the dimensions are at the nanoscale; therefore, these nanomaterials are known as dimensionless nanomaterials. Examples of 0-D CBNs are fullerene and quantum dots. The 1-D CBNs such as CNTs, nanoscrolls, and nanoribbons have one of their dimensions above the nanoscale; consequently, two of their dimensions are at the nanoscale. The 2-D CBNs have one of their dimensions below the nanoscale, for example, graphene, GO. Similarly, the 3-D CBNs, such as graphite and nanodiamond (ND), do not have any of their dimension at the nanoscale. The structural and physicochemical features of these CBNs are elaborated subsequently.

1.2.1 ZERO-DIMENSIONAL

1.2.1.1 Fullerene

The first fullerene, C_{60}, was discovered in 1985, but the family of fullerenes also comprises a large variety of other carbon-based compounds with various symmetries and atom counts. The most prevalent fullerene, also known as "Buckminsterfullerene," is made up of 60 carbon atoms organized in 20 hexagons and 12 pentagons, giving it the shape of a hollow sphere. The extremely stable and symmetrical structure of C_{60} garnered a lot of attention. Zero-dimensional fullerenes are thought to have highly intriguing chemical and physical characteristics for medical and technological purposes [24].

The primary function of fullerenes is to serve as a photosensitizer for the photoproduction of singlet oxygen ($^1O_2$) ROS; as a result, they are used in photodynamic treatment (PDT) and blood sterilization [25–27]. Unfortunately, fullerene dispersibility is a significant barrier to its utilization in nanomedicine. The fundamental issue is their limited solubility in many solvents, particularly water, where singlet oxygen has a prolonged lifespan. To increase fullerenes' solubility in water, a number of techniques have been devised to functionalize them with hydrophilic groups [28,29]. The ability of fullerene to scavenge free radicals like reactive oxygen species (ROS) and reactive nitrogen species (RNS) and serve as an antioxidant has boosted its adoption in biological applications. Cells can be shielded against nitric oxide-induced apoptosis with the use of derivatives of glutathione C_{60} [30]. The IgE-dependent mediator produced in human mast cells (hMCs) and peripheral blood basophils was substantially suppressed when pre-incubated with C_{60}, confirming the function of fullerenes as a potent inhibitor of allergic reaction [31]. Fullerenes may potentially act as photosensitizers. Based on the polarity of the media, they can absorb photons in the visible and UV range, producing photo-excited fullerene molecules in the triplet state and, in some cases, singlet oxygen or ROS. Moreover, to boost the quantum yield (QY) of ROS generation, fullerenes could be integrated with light-harvesting antennas. The utilization of fullerenes in PDT can thus be exploited to cure cancer and eradicate germs. The fabrication of molecular or particulate structures with one or even more organic compounds covalently linked to the fullerene cage surface in a geometrically regulated fashion is made possible by the cage-like nanoscale structure of fullerenes. Targeted drug transport across biological membranes and receptor ligands for antagonizing cellular and enzymatic activities are appropriate in this situation. An alternate method of preparing fullerenes for use in pharmaceutical applications, with improved dispersion, absorption, and delivery efficiency, is the liposome encapsulation [18].

Significant scientific advancements have been made in the field of fullerene therapeutics, although the lack of success in clinical investigations is a consequence of concerns about the long-term safety and toxicity of fullerenes. On the other hand, fullerene-based cosmetics have long been used in human skincare and have undergone clinical testing, indicating that, at minimum, external usage of fullerenes is acceptable [32,33]. Ample capacity is also offered for the encapsulation of atoms, compounds, and particles owing to the robust cage-like structure of fullerenes. For instance, water-soluble gadolinium metallofullerenes (gadofullerenes), which have a high relaxivity, are extremely intriguing MRI contrast agents. Fullerenes have the ability to self-assemble into fullerosomes, which can function as multivalent drug delivery systems (DDSs) with the potential for various targeting characteristics [34].

1.2.1.2   Quantum dots

Graphene quantum dots (GQDs) may be produced by slicing graphene into tiny fragments with diameters of a few nanometers (2–20 nm). The quantum confinement and edge effects increase with decreasing size, as has been demonstrated with graphene nanoribbons (GNRs), especially after their diameters fall underneath the 10 nm barrier [35]. This indicates that GQDs exhibit nonzero band gaps, in contrast to graphene sheets, which have a band gap of zero width and are less helpful in electrical and optoelectronic applications [36]. The key factors driving the rise in popularity of GQDs are their ease of synthesis from a virtually infinite variety of organic precursors (such as sugar, proteins, enzymes, etc.) and their robust photoluminescence (PL), which fluctuates in tandem with variations in band gap size [37,38]. Additionally, it has been proven that the chemical modification of GQDs has an impact on their PL and band gaps [35]. A strong emission band between 400 and 600 nm may be detected in their PL spectra. Moreover, GQDs are being researched to provide low-toxicity, environmentally acceptable substitutes that possess identical and desirable performance attributes as hazardous conventional (CdSe) QDs [39]. Although this issue is outside the purview of this book, it is essential to note that there is a large family of carbon quantum dots (CQDs) with outstanding PL characteristics [40,41].

CQD nanoparticles are made of carbon that is smaller than 10 nm in size. Sun et al. (2007) released the very first study on quantum-sized bright and colorful photoluminescence CQDs using laser ablation of a carbon target and a surface passivation approach [42]. CQDs have recently undergone substantial research to obtain high fluorescence QY utilizing simple synthesis techniques [43]. Natural polymers and other organic materials have often been used to produce CQDs.

CQDs have also been produced using amino acids [44], grape peel [45], apple juice [46], and vegetables [47]. Additionally, a number of straightforward and relatively inexpensive procedures have been devised for the synthesis of CQD, such as chemical and electrochemical oxidation [48], combustion/thermal microwave heating, hydrothermal carbonization [49], and pyrolysis [50]. Second, utilizing a one-step solvothermal technique and nitrogen-rich solvents like dimethyl-imidazolidinone (DMEU) and N-methyl-2-pyrrolidone (NMP), homogenous nitrogen-doped CQDs can be produced [51]. Recent advances in chemistry have made it simple to achieve -C(O)OH-modified CQDs, which is thought to be a novel approach to the acid assault on CNTs [52]. The fluorescence characteristics of the CQDs have also been tuned by incorporating surface flaws, adjusting their size, and implementing chemical functionalization.

1.2.2 ONE-DIMENSIONAL

1.2.2.1 Carbon Nanotubes

Carbon nanotubes (CNTs) are one-dimensional graphitic morphologies developed by rolling graphite/graphene sheets, which, along with graphite and fullerenes, may form a variety of carbon allotropes. Theoretically, a carbon nanotube is distinct because it is formed from a graphene sheet that has been rolled up and can have one or more walls [53]. The CNTs are mainly classified as SWCNT and MWCNT based on the existence of the number of graphene sheets within the nanotubes and the type of chirality. Single-wall carbon nanotubes (SWCNTs) are a kind of nanotube with a single wall that was first discovered in 1993 [54]. In contrast, those having numerous walls are known as multiwall carbon nanotubes (MWCNTs), and Iijima made this discovery in 1991 [55].

CNTs are cylindrical nanotubes that resemble buckytubes and have special features that make them useful in a variety of practical applications. CNTs display superior mechanical, electrical, thermal, and optical characteristics. Nanotubes have exceptional rigidity and toughness, as well as reversible folding and collapsing. CNTs are one of the stiffest substances known, but they have the ability to deform after being compressed. This is owing to the hexagonal network's high C-C bond stiffness, which results in an axial Young's modulus (E) of 1 TPa and tensile strength (σ) of 150 GPa [11]. In addition to simple elements, these carbon assemblages may generate a variety of configurations and forms. Beneath high pressure, nanotubes can merge, exchanging numerous sp^2 links for sp^3 bonds, allowing high-pressure nanotube linking to produce strong, infinite-length wires [11,56].

SWCNTs come in a variety of configurations and may be trundled up in several types of seamless tubes. Depending on their chirality and diameter, SWCNTs may be able to operate in this arrangement more clearly as a semiconducting, semimetallic, or metallic structure [57]. New techniques for synthesizing an array or tightly packed bundle of SWCNTs that meet reaction parameters that are economically possible and have ideal diameters less than 0.2 μm were disclosed in one of the US patents for the manufacturing of SWCNTs [58]. The lengths of SWCNT generally fall within the micrometers range, with diameters ranging from 0.4 to 2 to 3 nm. SWCNTs may often be bundled together and can be arranged hexagonally to produce a crystal-like

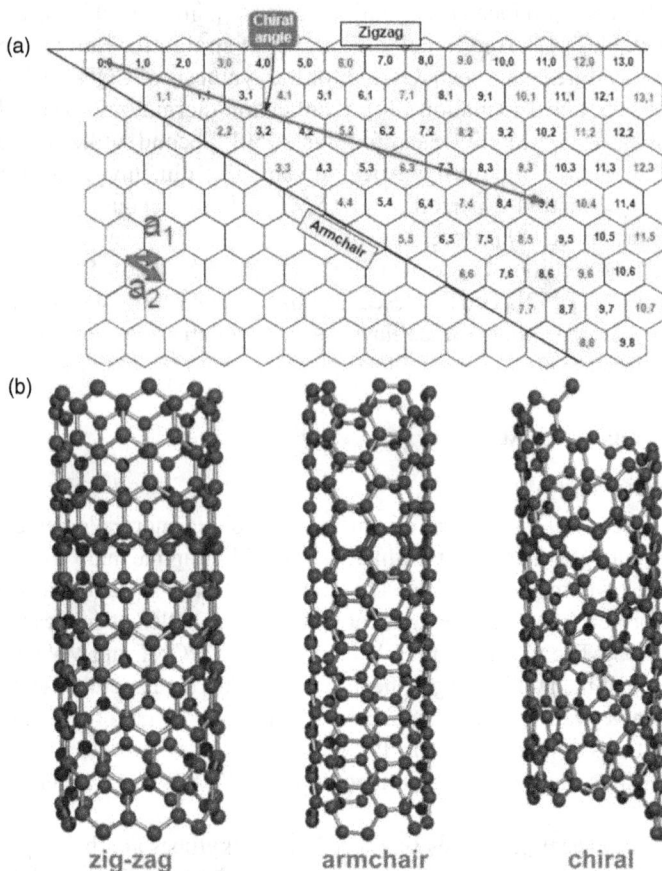

FIGURE 1.1 (a) The Chiral Vector C and Chiral Angle θ Defining a Nanotube on a Graphene Sheet [2], (b) Classification of SWCNTs Based on the Chirality. [Reprinted with permission from *N. Grobert (2007)*] [59].

structure. As shown in **Figure 1.1** [53,59], The SWCNTs are further divided into three different types based on how they are wrapped into cylindrical configurations, namely, armchair, chiral, and zigzag. A pair of indices (n, m) used to specify the configuration of an SWCNT are used to characterize the chiral vectors and their direct influence on the electrical properties of nanotubes. The graphene honeycomb crystal structure's number of unit vectors across two orientations is defined by the integers n and m. According to popular belief, nanotubes are zigzag nanotubes if m = 0, armchair nanotubes if n = m, and chiral in other states [53].

The diameter of MWCNTs, which varies based on the number of tubes rolled together, ranges from 2 to 50 nm. MWCNTs are composed of multilayered graphene nanosheets that have been wrapped around one another. In contrast to SWCNTs, MWCNTs may be produced without a catalyst and have both a complex structure and a pure form. Additionally, the MWCNTs are challenging to twist and frequently take the appearance of granules or a black, fluffy powder [54]. The interlayer spacing in these tubes is roughly 0.34 nm [11,53]. The Russian Doll and Parchment models are two important structural models for MWCNTs. The Russian Doll model is present when a carbon nanotube has other nanotubes beneath it, and the outer nanotube is thicker than the inner one. The Parchment model, in contrast, describes a single graphene sheet being wrapped around itself several times to resemble a scroll of paper. MWCNTs and SWCNTs have comparable properties. Due to their multilayer structure, MWCNTs exhibit strong tensile strength properties that SWCNTs lack while protecting the inner carbon nanotubes from chemical reactions with exterior pollutants [53,60]. Additionally, there is another variety of CNTs that resembles SWCNTs in terms of structure. These nanotubes, often referred to as dual or double-walled carbon nanotubes, are composed of two concentric sheets that enclose an inner cylindrical tube inside an outer tube (CNTs) [61].

CNTs have been widely used as drug delivery in pharmaceutical and medicinal applications since the turn of the 21st century. They are distinguished from bulk equivalents of the same composition (in microscale) by their very tiny size, high reactivity, needle-like shape, substantial strength, adaptive interaction with the cargo, greater drug loading efficiency, remarkable electrical and optical characteristics, good stability, biocompatibility, and capacity to deliver therapeutic molecules at particular or targeted locations. They also stand out owing to their high surface area to mass ratio and capability to deliver therapeutic molecules at specific or targeted sites [56,62]. Furthermore, because CNTs immediately penetrate cells and keep drug molecules intact throughout delivery without metabolizing them, they have been found to be an efficient drug delivery vehicle. Several therapeutic compounds, such as drugs, antibodies, nucleic acids, proteins, and enzymes, can be conjugated to or absorbed by CNTs, such as SWCNT and MWCNT. CNTs display toxicity and biodegradability-related problems, which further restricts their use for biomedical applications even if these traits are associated with highly desirable characteristics. However, despite several limitations, CNTs continue to exhibit excellent performance in the field of health care, notably in the fields of drug delivery, gene therapy, bioimaging, and biosensors. [11,62].

Lack of solubility, dispersibility, biodistribution, bioactivity, biodegradability, and toxicity are the main obstacles to the use of CNTs in biomedical domains. The hydrophobic structure, van der Waals interactions, the length of the CNTs, as well as the nonuniformity in their surface properties are mostly responsible for these deficiencies. However, these difficulties can be solved by functionalizing CNTs with hydrophilic and more biocompatible functional components like biopolymers and targeting ligands. Numerous biological applications, including biosensing, disease diagnosis, and therapy, have benefited greatly from functionalized CNTs [63]. They provide biomedical imaging, enable the detection of diverse biological targets, and deliver therapeutic materials, such as drugs and genes [64,65]. Their inherent spectroscopic characteristics, including photoluminescence and Raman scattering, can offer useful tools for monitoring, identifying, and imaging disorders. They can also aid in tracking the state of *in-vivo* treatment, pharmacodynamic behavior, and drug delivery effectiveness.

1.2.2.2 Graphene nanoribbons

Graphene nanoribbons (GNRs) are thin strips of graphene made of alternating hexagonal carbon cells that can be up to 50 nm broad and dozens of micrometers long based on the production process [66]. To examine the edge and nanoscale effects of graphene, Fuhita et al. (1996) computationally interpreted GNRs in 1996 [67,68]. GNRs are notably different compared to the more well-known 2-D graphene nanosheets owing to their quasi-1-D structure [69]. GNRs are very precise tools that hold promise for nanoelectronic components, incredibly sensitive mechanical and chemical sensors, etc. [70–72]. They are virtually perfect nanowires or nanotags.

Additionally, the synthesis technique has a substantial impact on the structure and physical characteristics of GNRs. GNRs exhibit a 1-D morphology with a substantial class of conjugated polymers, whose performance parameters are determined by the conditions of synthesis and the technique used to form films [73,74]. Since the structure, width, and orientation of the crystal's edge are extremely important to the electrical and optical characteristics of GNRs, their structural perfection is a key issue [66]. The "armchair" or AGNRs, "zigzag" or GNRs with zigzag edges (ZGNRs), and "cove" edge configurations are the three most often researched varieties of GNRs edge structures [75]. The most typical GNRs have zigzag and armchair-style edges. Although ZGNRs are anticipated to have lower band gaps with confined magnetic edge states and enormous prospective for spintronic applications, AGNRs are distinguished by a large band gap that modulates with their width [76–78]. Cove-type GNRs may have their edges altered to smoothly decrease energy band gaps, albeit at the cost of conjugation breakdowns and higher morphological spreading [79].

The sp^2 hybridized carbon's interaction with other molecules causes GNRs to assemble readily in both their solid and liquid forms. The easiest way to reduce such "π-π" interaction in the solution is to include different functional groups. As a result, the additional functional groups might lessen π-π interaction while maintaining the aromatic structure. For this goal, three techniques have been described so far: introducing alkyl heteroatoms [80], functionalizing with polymers of high molecular weight [81], and introducing bulky 3-D heteroatoms to the surface of GNRs [82]. The term "graphene oxide nanoribbons" (GONRs) refers to oxygenated derivatives of GNRs that are amphiphilic carbon nanostructures. The high specific surface area of GNRs allows for the loading of a significant amount of drug molecules. The functionalization of GONRs with various biomolecules is caused by oxygen-containing functionalities, which improves their applicability in biomedical fields [83]. GNRs have a flexible and distinctive characteristic that allows them to go from having semiconducting properties to semimetal properties through simply altering their width [84]. Additionally, the reduction processes, including electrochemical, thermal, and chemical ones, can convert GONRs into reduced GONRs (rGONRs). GNRs offer strong mechanical strength, good thermal and electrical conductance, and chemical stability. Due to their oxygenated functional groups, GONRs are more biocompatible than other derivatives. This characteristic enables the utilization of GONRs for applications such as drug delivery [85], bone regeneration [86], antibacterial [87], photothermal, biosensing, and bioimaging [88]. Chemical and other modifications are necessary to broaden the variety of applications afforded by GNRs [89]. GNRs are the most effective carriers for anticancer drugs, certain highly aromatic pharmaceuticals, and other biomolecules.

1.2.2.3 Graphene Nanoscrolls

Graphene and CNTs are among the most intriguing nanomaterials in the carbon family owing to their perfect 1- and 2-dimensional forms. They were discovered in 2004 and 1991, correspondingly, and since then have sparked a lot of attention due to their remarkable physicochemical characteristics [90–92] and substantial applications [18,93,94]. The characteristics of CNTs have been thoroughly studied over the past few years, and graphene research is now quickly gaining ground alongside CNTs. Lately, the development of unique nanostructures has been presented through folding and curling graphene nanosheets, which have undergone extensive investigations [95]. This has led to the development of the intriguing carbon nanomaterial known as the graphene nanoscroll (GNS) or carbon nanoscroll (CNS). According to the size of graphene nanosheets and rolling orientation, a continuous graphene sheet of varied chirality and diameter has been rolled up to study the GNS structure [96]. GNSs are intriguing nanostructures that, although predicted to display distinct characteristics, combine some of the comprehensive and individual mechanical and electrical properties demonstrated by graphene and CNTs. Due to the peculiar morphology of GNSs, several theoretical studies have predicted their remarkable electronic and optical properties [97,98]. Since the GNSs do not have a closed-end morphology like CNTs, their diameter can be easily adjusted. These characteristics may be used for a variety of scientific applications, including chemical doping, hydrogen storage, and nanoactuators in nanomechanical systems [98,99].

Similar to GNS, its oxidized derivative graphene oxide nanoscrolls (GONS) have also been studied for numerous applications, including methanol oxidation, supercapacitor, and drug delivery [100,101]. A prospective 1-D nanomorphology of GONS was established by the researchers Amadei et al. (2016) [102] and Fan et al. (2015) [103] by scrolling the single-atomic thin GO nanosheets into a spiral configuration. They took their inspiration from the structure of CNS and CNT. As illustrated in **Figure 1.2c** [100], the GONS has an analogous 1D shape as CNT, although with configurable interlayer spacing and additionally accessible inter-wall region. GNS/CNS and GONS vary significantly from each other due to the inclusion of oxygenated functional groups in GONS. Despite the fact that GONS has a poorer electric conductivity, the reduced form of GONS demonstrated superior electrochemical performance and electric conductivity [100,103]. The aggregation tendency of GO sheets, their instability in the organic solvent, less porous structure, and closed-end morphology of CNT are the driving forces underlying the investigations associated with GONS. Moreover, the structural and morphological alteration of GONS combined with the comparative physicochemical characteristics of GO makes it more viable to employ in real-world applications [104]. Furthermore, the effective and rapid fabrication of GONS was aided by recent advancements in the techniques for the synthesis of CNS.

The GONS can be fabricated through advanced synthesis approaches such as ultrasonication, lyophilization, vertex fluidic device, molecular combing, and solvent-induced self-assembly methods [100]. Out of which, the ultrasonication treatment is the most common approach employed for the synthesis of GONS of tunable dimensions. The length of nanoscrolls can be adjusted by altering the sonication parameters [104]. GO nanoscrolls exhibit higher specific surface area and surface-to-volume ratio than GO nanosheets. Furthermore, the one-dimensional nanomorphology of

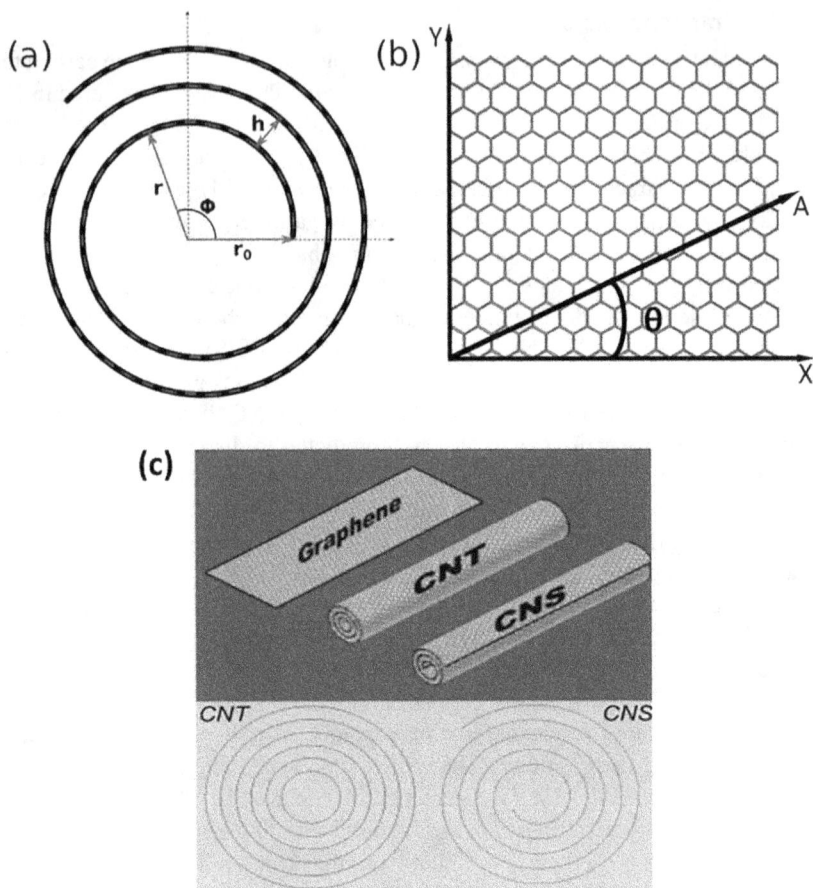

FIGURE 1.2 (a) Scheme Demonstrating a Cross-Section of GONS Relationship between r, ro, h, and φ. (b) Scheme for Rolling Up GO Nanosheets along with Axis A and Angle θ. (c) Structural Comparison of MWCNT and GONS. [Reproduced with permission] [100].

GONS with deagglomeration tendency, suitable aqueous stability, enriched oxygen functional groups, functionalization ability, smaller and adjustable lengths, and better biocompatibility provide significant advantages for their application in drug delivery systems [101].

1.2.3 Two-Dimensional

1.2.3.1 Graphene

Graphene, a unique carbon allotrope, has significantly revolutionized a number of disciplines, notably materials science, electronics, quantum physics, biomedicine, and energy systems. Since its discovery in 2004, several investigations have been made to understand its physicochemical properties. During the past ten years, research into the use of graphene and its derivatives in the biomedical sector has drawn a lot of attention, notably in the fields of tissue engineering and drug and gene delivery for the treatment of cancer. The 2-D honeycomb crystal structure of graphene is made up of a single layer of densely packed carbon atoms. The name "graphene" is made up of the prefix "graph" for graphite and the suffix "-ene" for the C-C double bond. Boehm, Setton, and Stumpp suggested the use of this phrase in 1994 [105,106]. Due to the absence of oxygen-containing groups, graphene is thought to be hydrophobic. Its structure resembles multiple connected benzene rings with hydrogen atoms replaced by carbon atoms (**Figure 1.3**) [107].

Graphene contains one π orbital and three perpendicular σ bonds to the plane. Although the out-of-plane π bonds control the interactions among graphene layers, the strong in-plane σ-bonds operate as the hexagonal stiff backbone chain. Modifications in graphitic layers are nearly always brought on by the absence of one or more sp^2 carbon atoms or even the introduction of one or more extra atoms through sp^3 hybridization [108]. Single sp^2-bonded carbon atom allotropes, which can exist in zero to three dimensions and include fullerene, graphene, nanotubes, and graphite, have indeed been incorporated into various polymeric composites over the past few decades due to their exceptional mechanical, thermal, electrical, and foldable properties [109].

A wider class of graphene-based nanomaterials (GBNs) includes few-layer graphene (FLG), GO, reduced GO (rGO), and nano GO. Although FLG is commonly referred to as graphene, it is composed of two to ten stacked layers of graphene and was initially created as a by-product of the manufacture of graphene [110]. A monolayer graphene nanosheet with oxygenated functional groups, including hydroxyl, carboxyl, and epoxide groups, all over its edges and surface makes up graphene in its oxidized state, also known as GO. When GO is reduced chemically and thermally in reducing conditions, the outcome is rGO, which has less oxygen composition. The term "NGO" and "graphene nanosheets" are both used to describe graphene having a lateral dimension of less than 100 nm.

Since the discovery of graphene in 2004, scientists have paid great attention to its unique physicochemical properties [110,111]. Recently, numerous studies and demonstrations of graphene applications in nanoelectronics, material science, and engineering have been undertaken [112,113]. Nevertheless, GO, a type of graphene

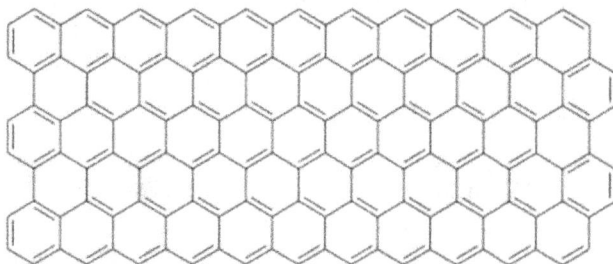

FIGURE 1.3 Structure of Graphene Nanosheet.

that has endured oxidation, has lately come to light as having significant potential in the biomedical field. Despite this renewed focus, graphene and GBN have previously been used in a variety of biomedical applications, including photothermal therapy (PTT), tissue engineering, biosensing, disease diagnostics, and drug delivery [114,115]. The properties of graphene, such as its high specific surface area attributable to the 2D flat structure of the nanosheets and the adaptable surface and morphological alterations leading to their enhanced biocompatibility, contributed to its rapid proliferation. The ability to bind or adsorb biomolecules or functional groups to both sides of the graphene surface, permitting high functionalization and drug-loading efficiencies, is a great value addition. All things considered, graphene nanoparticles show considerably greater promise than CNTs. Although GBNs are excellent for innovative drug delivery systems (DDSs) due to their considerable surface characteristics and improved drug loading capacity, their poor aqueous stability, biocompatibility, biodistribution, and toxicity are the main obstacles to their use in the biomedical field [116].

Due to its hydrophobic nature, graphene must be functionalized to be processed and dispersed in aqueous and organic solutions [117,118]. To integrate graphene's outstanding properties with biological activity, a graphene surface may also be functionalized physically or chemically to accommodate biological moieties [119]. Both covalent and non-covalent functionalization have previously been widely used to enhance the properties of graphene [120,121]. It has also been proven that combining covalent and non-covalent functionalization is a viable approach. Covalent functionalization often entails GO or rGO that has been chemically produced by the cross-linking of hydrophilic polymers or nucleic acids (NAs), the amine-to-carboxylate group coupling reaction, or sulfonating methods. Nevertheless, the non-covalent modifications rely on the stabilizing properties of surfactants that attach toward the surface through hydrophobic forces or π–π interactions on a graphene surface to establish colloidal dispersions of graphene nanosheets [122].

Functionalization with oxygenated functional groups through the formation of GO has multiplied the adaptability of graphene in drug delivery, cancer therapeutics, and other biomedical applications. Furthermore, the widening of the graphene band gap induced by doping and intercalation might aid in the development of effective nanoelectronics components. The graphene-based nanomaterials potentially provide a gateway to new domains of biotechnology unless they were biofunctionalized with certain biomolecules such as proteins, nucleic acids, enzymes, and peptides [123]. In addition, due to its aptitude to quench a variety of chemical dyes, quantum dots (QDs), and rapid DNA sequencing, graphene has recently been recognized as a viable element in the design of fluorescence resonance energy transfer (FRET) biosensors [124].

1.2.3.2 Graphene oxide

Since its discovery, graphene has achieved extensive utility in battery electrodes [125], biosensors [126], hydrogen storage [127,128], and supercapacitors [125,126] due to its remarkable electrical, optical, mechanical, and thermal characteristics. Specifically, graphene nanomaterials' significantly larger surface area and optical characteristics have sparked a lot of intrigue in biological applications such as biosensing and drug and gene delivery [129,130]. Nevertheless, graphene's low water solubility owing to π-π staking hinders its application in biomedical fields. In the past, the parent material graphene underwent additional morphological changes and functionalization to enhance its surface properties and prospects for a wide range of practical applications.

Certainly, the oxidative and hydrophilic graphene derivatives GO and rGO are enriched in hydroxyl, carboxyl, and epoxy functional entities, which improve their stability and water dispersibility as well as their potential to emit infrared and visible light [131]. In addition to its fundamental physicochemical properties, graphene and its derivative GO are presently the subject of comprehensive research due to their exciting prospects for application in a variety of biomedical engineering fields, including drug delivery, cancer therapeutics, biosensing, and tissue engineering [132]. For many different applications, the modification of defects in nanomaterials based on graphene is directly relevant. GO and rGO are regarded as general nanomaterials within the family of graphene-derived materials [133,134]. GO produced by oxidizing graphene exhibits a range of physicochemical properties. It is a hydrophilic graphene derivative and resembles a single atomic thick, two-dimensional honeycomb structure [135]. The adjustable morphology [136] and low cytotoxicity of GO, among other qualities, make it beneficial for biological applications. It shows fluorescence in the infrared and visible portions of the electromagnetic spectrum and Raman signals in the D, G, and 2D areas, making it suitable for bioimaging and biosensing [136]. The oxygen-containing functional units are situated in the base and edging planes of the GO nanosheets, as shown in **Figure 1.4** [137].

Although the fundamental structure of GO and rGO is comparable to that of graphene, they additionally contain oxygenated functional groups in varying amounts [135,138]. The GO has exceptional hydrophilicity because it is composed of single-layer nanostructures that are stuffed with functional groups rich in oxygen.

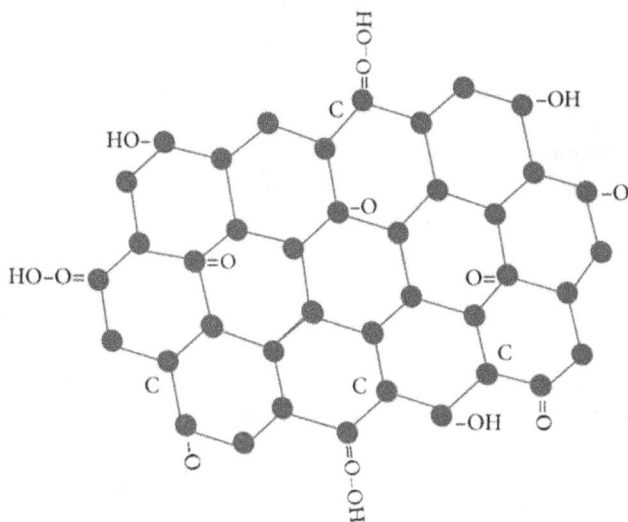

FIGURE 1.4 Chemical Structure of GO. [Replicated with permission from *Song et al. (2014)*].

A traditional Hummers process and its variations are frequently used for the production of GO. Strong acids and oxidants are used in the GO production process to introduce oxygenated functional units into the GO. The earliest approach was reported by Brodie (1859) [139], and it was followed by Staudenmaier (1898) [140], Hummers (1958) [141], Tour (2010) [142], Sun (2013) [143], and Peng (2015) [144]. Some of the disadvantages of these technologies include the low degree of oxidation, complicated reaction conditions, poisonous gas emissions, the requirement for purification processes, and high production costs. However, the Hummers method and its adaptations have substantially mitigated many of these restrictions. Because of its functional groups, GO has a superior water solubility than other compounds; however, without surface functionalization, these functional groups are inadequate for biological applications. Crucially, these oxygen-containing functional units provide a variety of active sites for doping the elements or grafting more functional entities to increase the surface properties of GO while maintaining its core properties [135,145].

Together with the previously mentioned characteristics, GO may be combined with polymers and other components to develop a range of hybrids. These additions can enhance GO's biocompatibility, loading capacity, structural features and targetability with polyacrylic acid (PAA), chitosan, polyethylene glycol (PEG), folic acid (FA), and other substances [146]. The hydrodynamic stability of GO is likewise a significant issue for its use in drug administration. Owing to nonspecific binding and electrostatic interactions, GO does have a tendency to aggregate in physiological solutions, including proteins and salt, which hinders the formation of biological probes [147,148]. The rigorous functionalization of GO improves its physiological solubility and makes it more suitable for biological applications. Also, due to its superior qualities, including a greater surface area, GO is one of the most well-liked and thoroughly studied nanomaterials for applications involving drug administration. However, a distinct graphene derivative, rGO, has also been used for a variety of practical purposes, such as drug administration, and it can be readily made by thermally or chemically reducing GO [132,149].

1.2.4 THREE-DIMENSIONAL

1.2.4.1 Diamond

Diamond, both natural and synthetic, is now being researched in a variety of industries. Diamond is frequently close to the top of any list describing the unique characteristics of a material [150]: crystalline diamond exhibits the largest atomic density of any bulk crystal, products with high modulus, and superior thermal conductivity. Broad band gap semiconductor diamond is highly translucent throughout the distant infrared to the ultraviolet region, making it an excellent material for optical applications [2]. Diamond is appealing because it is an sp^3-hybridized material that may be transformed into a variety of topologies and configurations. Moreover, tweaking the growth conditions leads to CVD diamond films that range from microcrystalline to ultra-nanocrystalline. Ultra-nanocrystalline films made of diamond offer the benefit of having smooth surfaces, less strain, and better-breaking resistance. Diamond domains with narrow sp^2 borders, measuring at least 10 nm in size, are a distinguishing feature of such films. The most intriguing types of diamond that have been investigated for use in drug delivery or clinical applications are nanoscale diamond particles (also known as nanodiamonds, NDs), and diamond nano-films. Diamond is typically regarded as a biocompatible material because of its chemical and biochemical impermeability, which means that it is chemically non-cytotoxic when in interaction with living cells [151]. As a result, diamond is a material that may be used to cover medical equipment, develop artificial tissues, or facilitate the development of living cells. For the development of various cell phenotypes, such as neurons, fibroblasts, osteoblasts, and several other cell lines, ND nanoparticles and nanoplatelets have been utilized as substrates [2]. Fluorescent nanodiamonds (FNDs) were employed by Guarina et al. (2018) to assess the functional effects of these materials on hippocampal neurons utilizing multielectrode array (MEA) recordings. Based on the embryonic stage of incubation with FNDs, the activation frequency of neurons was influenced differentially (seven versus 14). During 14 days *in-vitro*, FNDs significantly decreased the frequency of neuronal activity [152].

Diamond consistently showed minimal detectable cytotoxicity, and in some situations, it even seemed to encourage cell adhesion and growth compared to more traditional substances like glass or cell culture polystyrene. Due to their unique chemical and electrical characteristics and resilience, NDs were utilized in neuroscience in addition to being used as a growing substrate to design biosensors for monitoring neural activity [153]. Nanowires made of diamond must also be taken into account. Diamond nanowires are thought to help with problems like selectivity and sensitivity that are relevant to enhancing the overall effectiveness of sensors [2,154]. Diamond-based materials provide special benefits over traditional substances in the domain of cellular detection [155], which subsequently results from the material's exceptional physicochemical characteristics, such as mechanical resilience, broad spectral transparency, and thermal conductivity [156]. Diamond-based platforms are cytocompatible and substantially better at supporting cell adhesion and proliferation than normal substrates, according to *in-vitro* testing [157]. However, the pure diamond surface's biochemical inertness does not prevent it from effectively chemically functionalizing when terminated with certain covalent bonds, which enables the attachment of a wide range of molecules, including DNA strands [158].

Although diamond-based substrates appear to have a bright future, it must be highlighted that their potential for biological applications, particularly in the domain of neurosciences, is currently constrained. Perhaps in the future, like in the instance of GO, appropriate tuning of the nanomaterial's physicochemical and morphological features will aid in overcoming its present significant limits.

1.3 CHARACTERIZATION TECHNIQUES FOR CBNS

The CBNs must be thoroughly investigated after synthesis to ensure the quality of the product (quality, defects, functional groups, morphology, and structure, etc.) and to clarify their composition. Several characterization approaches may be used to explore the attributes of CBNs and CBN-based nanocomposites. These methods comprise electron microscopy (SEM and TEM), Fourier transform infrared spectroscopy (FTIR), UV-Vis spectroscopy, atomic force microscopy (AFM), X-ray photoelectron spectroscopy (XPS), energy dispersive X-ray analysis (EDX), Raman spectroscopy, and X-ray diffraction (XRD). For a thorough characterization, many approaches must be used as they each give diverse morphological, physical, and chemical characteristics. The significance and details of some of these characterization techniques related to CBNs are provided subsequently.

1.3.1 ELECTRON MICROSCOPY

The morphological investigation of CBNs and other nano-morphology may be carried out with the use of electron microscopic imaging techniques, including TEM and SEM. The dimensionalities and morphological configurations, and orientations of carbon-based nanomaterials, including graphene and its derivatives, CNTs, quantum dots and nanodiamonds, can be observed at the initial stages through these microscopical investigations. Higher resolution and the most comprehensive morphological, crystal, and topographic assessment are possible with high-resolution (HR) TEM. To determine the elemental composition of the CBNs, energy dispersive X-ray analysis (EDX) is frequently used in conjunction with electron microscopy. The orientation/alignment of CNTs and the patterned surfaces resulting from the various CNT growing processes were visualized using SEM. SWCNTs and MWCNTs may be differentiated, and their diameters measured using HRTEM. Moreover, HRTEM-EDX is capable of detecting and identifying the existence of carbon-containing and catalytic nanoparticles [35,159]. The potential of HRTEM to determine the chiral indices of SWCNTs is more intriguing.

Moreover, it made it possible to recognize fullerenes (C_{60}) within SWCNTs (peapod structures) [160] and even to see the deformation of tiny hydrocarbon molecules that were contained within carbon nanotubes [161].

1.3.2 FTIR SPECTROSCOPY

The existence of various functional groups in pristine and functionalized CBNs can be validated through FTIR spectroscopic analysis. In the case of GO, the existence of oxygenated functional groups such as hydroxyl, carboxyl, and epoxy groups was confirmed by FTIR. Although FTIR spectroscopy was widely employed for functionalized CBNs, the intensity signals from FTIR spectroscopy are often weak. Therefore, other methods, like Raman spectroscopy and XPS, are more suited for assessing pristine carbon nanomaterials [35].

1.3.3 UV-VIS SPECTROSCOPY

UV-Vis spectroscopy was frequently employed to evaluate the absorption bands of numerous nanomaterials and nanocomposites, especially the materials that describe photoactivity. A π-π^* transition of aromatic C = C interactions may be seen in graphene and CNTs, which exhibit a significant absorption band at about 230 nm [162]. Incidentally, graphene has a smaller percentage of sp^2 carbons as compared to GO, which illustrates how it is less transparent in the UV-visible spectrum. Such distinct characteristic was utilized to analyze reduction reactions or determine the degree of GO oxidation [163]. Also, as the quantity of layers in graphene climbs, the absorbance of the material increases. Using this property, Sun et al. (2010) computed the number of layers of graphene using UV-visible absorbance at 550 nm [164].

UV-vis spectrophotometry was utilized in the instance of CNTs to evaluate the dispersion strategies of SWCNTs and MWCNTs since the intensity of the absorbance rises as the dispersion is enhanced. Furthermore, UV-vis absorbance may be used to estimate the concentration of CNTs that exist in a solution [35,165].

1.3.4 RAMAN SPECTROSCOPY

The most adaptable tool for characterizing carbon-based nanomaterials is recognized as the Raman spectroscopy investigation. Such a nondestructive characterization method, which is widely employed for carbonaceous materials, yields critical fragments of information. This characterization technique enables one to examine functionalization, structure, and purity, among the other features of CBNs. According to Raman spectroscopy, the D, G, and 2D peaks, which are located about 1350, 1580, and 2700 cm^{-1}, correspondingly, are where carbon allotropes may be distinguished. The D-band (D-disorder) results from the out-of-plane vibrational modes, and it is evidence of the inclusion of sp^3 carbon, whereas the G-band (G-graphite) belongs to the axially stretched (E$_{2g}$) phase of graphite. As a result, the sp^2-hybridized carbon atoms become disordered, which results in the structural aberrations observed in the twisted graphene sheet and/or tube ends. The second-order Raman scattering mechanism is the source of the 2D band, which has almost twice the frequency of the D band [35,166].

The intensity of the G-band of graphene increases with the increase in the number of sheets. Moreover, this expansion broadens the 2D band in the plane of higher wavenumber [166]. This phenomenon was used by Ferrari et al. (2006) to design a system for estimating the layers within graphene specimens [167]. The ratio of peak intensities I_D/I_G is another intriguing statistic since it could be employed to assess the degree of disorder in graphene. When the defects are identified, two distinct phases have been outlined: the first stage depicts the transformation from pure graphite to nanocrystalline graphite with lower defect density, while the second stage accounts for the shift from nanocrystalline graphite to mostly sp^2 amorphous carbon of higher defect density [168].

The I_D/I_G ratio is another tool for evaluating the purity of CNTs, although it is relatively simple to comprehend. The proportion of defects increases as the I_D/I_G ratio rises. In addition to the D and G bands, the radial breathing modes (RBMs) provide another intriguing band, which may be detected at lower wavenumbers ranging from 160 to 350 cm^{-1} [169]. These modes are produced through symmetric contraction and expansion of the tubes along the tube's axis. RBM could be employed to investigate the electronic framework via its intensity (I_{RBM}) and to evaluate the nanotube diameter (d$_t$) via its frequency (ω_{RBM}). It could also be utilized to carry out an (n, m) attribution of a solitary isolated SWCNT through the evaluation of both dt and I_{RBM}. Additionally, the identification of the RBM spectrum provides a clear indication of the existence of SWCNTs. In the case of MWCNTs, the RBM signal is barely perceptible. The reason for this is that the RBM band of wide-diameter tubes is often too weak, and the ensemble median of the inner tube diameter enhances the signal. The inverse relationship between RBM's frequency and tube diameter is one of its most appealing characteristics [35].

1.3.5 X-ray Photoelectron Spectroscopy (XPS)

An effective qualitative investigation of the nanomaterials as well as the surface chemistry of CBNs can be performed using the nondestructive characterization method known as XPS. It serves as the most trustworthy characterization method for determining the elemental composition, chemical state, and electronic state, along with the functional groups present within the CBNs. The sp^2 carbon (C-C), epoxy (C-O), hydroxyl (C-OH), and carboxyl (COO) peaks in the XPS spectra (C1s) for GO and GONS are located at binding energies of 285, 287, and 290 eV, correspondingly [100,170]. XPS examination was extensively used to evaluate variations in oxygenated functional entities in GO and rGO.

1.3.6 X-ray Diffraction

The XRD techniques play a significant role in the assessment of amorphous and crystalline materials by offering insights about phase recognition, lattice structure, and qualitative evaluation. This method can estimate interlayer spacing and is effective for describing and identifying polycrystalline phases. Because of these factors, XRD has been extensively used to track the oxidation of graphite and the subsequent exfoliation of graphite oxide to graphene oxide. According to the XRD pattern, pure graphite has a basal reflection (002) peak at 2θ = 26° (interlayer spacing 0.34 nm), while graphite oxide was found at 2θ = 12° (interlayer distance 0.7 nm). An interlayer extension in graphite oxide is caused by the complexation of oxygen species among the graphite layers. As oxidation progressed, the (0 0 2) diffraction line's strength progressively faded until it eventually vanished. Simultaneously, oxidation enhanced the strength of the diffraction peak at 12°. The peak at 12° vanished after complete exfoliation of the graphite oxide [102,171,172]. The literature's diverse research concluded that the peak emerged in the region 2θ = 23.0–23.5°, which reflects the rGO of (0 0 2) plane. The XRD pattern in range 2θ = 9–11.20°, on the other hand, reflects the (0 0 1) plane of GO. Due to the addition of hydrophilic groups brought about via oxidation and GO synthesis, there is an increase in the interlayer spacing in the crystallographic planes of graphite [100].

In comparison to CNTs, as-produced SWCNTs have the propensity to form crystalline frameworks that exhibit a peak at 2θ = 6° in the XRD spectra [173]. This method makes it possible to determine the number of SWCNTs present within every bundle [159]. A (0 0 2) plane for a peak of graphite is visible in MWCNTs at 2θ = 26°. The growth of the MWCNTs has been demonstrated using these signals [35].

1.4 APPLICATIONS OF CBNS

The development of unique nanomaterials with extraordinary functionalities has resulted in the expansion of nanotechnology in almost all commercial areas in recent years. CBNs have potential applications as nanomaterials in a variety of fields, including biomedical, energy, electronics, and environmental remediation. The enormous potential of these materials should continue to pique scientific interest, and any use of the new technology is anticipated to transform human civilization. Herein, we briefly cover studies on and applications for carbon-based nanomaterials and nano-composites in therapeutics and environmental remediation.

1.4.1 THERAPEUTICS

The human race has been provided with a variety of nano-enabled commodities or nanosystems, which are now used for a variety of biomedical applications. In the realm of nanostructure purview, such nano-constructs and combinations with pharmaceuticals, enzymes, nucleic acids, viruses, proteins, cellular lipid bilayers, cellular receptor sites, and antigens (crucial for immunotherapy) are multidimensional [174]. A group of nanosystems that have been extensively investigated for drug delivery and other biomedical applications is the CBNs. Recently, they have demonstrated effectiveness in fields including theranostics [175], cancer treatment [10,176], and regenerative medicine [177]. **(See Figure 1.5)**[178].

Certain characteristics of carbon nanomaterials, including their large surface areas and outstanding electrical and mechanical characteristics, encourage their utilization in the diagnostic and therapeutic domains as well. The major advantages over the utilization of CBNs in the field of therapeutics and diagnostics are:

1. They may absorb a significant amount of drug due to their supramolecular "π–π stacking" characteristic.
2. CBNs can be used as novel therapeutic components due to their distinct optical properties and easy fusion with illuminating components.

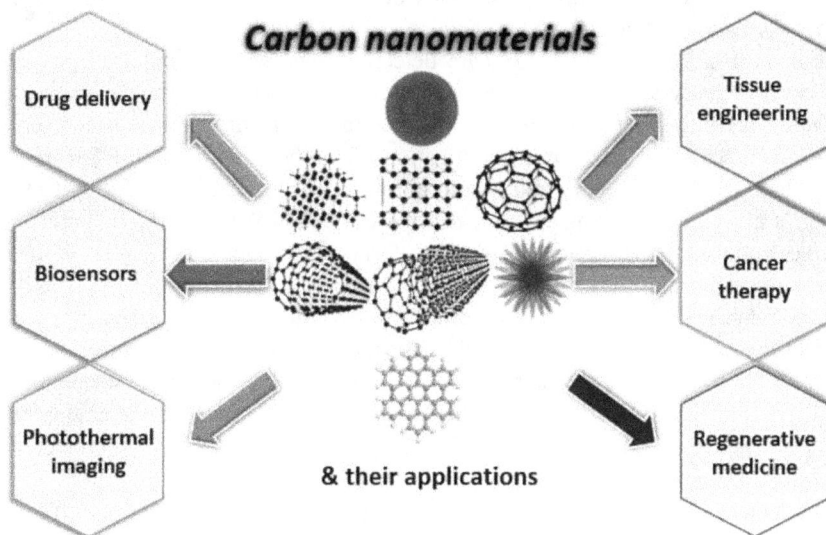

FIGURE 1.5 The Biomedical Application of Carbon-Based Nanomaterials. [Replicated with permission from *Mahor et al. (2021)*] [178].

3. CBNs have outstanding near-infrared (NIR) heat conversion competence that makes them a good choice for photothermal treatment (PTT).
4. Therapeutic agents can be released under regulated conditions using tunable surface chemistry.

The deployment of CBNs in the biomedical field is hindered by their colloidal stability in organic or aqueous environments [20]. Nevertheless, this could be resolved by stimulating the surface of CBNs using functionalization via covalent and non-covalent approaches. One such inevitable stage that modulates the surface by incorporating distinct functional entities is the functionalization of CBNs. There are several methods for covalent functionalization, including oxidation, plasma treatments, dehydrogenation, etc. [178]. Due in significant part to the surface modification of CBNs, which allows them to, for example, penetrate biological membranes, they have been widely used in the administration of drugs. The therapeutic efficacy of CBNs-assisted DDSs can be improved through their functionalization with certain targeting ligands such as aptamers and folic acid (FA), which also reduces their cytotoxicity toward healthy cells.

Modest targeting molecules, such as FA [179], which targets folate receptors espoused on the exterior of a range of robust cancerous cells, ligands with an affinity for a particular receptor overexpressed on a particular malignant tumor [10,180], a monoclonal antibody that recognizes tumor-associated antigens [181], and magnetic nanoparticles [100], can also be incorporated with the drug-loaded CBNs. Such techniques allow for targeted delivery by receptor-mediated endocytosis or drug aggregation at the target region with the use of an externally applied magnetic field. As a result, functionalized CBNs have found use in the transport of proteins, enzymes, nucleic acids, and biomolecules. CBNs have been used to administer anticancer drugs, fluorescent markers for tumor identification, PTT, and other theranostics [100,178].

For the functions like point-of-care detection, the design of precise biosensors is essential. Early and accurate diagnosis of conditions like cancer can increase a patient's likelihood of surviving [182]. Bioimaging is a technique that allows for the molecular characterization and investigation of biological processes [183]; it may examine a treatment plan in addition to aiding in illness detection. Owing to their superior attributes of having a large surface area, being robust, and having outstanding electronic attributes, graphene-based materials were extensively employed in bioimaging and biosensing applications [182]. The capacity to transport electrons and the amphiphilicity of these nanomaterials are two important properties that might affect their potential for biosensing [184]. The flaws in GO facilitate electron transfer, whereas the functional groups enable surface modification and luminescent component binding [185]. Proteins, oligonucleotides, and antigens are typical examples of detection molecules [186]. These can be covalently or non-covalently connected to the horizon of graphene derivatives.

To detect CD59, a lung cancer biomarker, Chauhan et al. (2020) loaded anti-CD59 antigens onto graphite electrodes to form an immunosensor. The graphite rods were coated with GO to increase their conductivity. The study provided a quick and noninvasive lung cancer diagnostic method [187]. A rapid and accurate method of detecting the lung cancer (NSCLC) biomarker CK19 in spiking human plasma was developed by Chiu et al. (2018) using a carboxyl-GO-modified biomaterial-based SPR biosensor. Such GO-COOH-based SPR chip, which has a positive linear range (0.001–100 pg/mL) with shorter response times than a conventional SPR chip, outperformed it in terms of detection limits. They later discovered that a biosensor system based on carboxyl-GO could identify CK19 at levels as low as 0.05 pg/mL in 10% serum proteins and 0.001 pg/mL in PBS solution [188].

CNTs have undergone extensive investigation toward the targeted and controlled delivery of anticancer agents due to their distinct properties. CNTs are drug carriers for several anticancer cancer medicines and efficient phototherapy stimulators due to their inherent optical characteristics. Because of their adaptability, CNTs can be used therapeutically for a variety of cancers. At this time, a lot of anticancer treatment strategies are aimed at eradicating tumor cells and the conditions that support them. Actively going after cancer cells can effectively remove their parenchyma, but treating the tumor microenvironment unswervingly can stop tumor cells from proliferating and spreading by upsetting their environment, which also indirectly kills cancer cells [189]. Recently, Zhou et al. (2022) synthesized multifunctional and PEGylated MWCNTs for the targeted delivery of the anticancer agent, Doxorubicin (DOX). Adipic acid (AA) was used as a cross-linking agent to bind the targeted ligand of folic acid (FA) to hyperbranched poly-L-lysine (HBPLL). Further, DOX was successfully integrated on the MWCNT-PEG-AA-HBPLL-FA nanocarrier, and the *in-vitro* release of drugs was examined using a UV-Vis spectrophotometer. The *in-vitro* cytotoxicity and anticancer capabilities of DOX-loaded nanocarrier were investigated in the human embryonic kidney (HEK293) and liver cancer (HepG2) cells. The presented nanocarrier demonstrated effective drug loading efficiency, pH-responsive and targeted drug release; this assessment is significant as it can get around some of the drawbacks of traditional cancer chemotherapy, like the simplicity through which obtained nanoparticles attach to cancerous cells receptors, which then quickly enter receptor-mediated endocytosis and deliver the drug to the affected regions. At acidic pH levels, intracellular endosome surroundings showed a significant proportion of drug release rate. The nanoparticles have been reported to have significant cytotoxicity for HepG2 cells and low cytotoxicity for HEK293 cells. [190]. A Novel SWCNTs-based DDS was designed by Yu et al. (2016) for the prolonged delivery of Paclitaxel (PTX). The sidewalls of SWCNTs were non-covalently linked with chitosan to improve their biocompatibility. To achieve the cell-targeting property, biodegradable hyaluronan was also added into the chitosan's outer surface. The results showed that PTX release depended on pH and was enhanced at lower pH values (pH 5.5). The improved SWCNTs drastically lowered intracellular reactive oxygen species (ROS), which may have boosted the activation of mitogen-activated protein kinases and greatly facilitated cellular damage. Western blotting results showed that apoptosis-related proteins were highly expressed in A549 cells. The vitality of the A549 cells was decreased by PTX-loaded SWCNTs, as evidenced by cell viability assays and a lactate dehydrogenase (LDH) release experiment [191].

In the family of CBNs, the graphene quantum dots (GQDs) are considered the smallest derivatives of graphene. Owing to their tiny size, GQDs are able to cross the blood-brain barrier (BBB) and deliver nucleic acid cargo to cell cytosols and nuclei. Due to their low toxicity, high solubility, and luminous properties that make it straightforward to track drug release, GQDs are a great option for gene carriers. Recently, Ghafary et al. (2017) established a distinctive nanoconjugate consisting of GQDs, the chimeric peptide MPG-2H1, and plasmid DNA (pDNA) that is capable of real-time monitoring and gene delivery [192]. The nanoconjugate was synthesized by non-covalent interactions between each component. The enhanced complex achieved transfection efficiency that was approximately eight times greater than the typical peptide-pDNA combination. The results of this study suggest that GQDs could perform well as a transfection vector for gene delivery applications. Due to the significant presence of the sp^2 domain and the possibility for "π-π stacking," GQDs provide greater drug loading in comparison to certain other nanomaterial drug carrier systems. Because these biomolecules must be covalently bonded to the edge groups, the active sites on the edge of GQDs are unfortunately restricted to ligands, making it doubtful that they will be exploited in gene delivery applications [192]. The promising outcomes of several studies on gene therapy employing CBNs have boosted the hopes of individuals seeking treatment. However, the regulatory clearances will take a long time, even though this is a very different notion because the technology and its implications for individuals seem mostly unstudied.

Carbon-based nanomaterials, with their superior mechanical and chemical properties, have displayed significant potential for tissue engineering applications. CNTs were effectively used in the development of medications for bone, cardiac, and neurological regeneration. Bone is capable of self-healing and rebuilding after mild trauma or fractures. Nevertheless, in pathogenic injuries, acute bone attrition, or core tumor excision, bone is no longer able to mend itself if the flaws are greater than a threshold size (5 mm) [193,194]. This case reported a variety of treatments, including xenografts, allografts, and autografts. Unfortunately, these methods have serious disadvantages, including limited availability and donor site morbidity for autografts, the risk of resistance and infection transmission for allografts, and the probability of immunogenicity and a poor clinical prognosis for xenografts [194]. Consequently, a novel and highly promising approach involving the use of 3D constructions known as tissue-engineered synthetic bone scaffolds has gained tremendous attention, which provides the support required for cell adhesion, growth, and transformation. Tanaka et al. (2017) developed a 3D block construction consisting of CNTs and compared its efficiency as a scaffold for bone regeneration to that of PET-reinforced gelatin. The artificial structure and rat femoral bone had compressive strengths of 62.1 MPa and 61.86 MPa, respectively, and mechanical analysis revealed no discernible differences. Cell adhesion occurred earlier on CNT scaffolds compared to collagen-reinforced PET scaffolds. Recombinant human BMP-2 was added, which boosted the ALP activity in the CNTs block and showed good osteogenesis properties [195].

Corresponding to this, multiple investigations have shown that GO-based nanocarriers may effectively be used for muscle, skin, and cardiac tissue regeneration [10]. Altogether, CBNs showed excellent efficacy and capacity for drug administration in regenerative medicine, gene therapy, and cancer treatments, which may indicate a flexible treatment option for diseased individuals. Despite the positive outcomes of CBNs biocompatibility trials, further research is needed to fully understand the harmful effects and toxicity of carbon-based nanocarriers.

1.4.2 ENVIRONMENTAL REMEDIATION

There are significant environmental degradation concerns as a result of the rise of modern civilization, the expansion of urbanization, the expansion of industrial output, and the intensification of transportation. Human productivity and routine everyday activities are increasingly causing environmental disruption. Antibiotics, pesticides, dyes, heavy metals, greenhouse gases, endocrine disruptors, and organic compounds are just a few of the toxic emissions that are released into groundwater, soil, and air, endangering both human health and the ecosystem [196]. According to the "UN Global Water Development Report, 2018," around 80% of effluent from urban and commercial operations is discharged into the environment without any pretreatment, which either directly or indirectly degrades the quality of the water [197]. Generally, effluent should be processed before being released into the environment because it includes hazardous proportions of metallic ions, organic compounds, dyes, and other cancer-causing substances [198]. Researchers have worked hard to identify a variety of compounds that may effectively eliminate contaminants from wastewater, including clay minerals, carbon-based materials, and both organic and inorganic nanomaterials [199].

Due to their outstanding physicochemical characteristics, CBNs have received a lot of interest in the domain of environmental remediation. These nanomaterials have higher specific surface areas, superior acid stability, and heat resistance [197]. It has been discovered that CBNs, with adsorption effectiveness > 80% and photocatalytic degradation efficiency > 98%, may efficaciously eliminate contaminants like heavy metals, nitric oxide, dyes, hydrogen sulfide, and pharmaceutical compounds from the surroundings [196]. Throughout the past ten years, studies regarding the utilization of CBNs in the remediation of pollutants have steadily increased (2012–2021). Porous frameworks and functional units are the major attributes of adsorbent in nature, which makes it possible to use CBNs in the prevention of environmental pollution. Particularly at lower concentrations, photodegradation is a useful method for the removal of organic compounds from contaminants. The optimum outcomes in the photocatalytic breakdown of organic compounds are the final products of carbon dioxide and water. In the case of heavy metal ions, in addition to their deposition on CBNs, metal ions may also be immobilized in the surroundings by the photocatalytic degradation of high-valent components to low-valent ones, followed by the production of in-situ precipitates [197].

Significant benefits and potential for application-driven investigation have been made possible by the distinct physicochemical characteristics of graphene and related materials, specifically through graphene oxide (GO). GO, with its 2D structure, higher surface area, oxygenated functional entities, and functionalization ability, delivered substantial potential for the removal of heavy metal ions, organic pollutants, radioactive pollutants, and agricultural pollutants like pesticides and herbicides. Nevertheless, the stability and propensity for aggregation of GO in aqueous environments result in a decline in its performance efficiency. The effective surface area of GO nanostructure tends to decrease with aggregation, which has an impact on the overall effectiveness of the water treatment process. These restrictions could be circumvented by functionalizing GO with inorganic nanomaterials as well as other functional groups. Recently, a unique nanocomposite based on GO and other functionalized nanostructures has been designed for rapid, inexpensive, and effective methods and used successfully to remove various types of contaminants [138].

To remove lead (Pb (II)) ions from an aqueous system, Zarenezhad et al. (2021) recently synthesized magnetic graphene oxide (MGO) and further functionalized it using MEA, melamine, and Ethylenediamine (EDA). For process improvement, the variables influencing the adsorption of Pb (II) ions were examined. A comparison of the adsorption performances for nanocomposites such as MEA-MGO, M-MGO and EDA-MGO revealed 97.65%, 96.34%, and 98% removal efficiency for lead ions, respectively. Moreover, 98% elimination of Pb (II) was seen under ideal circumstances (Co = 20 ppm, X = 40 mg, pH = 4, t = 10 min) [200]. Utilizing the free radical reaction approach, Pashaei-Fakhri et al. (2021) were able to effectively produce a nanocomposite hydrogel, particularly acrylamide/GO-bonded sodium alginate (AM-GO-SA) and acrylamide bonded sodium alginate (AM-SA) hydrogel. The effectiveness of the developed hydrogel composites was assessed for the adsorption of crystal violet dyes. It was discovered that AM-SA and AM-GO-SA each had the highest capacity for adsorption at 62.07 mg/g and 100.30 mg/g, correspondingly [201]. In a single step, Chen et al. (2019) demonstrated an entirely novel bio-adsorbent for simultaneous photochemical reduction and dye adsorption. The bio-adsorbent was synthesized using GO, titanium dioxide (TiO_2), and corn straw pith (CSP). The GO and CSP serve as coats and stents, respectively. Nevertheless, TiO_2 nanoparticles are affixed to the adsorbent's surface and serve as both an adsorbent with enhanced hydrophilicity and a photochemical dye degradation agent. The direct use of the adsorbent maize straw pith during pyrolysis offered a valuable and economical utilization for the agricultural commodity. The adsorption process was accomplished via non-covalent interactions, including π–π stackings and electrostatic interaction. The configuration and structure of the GO loading with 5 weight percent and 20 weight percent TiO_2 were excellent, with significant removal efficiency for pollutants [202]. The potential use of GO nanoplatelets for the elimination of carbamazepine was examined by Bhattacharya et al. in 2020. Response surface methodology (RSM) Artificial Neural Network modeling was used to significantly improve the adsorption system for the dosage of adsorbent, initial amount of carbamazepine, temperature, and pH. At adsorbent dosage of 1g/L, pH 2, and 120 minutes of adsorption process, the highest adsorption capacity was reported to be 9.2 mg/g and removal efficiency of 99%. [203].

In addition, to GO, other CBNs such as carbon quantum dots (CQDs) [204], CNTs [197], and fullerene [24] have also been extensively utilized for environmental remediation applications. For instance, with their distinct PL attributes and significant conversion abilities, CQDs have delivered tremendous potential for the degradation of dyes and other organic contaminants along with active pharmaceutical agents [205]. Recently, Zhou et al. (2019) used a microwave-assisted technique to produce carbon dots (CDs), which were then divided into three distinct size fractions using size exclusion chromatography. The lack of a link between CD size and PL emission wavelength demonstrates that the PL process is not dependent on quantum size. The light absorption characteristics and band gap of the CDs altered with particle size, as evidenced by UV/vis absorption and diffuse reflectance spectrometry. The photodegradation of organic dyes was carried out independently using each of the three CDs segments beneath simulated sunlight exposure. It was discovered that as the dimension of the particles reduced, the reactivity of the CDs was increased. The 2-nm CDs were able to completely degrade both methylene blue (MB) and rhodamine B (RhB) in 150 minutes. The scavenger experiments revealed that the major components engaged in the photodegradation of the dyes by the 2-nm CDs are superoxide radicals and holes. Throughout the several cycles of dye degradation, these CDs demonstrated excellent stability. The 2-nm CDs have also demonstrated decent p-nitrophenol photodegradation. For the first time, the findings of this study described that bare carbon dots might be used to degrade environmental pollutants [206].

A study done by Qi et al. (2016) described that a facile solution-phase approach could be used to effectively synthesize a variety of fullerene (C_{60})-modified anatase TiO_2 (a-TiO_2) nanostructures of varied C_{60} proportions. Under UV-A light irradiation, the photodegradation of MB by pristine a-TiO_2 and C_{60}@a-TiO_2 nanostructures was evaluated, revealing that C_{60} significantly improves the photocatalytic performance of a-TiO_2 nanoparticles with an ideal level of 2.0 wt%. They looked into the electronic configuration of the C_{60}@a-TiO_2 hetero-interfaces in conjunction with the density functional theory (DFT) computations to unveil the fundamental mechanism of the C_{60} stacking on the photocatalytic performance. It was discovered that introducing C_{60} to the interface of a-TiO_2 not only reduced the energy gap but also established a new doping state across the valance and conduction band. As a consequence, the C_{60}@a-TiO_2 nanocomposites would exhibit better photocatalytic activity due to the effective charge separation and greater light adsorption caused by the existence of a transitional electronic state [207].

The photocatalytic breakdown of organic contaminants is still a "black box" technique, particularly in terms of the study of reactive component activity and the determination of intermediate compounds, both of which are useful in evaluating the catalytic characteristics of nanomaterials. The quantitative measurements of intermediates online remain quite challenging. Future research may focus on developing quick online analysis to comprehend how organic contaminants degrade through photocatalysis. The majority of nanostructures are still being developed in laboratories and are thus difficult to produce and utilize on a large scale. CBNs continue to struggle with high manufacturing costs and challenges with large-scale production. To safeguard the homeland of mankind, environmental remediation is receiving a growing amount of attention worldwide. In the future, mass manufacturing and cost-reduction strategies will likely receive increased emphasis in the R&D of CBNs. The advancement of methodologies might enable the mass production of inexpensive CBNs. Since CBNs are eventually discharged into the ecosystem, their toxicity in the natural surroundings must additionally be taken into account [197].

It is unavoidable that a certain amount of CBNs would be discharged into the atmosphere through their production operations when those are employed for environmental remediation; hence, environmental nanoparticle residues need to be factored in. Despite the fact that the study on the toxicity of nanostructures in the ecosystem is still in its early stages, it is important to consider the toxicity of CBNs.

1.5 SUMMARY

Extensive research on carbon-based nanomaterials, including 1-D, 2-D, and 3-D configured derivatives over the past 20 years, have revealed their perspective for use in a range of fields, including biomedical applications, environmental remediation, and catalysis. CBNs are highly suited for their wide range of applications due to their distinctive structural features, chemical inertness, opto-electronic capabilities, and surface tunability. The advancement of CBNs has been accelerated, especially for diagnostic and therapeutic applications, as a result of recent concerns about world health and the essential need to alleviate debilitating diseases. Multimodal surveillance, light-mediated treatment, and diagnostics are made possible by the optical characteristics of CBNs, which include fluorescence and luminescence. As intriguing nanoplatforms for the combined strategy of drug administration and diagnostics in the mitigation of conditions like cancer, CBNs' low dimensionality, high surface-to-volume ratio, adjustable surface characteristics, and reasonable biocompatibility represent a few of their other significant advantages.

In addition, the porous structure and functionalization ability of CBNs have demonstrated significant advantages for their application of environmental remediations. The CBNs are primarily utilized for the adsorption and photocatalytic degradation of organic pollutants, along with the separation of heavy metal ions, radionuclides, and agricultural pollutants. The opto-electronic attributes of CBNs, especially CQDs, have demonstrated their potential application in sensing trace molecules, gas, and other contaminants.

In the present chapter, we have highlighted the fundamental characteristics of CBNs, including their structure, surface characteristics, and potential applications. The characterization techniques have been demonstrated to validate and investigate the structural, morphological, and functional attributes of CBNs, including graphene, GO, CNTs, and CQDs. It is believed that the fundamental understanding of CBNs may contribute to the advancements of these nanomaterials and open up new avenues for their application in drug delivery systems.

REFERENCES

[1] G.A. Silva, Nanotechnology approaches to crossing the blood-brain barrier and drug delivery to the CNS, Curr. Res. Pharm. Technol. 4 (2011) 81–84. doi:10.1201/b13128-27.

[2] R. Rauti, M. Musto, S. Bosi, M. Prato, L. Ballerini, Properties and behavior of carbon nanomaterials when interfacing neuronal cells: How far have we come? Carbon. 143 (2019) 430–446. doi:10.1016/j.carbon.2018.11.026.

[3] D. Pantarotto, J.P. Briand, M. Prato, A. Bianco, Translocation of bioactive peptides across cell membranes by carbon nanotubes, Chem. Commun. 4 (2004) 16–17. doi:10.1039/b311254c.

[4] Q. Li, J. Song, F. Besenbacher, M. Dong, Two-dimensional material confined water, Acc. Chem. Res. 48 (2015) 119–127. doi:10.1021/ar500306w.

[5] D. Yu, K. Goh, H. Wang, L. Wei, W. Jiang, Q. Zhang, L. Dai, Y. Chen, Scalable synthesis of hierarchically structured carbon nanotube–graphene fibres for capacitive energy storage, Nat. Nanotechnol. 9 (2014) 555–562. doi:10.1038/nnano.2014.93.

[6] R. Singh, V.S.K. Yadav, M.K. Purkait, Cu2O photocatalyst modified antifouling poly-sulfone mixed matrix membrane for ultrafiltration of protein and visible light driven photocatalytic pharmaceutical removal, Sep. Purif. Technol. 212 (2019) 191–204. doi:10.1016/j.seppur.2018.11.029.

[7] C. Ge, J. Du, L. Zhao, L. Wang, Y. Liu, D. Li, Y. Yang, R. Zhou, Y. Zhao, Z. Chai, C. Chen, Binding of blood proteins to carbon nanotubes reduces cytotoxicity, Proc. Natl. Acad. Sci. 108 (2011) 16968–16973. doi:10.1073/pnas.1105270108.

[8] Y. Liu, X. Dong, P. Chen, Biological and chemical sensors based on graphene materials, Chem. Soc. Rev. 41 (2012) 2283–2307. doi:10.1039/C1CS15270J.

[9] C. Lee, X. Wei, J.W. Kysar, J. Hone, Measurement of the elastic properties and intrinsic strength of monolayer graphene, Sci. 321 (2008) 385–388. doi:10.1126/science.1157996.

[10] A.D. Sontakke, S. Tiwari, M.K. Purkait, A comprehensive review on graphene oxide-based nanocarriers: Synthesis, functionalization and biomedical applications, FlatChem. 38 (2023) 100484. doi:10.1016/j.flatc.2023.100484.

[11] R. Jha, A. Singh, P.K. Sharma, N.K. Fuloria, Smart carbon nanotubes for drug deliv-ery system: A comprehensive study, J. Drug Deliv. Sci. Technol. 58 (2020) 101811. doi:10.1016/j.jddst.2020.101811.

[12] K.I. Bolotin, K.J. Sikes, Z. Jiang, M. Klima, G. Fudenberg, J. Hone, P. Kim, H.L. Stormer, Ultrahigh electron mobility in suspended graphene, Solid State Commun. 146 (2008) 351–355. doi:10.1016/j.ssc.2008.02.024.

[13] C.-H. Liu, Q. Chen, C.-H. Liu, Z. Zhong, Graphene ambipolar nanoelectronics for high noise rejection amplification, Nano Lett. 16 (2016) 1064–1068. doi:10.1021/acs.nanolett.5b04203.

[14] L. Gomez De Arco, Y. Zhang, C.W. Schlenker, K. Ryu, M.E. Thompson, C. Zhou, Con-tinuous, highly flexible, and transparent graphene films by chemical vapor deposition for organic photovoltaics, ACS Nano. 4 (2010) 2865–2873. doi:10.1021/nn901587x.

[15] S. Wang, P.K. Ang, Z. Wang, A.L.L. Tang, J.T.L. Thong, K.P. Loh, High mobility, printable, and solution-processed graphene electronics, Nano Lett. 10 (2010) 92–98. doi:10.1021/nl9028736.

[16] T.S. Sreeprasad, S.M. Maliyekkal, K.P. Lisha, T. Pradeep, Reduced graphene oxide–metal/metal oxide composites: Facile synthesis and application in water purification, J. Hazard. Mater. 186 (2011) 921–931. doi:10.1016/j.jhazmat.2010.11.100.

[17] P.R. Supronowicz, P.M. Ajayan, K.R. Ullmann, B.P. Arulanandam, D.W. Metzger, R. Bizios, Novel current-conducting composite substrates for exposing osteoblasts to alter-nating current stimulation, J. Biomed. Mater. Res. 59 (2002) 499–506. doi:10.1002/jbm.10015.

[18] K.D. Patel, R.K. Singh, H.W. Kim, Carbon-based nanomaterials as an emerging plat-form for theranostics, Mater. Horizons. 6 (2019) 434–469. doi:10.1039/c8mh00966j.

[19] W. Tao, D. Ni, G. Liu, P. Huang, X. Mou, K. Yang, D. Maiti, X. Tong, Carbon-based nanomaterials for biomedical applications: A recent study, Front. Pharmacol. (2019). doi:10.3389/fphar.2018.01401.

[20] D. Konios, M.M. Stylianakis, E. Stratakis, E. Kymakis, Dispersion behaviour of graphene oxide and reduced graphene oxide, J. Colloid Interface Sci. 430 (2014) 108–112. doi:10.1016/j.jcis.2014.05.033.

[21] A.M. Pinto, I.C. Gonçalves, F.D. Magalhães, Graphene-based materials biocompatibil-ity: A review, Colloids Surf. B. 111 (2013) 188–202. doi:10.1016/j.colsurfb.2013.05.022.

[22] P. Yang, S. Gai, J. Lin, Functionalized mesoporous silica materials for controlled drug delivery, Chem. Soc. Rev. 41 (2012) 3679. doi:10.1039/c2cs15308d.

[23] A. Schinwald, F.A. Murphy, A. Jones, W. MacNee, K. Donaldson, Graphene-based nanoplatelets: A new risk to the respiratory system as a consequence of their unusual aerodynamic properties, ACS Nano. 6 (2012) 736–746. doi:10.1021/nn204229f.

[24] Y. Pan, X. Liu, W. Zhang, Z. Liu, G. Zeng, B. Shao, Q. Liang, Q. He, X. Yuan, D. Huang, M. Chen, Advances in photocatalysis based on fullerene C60 and its derivatives: Properties, mechanism, synthesis, and applications, Appl. Catal. B Environ. 265 (2020) 118579. doi:10.1016/j.apcatb.2019.118579.

[25] S.S. Lucky, K.C. Soo, Y. Zhang, Nanoparticles in photodynamic therapy, Chem. Rev. 115 (2015) 1990–2042. doi:10.1021/cr5004198.

[26] G. Accorsi, N. Armaroli, Taking advantage of the electronic excited states of [60]-fullerenes, J. Phys. Chem. C. 114 (2010) 1385–1403. doi:10.1021/jp9092699.

[27] L. Yin, H. Zhou, L. Lian, S. Yan, W. Song, Effects of C 60 on the photochemical formation of reactive oxygen species from natural organic matter, Environ. Sci. Technol. 50 (2016) 11742–11751. doi:10.1021/acs.est.6b04488.

[28] Y. Fan, H. Liu, R. Han, L. Huang, H. Shi, Y. Sha, Y. Jiang, Extremely high brightness from polymer-encapsulated quantum dots for two-photon cellular and deep-tissue imaging, Sci. Rep. 5 (2015) 9908. doi:10.1038/srep09908.

[29] A. Herreros-López, M. Carini, T. Da Ros, T. Carofiglio, C. Marega, V. La Parola, V. Rapozzi, L.E. Xodo, A.A. Alshatwi, C. Hadad, M. Prato, Nanocrystalline cellulose-fullerene: Novel conjugates, Carbohydr. Polym. 164 (2017) 92–101. doi:10.1016/j.carbpol.2017.01.068.

[30] Z. Hu, C. Zhang, P. Tang, C. Li, Y. Yao, S. Sun, L. Zhang, Y. Huang, Protection of cells from nitric oxide-mediated apoptotic death by glutathione C 60 derivative, Cell Biol. Int. 36 (2012) 677–681. doi:10.1042/CBI20110566.

[31] J.J. Ryan, H.R. Bateman, A. Stover, G. Gomez, S.K. Norton, W. Zhao, L.B. Schwartz, R. Lenk, C.L. Kepley, Fullerene nanomaterials inhibit the allergic response, J. Immunol. 179 (2007) 665–672. doi:10.4049/jimmunol.179.1.665.

[32] T.M. Benn, P. Westerhoff, P. Herckes, Detection of fullerenes (C60 and C70) in commercial cosmetics, Environ. Pollut. 159 (2011) 1334–1342. doi:10.1016/j.envpol.2011.01.018.

[33] S.-R. Chae, E.M. Hotze, Y. Xiao, J. Rose, M.R. Wiesner, Comparison of methods for fullerene detection and measurements of reactive oxygen production in cosmetic products, Environ. Eng. Sci. 27 (2010) 797–804. doi:10.1089/ees.2010.0103.

[34] M. Wang, V. Nalla, S. Jeon, V. Mamidala, W. Ji, L.-S. Tan, T. Cooper, L.Y. Chiang, Large femtosecond two-photon absorption cross sections of fullerosome vesicle nanostructures derived from a highly photoresponsive amphiphilic C 60-light-harvesting fluorene dyad, J. Phys. Chem. C. 115 (2011) 18552–18559. doi:10.1021/jp207047k.

[35] A.G. Crevillen, A. Escarpa, C.D. García, Carbon-Based Nanomaterials in Analytical Chemistry, The Royal Society of Chemistry, Cambridge (2018): pp. 1–36. doi:10.1039/9781788012751-00001.

[36] V. Georgakilas, J.A. Perman, J. Tucek, R. Zboril, Broad family of carbon nanoallotropes: classification, chemistry, and applications of fullerenes, carbon dots, nanotubes, graphene, nanodiamonds, and combined superstructures, Chem. Rev. 115 (2015) 4744–4822. doi:10.1021/cr500304f.

[37] G.M. Durán, T.E. Benavidez, A.M. Contento, A. Ríos, C.D. García, Analysis of penicillamine using Cu-modified graphene quantum dots synthesized from uric acid as single precursor, J. Pharm. Anal. 7 (2017) 324–331. doi:10.1016/j.jpha.2017.07.002.

[38] J. Peng, W. Gao, B.K. Gupta, Z. Liu, R. Romero-Aburto, L. Ge, L. Song, L.B. Alemany, X. Zhan, G. Gao, S.A. Vithayathil, B.A. Kaipparettu, A.A. Marti, T. Hayashi, J.-J. Zhu, P.M. Ajayan, Graphene quantum dots derived from carbon fibers, Nano Lett. 12 (2012) 844–849. doi:10.1021/nl2038979.

[39] J. Shen, Y. Zhu, X. Yang, C. Li, Graphene quantum dots: Emergent nanolights for bioimaging, sensors, catalysis and photovoltaic devices, Chem. Commun. 48 (2012) 3686. doi:10.1039/c2cc00110a.

[40] G. Gedda, V.L.N. Balaji Gupta Tiruveedhi, G. Ganesh, J. Suribabu, Recent advancements of carbon dots in analytical techniques, in: S.K. Kailasa, A.C. Hussain (Eds.), Carbon-Based Nanomaterials in Analytical Chemistry, Elsevier, Cambridge (2023): pp. 137–147. doi:10.1016/B978-0-323-98350-1.00017-7.

[41] S.-L. Ye, J.-J. Huang, L. Luo, H.-J. Fu, Y.-M. Sun, Y.-D. Shen, H.-T. Lei, Z.-L. Xu, Preparation of carbon dots and their application in food analysis as signal probe, Chinese J. Anal. Chem. 45 (2017) 1571–1581. doi:10.1016/S1872-2040(17)61045-4.

[42] Y.-P. Sun, B. Zhou, Y. Lin, W. Wang, K.A.S. Fernando, P. Pathak, M.J. Meziani, B.A. Harruff, X. Wang, H. Wang, P.G. Luo, H. Yang, M.E. Kose, B. Chen, L.M. Veca, S.-Y. Xie, Quantum-sized carbon dots for bright and colorful photoluminescence, J. Am. Chem. Soc. 128 (2006) 7756–7757. doi:10.1021/ja062677d.

[43] J.-H. Liu, L. Cao, G.E. LeCroy, P. Wang, M.J. Meziani, Y. Dong, Y. Liu, P.G. Luo, Y.-P. Sun, Carbon "quantum" dots for fluorescence labeling of cells, ACS Appl. Mater. Interfaces. 7 (2015) 19439–19445. doi:10.1021/acsami.5b05665.

[44] P. Karfa, E. Roy, S. Patra, S. Kumar, A. Tarafdar, R. Madhuri, P.K. Sharma, Retracted article: Amino acid derived highly luminescent, heteroatom-doped carbon dots for label-free detection of Cd 2+ /Fe 3+, cell imaging and enhanced antibacterial activity, RSC Adv. 5 (2015) 58141–58153. doi:10.1039/C5RA09525E.

[45] J. Zhou, Z. Sheng, H. Han, M. Zou, C. Li, Facile synthesis of fluorescent carbon dots using watermelon peel as a carbon source, Mater. Lett. 66 (2012) 222–224. doi:10.1016/j.matlet.2011.08.081.

[46] V.N. Mehta, S. Jha, H. Basu, R.K. Singhal, S.K. Kailasa, One-step hydrothermal approach to fabricate carbon dots from apple juice for imaging of mycobacterium and fungal cells, Sens. Actuators B Chem. 213 (2015) 434–443. doi:10.1016/j.snb.2015.02.104.

[47] A. Sachdev, P. Gopinath, Green synthesis of multifunctional carbon dots from coriander leaves and their potential application as antioxidants, sensors and bioimaging agents, Analyst. 140 (2015) 4260–4269. doi:10.1039/C5AN00454C.

[48] Y. Dong, N. Zhou, X. Lin, J. Lin, Y. Chi, G. Chen, Extraction of electrochemiluminescent oxidized carbon quantum dots from activated carbon, Chem. Mater. 22 (2010) 5895–5899. doi:10.1021/cm1018844.

[49] Z. Zhang, J. Hao, J. Zhang, B. Zhang, J. Tang, Protein as the source for synthesizing fluorescent carbon dots by a one-pot hydrothermal route, RSC Adv. 2 (2012) 8599. doi:10.1039/c2ra21217j.

[50] X. Zhai, P. Zhang, C. Liu, T. Bai, W. Li, L. Dai, W. Liu, Highly luminescent carbon nanodots by microwave-assisted pyrolysis, Chem. Commun. 48 (2012) 7955. doi:10.1039/c2cc33869f.

[51] Z. Lei, S. Xu, J. Wan, P. Wu, Facile synthesis of N-rich carbon quantum dots by spontaneous polymerization and incision of solvents as efficient bioimaging probes and advanced electrocatalysts for oxygen reduction reaction, Nanoscale. 8 (2016) 2219–2226. doi:10.1039/C5NR07335A.

[52] C. Li, Z. Yan, L. Chen, J. Jin, D. Li, Desmin detection by facile prepared carbon quantum dots for early screening of colorectal cancer, Medicine (Baltimore). 96 (2017) e5521. doi:10.1097/MD.0000000000005521.

[53] A. Eatemadi, H. Daraee, H. Karimkhanloo, M. Kouhi, N. Zarghami, A. Akbarzadeh, M. Abasi, Y. Hanifehpour, S.W. Joo, Carbon nanotubes: Properties, synthesis, purification, and medical applications, Nanoscale Res. Lett. 9 (2014) 393. doi:10.1186/1556-276X-9-393.

[54] S. Iijima, T. Ichihashi, Single-shell carbon nanotubes of 1-nm diameter, Nature. 363 (1993) 603–605. doi:10.1038/363603a0.

[55] S. Iijima, Helical microtubules of graphitic carbon, Nature. 354 (1991) 56–58. doi:10.1038/354056a0.

[56] M. Lamberti, P. Pedata, N. Sannolo, S. Porto, A. De Rosa, M. Caraglia, Carbon nanotubes: Properties, biomedical applications, advantages and risks in patients and occupationally-exposed workers, Int. J. Immunopathol. Pharmacol. 28 (2015) 4–13. doi:10.1177/0394632015572559.

[57] M.S. Dresselhaus, G. Dresselhaus, J.C. Charlier, E. Hernández, Electronic, thermal and mechanical properties of carbon nanotubes, Philos. Trans. R. Soc. London. Ser. A Math. Phys. Eng. Sci. 362 (2004) 2065–2098. doi:10.1098/rsta.2004.1430.

[58] X. Zhang, J. Ma, H. Tennent, R. Hoch, Method for Preparing Single Walled Carbon Nanotubes (2012). https://patents.justia.com/patent/8287836.

[59] N. Grobert, Carbon nanotubes—becoming clean, Mater. Today. 10 (2007) 28–35. doi:10.1016/S1369-7021(06)71789-8.

[60] R.L. Vander Wal, G.M. Berger, T.M. Ticich, Carbon nanotube synthesis in a flame using laser ablation for in situ catalyst generation, Appl. Phys. A Mater. Sci. Process. 77 (2003) 885–889. doi:10.1007/s00339-003-2196-3.

[61] A. Aqel, K.M.M.A. El-Nour, R.A.A. Ammar, A. Al-Warthan, Carbon nanotubes, science and technology part (I) structure, synthesis and characterisation, Arab. J. Chem. 5 (2012) 1–23. doi:10.1016/j.arabjc.2010.08.022.

[62] H. Zare, S. Ahmadi, A. Ghasemi, M. Ghanbari, N. Rabiee, M. Bagherzadeh, M. Karimi, T.J. Webster, M.R. Hamblin, E. Mostafavi, Carbon nanotubes: Smart drug/gene delivery carriers, Int. J. Nanomedicine. 16 (2021) 1681–1706. doi:10.2147/IJN.S299448.

[63] D. Tasis, N. Tagmatarchis, A. Bianco, M. Prato, Chemistry of carbon nanotubes, Chem. Rev. 106 (2006) 1105–1136. doi:10.1021/cr050569o.

[64] M. Karimi, N. Solati, A. Ghasemi, M.A. Estiar, M. Hashemkhani, P. Kiani, E. Mohamed, A. Saeidi, M. Taheri, P. Avci, A.R. Aref, M. Amiri, F. Baniasadi, M.R. Hamblin, Carbon nanotubes part II: A remarkable carrier for drug and gene delivery, Expert Opin. Drug Deliv. 12 (2015) 1089–1105. doi:10.1517/17425247.2015.1004309.

[65] S. Prakash, M. Malhotra, W. Shao, C. Tomaro-Duchesneau, S. Abbasi, Polymeric nanohybrids and functionalized carbon nanotubes as drug delivery carriers for cancer therapy, Adv. Drug Deliv. Rev. 63 (2011) 1340–1351. doi:10.1016/j.addr.2011.06.013.

[66] O.V. Zakharova, E.E. Mastalygina, K.S. Golokhvast, A.A. Gusev, Graphene nanoribbons: Prospects of application in biomedicine and toxicity, Nanomater. 11 (2021) 2425. doi:10.3390/nano11092425.

[67] K. Nakada, M. Fujita, G. Dresselhaus, M.S. Dresselhaus, Edge state in graphene ribbons: Nanometer size effect and edge shape dependence, Phys. Rev. B. 54 (1996) 17954–17961. doi:10.1103/PhysRevB.54.17954.

[68] K. Wakabayashi, M. Fujita, H. Ajiki, M. Sigrist, Electronic and magnetic properties of nanographite ribbons, Phys. Rev. B. 59 (1999) 8271–8282. doi:10.1103/PhysRevB.59.8271.

[69] Y. Yang, R. Murali, Impact of size effect on graphene nanoribbon transport, IEEE Electron Device Lett. 31 (2010) 237–239. doi:10.1109/LED.2009.2039915.

[70] N. Harada, S. Sato, Electronic properties of NH4-adsorbed graphene nanoribbon as a promising candidate for a gas sensor, AIP Adv. 6 (2016) 055023. doi:10.1063/1.4952965.

[71] M. Berahman, M.H. Sheikhi, Hydrogen sulfide gas sensor based on decorated zig-zag graphene nanoribbon with copper, Sens. Actuators B Chem. 219 (2015) 338–345. doi:10.1016/j.snb.2015.04.114.

[72] M. Shekhirev, A. Lipatov, A. Torres, N.S. Vorobeva, A. Harkleroad, A. Lashkov, V. Sysoev, A. Sinitskii, Highly selective gas sensors based on graphene nanoribbons grown by chemical vapor deposition, ACS Appl. Mater. Interfaces. 12 (2020) 7392–7402. doi:10.1021/acsami.9b13946.

[73] X. Guo, M. Baumgarten, K. Müllen, Designing π-conjugated polymers for organic electronics, Prog. Polym. Sci. 38 (2013) 1832–1908. doi:10.1016/j.progpolymsci.2013.09.005.

[74] A. Celis, M.N. Nair, A. Taleb-Ibrahimi, E.H. Conrad, C. Berger, W.A. de Heer, A. Tejeda, Graphene nanoribbons: fabrication, properties and devices, J. Phys. D. Appl. Phys. 49 (2016) 143001. doi:10.1088/0022-3727/49/14/143001.

[75] A. Narita, X.-Y. Wang, X. Feng, K. Müllen, New advances in nanographene chemistry, Chem. Soc. Rev. 44 (2015) 6616–6643. doi:10.1039/C5CS00183H.

[76] G.Z. Magda, X. Jin, I. Hagymási, P. Vancsó, Z. Osváth, P. Nemes-Incze, C. Hwang, L.P. Biró, L. Tapasztó, Room-temperature magnetic order on zigzag edges of narrow graphene nanoribbons, Nature. 514 (2014) 608–611. doi:10.1038/nature13831.

[77] W.-X. Wang, M. Zhou, X. Li, S.-Y. Li, X. Wu, W. Duan, L. He, Energy gaps of atomically precise armchair graphene sidewall nanoribbons, Phys. Rev. B. 93 (2016) 241403. doi:10.1103/PhysRevB.93.241403.

[78] N. Merino-Díez, A. Garcia-Lekue, E. Carbonell-Sanromà, J. Li, M. Corso, L. Colazzo, F. Sedona, D. Sánchez-Portal, J.I. Pascual, D.G. de Oteyza, Width-dependent band gap in armchair graphene nanoribbons reveals fermi level pinning on Au(111), ACS Nano. 11 (2017) 11661–11668. doi:10.1021/acsnano.7b06765.

[79] T. de Sousa Araújo Cassiano, F.F. Monteiro, L. Evaristo de Sousa, G. Magela e Silva, P.H. de Oliveira Neto, Smooth gap tuning strategy for cove-type graphene nanoribbons, RSC Adv. 10 (2020) 26937–26943. doi:10.1039/D0RA02997A.

[80] A. Narita, X. Feng, Y. Hernandez, S.A. Jensen, M. Bonn, H. Yang, I.A. Verzhbitskiy, C. Casiraghi, M.R. Hansen, A.H.R. Koch, G. Fytas, O. Ivasenko, B. Li, K.S. Mali, T. Balandina, S. Mahesh, S. De Feyter, K. Müllen, Synthesis of structurally well-defined and liquid-phase-processable graphene nanoribbons, Nat. Chem. 6 (2014) 126–132. doi:10.1038/nchem.1819.

[81] Y. Huang, Y. Mai, U. Beser, J. Teyssandier, G. Velpula, H. van Gorp, L.A. Straasø, M.R. Hansen, D. Rizzo, C. Casiraghi, R. Yang, G. Zhang, D. Wu, F. Zhang, D. Yan, S. De Feyter, K. Müllen, X. Feng, Poly(ethylene oxide) functionalized graphene nanoribbons with excellent solution processability, J. Am. Chem. Soc. 138 (2016) 10136–10139. doi:10.1021/jacs.6b07061.

[82] Y. Huang, F. Xu, L. Ganzer, F.V.A. Camargo, T. Nagahara, J. Teyssandier, H. Van Gorp, K. Basse, L.A. Straasø, V. Nagyte, C. Casiraghi, M.R. Hansen, S. De Feyter, D. Yan, K. Müllen, X. Feng, G. Cerullo, Y. Mai, Intrinsic properties of single graphene nanoribbons in solution: Synthetic and spectroscopic studies, J. Am. Chem. Soc. 140 (2018) 10416–10420. doi:10.1021/jacs.8b06028.

[83] U. Rajaji, Graphene nanoribbons in electrochemical sensors and biosensors: A review, Int. J. Electrochem. Sci. 13 (2018) 6643–6654. doi:10.20964/2018.07.51.

[84] Y. Zhu, A.L. Higginbotham, J.M. Tour, Covalent functionalization of surfactant-wrapped graphene nanoribbons, Chem. Mater. 21 (2009) 5284–5291. doi:10.1021/cm902939n.

[85] S.M. Chowdhury, C. Surhland, Z. Sanchez, P. Chaudhary, M.A. Suresh Kumar, S. Lee, L.A. Peña, M. Waring, B. Sitharaman, M. Naidu, Graphene nanoribbons as a drug delivery agent for lucanthone mediated therapy of glioblastoma multiforme, Nanomed. Nanotechnol. Biol. Med. 11 (2015) 109–118. doi:10.1016/j.nano.2014.08.001.

[86] M. Mahmood, H. Villagarcia, E. Dervishi, T. Mustafa, M. Alimohammadi, D. Casciano, M. Khodakovskaya, A.S. Biris, Role of carbonaceous nanomaterials in stimulating osteogenesis in mammalian bone cells, J. Mater. Chem. B. 1 (2013) 3220. doi:10.1039/c3tb20248h.

[87] J. Chen, H. Peng, X. Wang, F. Shao, Z. Yuan, H. Han, Graphene oxide exhibits broad-spectrum antimicrobial activity against bacterial phytopathogens and fungal conidia by intertwining and membrane perturbation, Nanoscale. 6 (2014) 1879–1889. doi:10.1039/C3NR04941H.

[88] A. Gizzatov, V. Keshishian, A. Guven, A.M. Dimiev, F. Qu, R. Muthupillai, P. Decuzzi, R.G. Bryant, J.M. Tour, L.J. Wilson, Enhanced MRI relaxivity of aquated Gd 3+ ions by carboxyphenylated water-dispersed graphene nanoribbons, Nanoscale. 6 (2014) 3059–3063. doi:10.1039/C3NR06026H.

[89] A.P. Johnson, H.V. Gangadharappa, K. Pramod, Graphene nanoribbons: A promising nanomaterial for biomedical applications, J. Control. Release. 325 (2020) 141–162. doi:10.1016/j.jconrel.2020.06.034.

[90] M.M.J. Treacy, T.W. Ebbesen, J.M. Gibson, Exceptionally high Young's modulus observed for individual carbon nanotubes, Nature. 381 (1996) 678–680. doi:10.1038/381678a0.

[91] J. Hu, X. Ruan, Y.P. Chen, Thermal conductivity and thermal rectification in graphene nanoribbons: A molecular dynamics study, Nano Lett. 9 (2009) 2730–2735. doi:10.1021/nl901231s.

[92] L. Zhang, L. Balzano, D.E. Resasco, Single-walled carbon nanotubes of controlled diameter and bundle size and their field emission properties, J. Phys. Chem. B. 109 (2005) 14375–14381. doi:10.1021/jp0510488.

[93] F. Schedin, A.K. Geim, S.V. Morozov, E.W. Hill, P. Blake, M.I. Katsnelson, K.S. Novoselov, Detection of individual gas molecules adsorbed on graphene, Nat. Mater. 6 (2007) 652–655. doi:10.1038/nmat1967.

[94] M.I. Katsnelson, Graphene: Carbon in two dimensions, Mater. Today. 10 (2007) 20–27. doi:10.1016/S1369-7021(06)71788-6.

[95] M.M. Fogler, A.H. Castro Neto, F. Guinea, Effect of external conditions on the structure of scrolled graphene edges, Phys. Rev. B. 81 (2010) 161408. doi:10.1103/PhysRevB.81.161408.

[96] Y. Chen, J. Lu, Z. Gao, Structural and electronic study of nanoscrolls rolled up by a single graphene sheet, J. Phys. Chem. C. 111 (2007) 1625–1630. doi:10.1021/jp066030r.

[97] H. Pan, Y. Feng, J. Lin, Ab initio study of electronic and optical properties of multiwall carbon nanotube structures made up of a single rolled-up graphite sheet, Phys. Rev. B. 72 (2005) 085415. doi:10.1103/PhysRevB.72.085415.

[98] D. Xia, J. Xie, H. Chen, C. Lv, F. Besenbacher, Q. Xue, M. Dong, Fabrication of carbon nanoscrolls from monolayer graphene, Small. 6 (2010) 2010–2019. doi:10.1002/smll.201000646.

[99] R. Rurali, V.R. Coluci, D.S. Galvão, Prediction of giant electroactuation for papyrus-like carbon nanoscroll structures: First-principles calculations, Phys. Rev. B. 74 (2006) 085414. doi:10.1103/PhysRevB.74.085414.

[100] A.D. Sontakke, M.K. Purkait, A brief review on graphene oxide Nanoscrolls: Structure, Synthesis, characterization and scope of applications, Chem. Eng. J. 420 (2021) 129914. doi:10.1016/j.cej.2021.129914.

[101] A.D. Sontakke, R. Fopase, L.M. Pandey, M.K. Purkait, Development of graphene oxide nanoscrolls imparted nano-delivery system for the sustained release of gallic acid, Appl. Nanosci. 12 (2022) 2733–2751. doi:10.1007/s13204-022-02582-8.

[102] C.A. Amadei, I.Y. Stein, G.J. Silverberg, B.L. Wardle, C.D. Vecitis, Fabrication and morphology tuning of graphene oxide nanoscrolls, Nanoscale. 8 (2016) 6783–6791. doi:10.1039/c5nr07983g.

[103] T. Fan, W. Zeng, Q. Niu, S. Tong, K. Cai, Y. Liu, W. Huang, Y. Min, A.J. Epstein, Fabrication of high-quality graphene oxide nanoscrolls and application in supercapacitor, Nanoscale Res. Lett. 10 (2015) 1–8. doi:10.1186/s11671-015-0894-3.

[104] A.D. Sontakke, M.K. Purkait, Fabrication of ultrasound-mediated tunable graphene oxide nanoscrolls, Ultrason. Sonochem. 63 (2020) 104976. doi:10.1016/j.ultsonch.2020.104976.

[105] H.P. Boehm, R. Setton, E. Stumpp, International union of pure and applied chemistry inorganic chemistry division commission on high temperature and solid state chemistry* nomenclature and terminology of graphite intercalation compounds, Pure Appl. Chem. 66 (1994) 1893–1901. doi:10.1351/pac199466091893.

[106] S. Baig, M. Ahmed, A. Batool, A. Bashir, S. Mumtaz, M. Ikram, M. Saeed, K. Shahzad, M. Umer Farooq, A. Maqsood, M. Ikram, Introductory chapter: Brief scientific description to carbon allotropes - technological perspective, in: Graphene - Recent Advances and Future Perspective, IntechOpen, Cambridge (2022): pp. 225–240. doi:10.5772/intechopen.107940.

[107] V. Georgakilas, M. Otyepka, A.B. Bourlinos, V. Chandra, N. Kim, K.C. Kemp, P. Hobza, R. Zboril, K.S. Kim, Functionalization of graphene: Covalent and non-covalent approaches, derivatives and applications, Chem. Rev. 112 (2012) 6156–6214. doi:10.1021/cr3000412.

[108] V.B. Mbayachi, E. Ndayiragije, T. Sammani, S. Taj, E.R. Mbuta, A. Ullah Khan, Graphene synthesis, characterization and its applications: A review, Results Chem. 3 (2021) 100163. doi:10.1016/j.rechem.2021.100163.

[109] G. Yang, L. Li, W.B. Lee, M.C. Ng, Structure of graphene and its disorders: A review, Sci. Technol. Adv. Mater. 19 (2018) 613–648. doi:10.1080/14686996.2018.1494493.

[110] K.S. Novoselov, A.K. Geim, S.V. Morozov, D. Jiang, Y. Zhang, S.V. Dubonos, I.V. Grigorieva, A.A. Firsov, Electric field effect in atomically thin carbon films, Sci. 80, 306 (2004) 666–669. doi:10.1126/science.1102896.

[111] A.K. Geim, Graphene: Status and prospects, Sci. 80, 324 (2009) 1530–1534. doi:10.1126/science.1158877.

[112] X. Huang, Z. Yin, S. Wu, X. Qi, Q. He, Q. Zhang, Q. Yan, F. Boey, H. Zhang, Graphene-based materials: Synthesis, characterization, properties, and applications, Small. 7 (2011) 1876–1902. doi:10.1002/smll.201002009.

[113] L. Dai, Functionalization of graphene for efficient energy conversion and storage, Acc. Chem. Res. 46 (2013) 31–42. doi:10.1021/ar300122m.

[114] M. Teimouri, A.H. Nia, K. Abnous, H. Eshghi, M. Ramezani, Graphene oxide–cationic polymer conjugates: Synthesis and application as gene delivery vectors, Plasmid. 84–85 (2016) 51–60. doi:10.1016/j.plasmid.2016.03.002.

[115] C. Spinato, C. Ménard-Moyon, A. Bianco, Chemical functionalization of graphene for biomedical applications, Funct. Graphene. 9783527335 (2014) 95–138. doi:10.1002/9783527672790.ch4.

[116] T.P. Dasari Shareena, D. McShan, A.K. Dasmahapatra, P.B. Tchounwou, A review on graphene-based nanomaterials in biomedical applications and risks in environment and health, Nano-Micro Lett. 10 (2018) 1–34. doi:10.1007/s40820-018-0206-4.

[117] D. Li, M.B. Müller, S. Gilje, R.B. Kaner, G.G. Wallace, Processable aqueous dispersions of graphene nanosheets, Nat. Nanotechnol. 3 (2008) 101–105. doi:10.1038/nnano.2007.451.

[118] Y. Si, E.T. Samulski, Synthesis of water soluble graphene, Nano Lett. 8 (2008) 1679–1682. doi:10.1021/nl080604h.

[119] C. Shan, H. Yang, D. Han, Q. Zhang, A. Ivaska, L. Niu, Water-soluble graphene covalently functionalized by biocompatible poly-l-lysine, Langmuir. 25 (2009) 12030–12033. doi:10.1021/la903265p.

[120] C.-T. Hsieh, W.-Y. Chen, Water/oil repellency and work of adhesion of liquid droplets on graphene oxide and graphene surfaces, Surf. Coatings Technol. 205 (2011) 4554–4561. doi:10.1016/j.surfcoat.2011.03.128.

[121] J. Park, M. Yan, Covalent functionalization of graphene with reactive intermediates, Acc. Chem. Res. 46 (2013) 181–189. doi:10.1021/ar300172h.

[122] N. Mohanty, V. Berry, Graphene-based single-bacterium resolution biodevice and DNA transistor: Interfacing graphene derivatives with nanoscale and microscale biocomponents, Nano Lett. 8 (2008) 4469–4476. doi:10.1021/nl802412n.

[123] S.K. Min, W.Y. Kim, Y. Cho, K.S. Kim, Fast DNA sequencing with a graphene-based nanochannel device, Nat. Nanotechnol. 6 (2011) 162–165. doi:10.1038/nnano.2010.283.

[124] Y. Wang, Z. Li, J. Wang, J. Li, Y. Lin, Graphene and graphene oxide: Biofunctionalization and applications in biotechnology, Trends Biotechnol. 29 (2011) 205–212. doi:10.1016/j.tibtech.2011.01.008.

[125] Y. Zhu, S. Murali, W. Cai, X. Li, J.W. Suk, J.R. Potts, R.S. Ruoff, Graphene and graphene oxide: Synthesis, properties, and applications, Adv. Mater. 22 (2010) 3906–3924. doi:10.1002/adma.201001068.

[126] W. Ren, H.M. Cheng, The global growth of graphene, Nat. Nanotechnol. 9 (2014) 726–730. doi:10.1038/nnano.2014.229.

[127] P. Dhar, S.S. Gaur, A. Kumar, V. Katiyar, Cellulose Nanocrystal templated graphene nanoscrolls for high performance supercapacitors and hydrogen storage: An experimental and molecular simulation study, Sci. Rep. 8 (2018) 1–15. doi:10.1038/s41598-018-22123-0.

[128] S.B. Singh, M. De, Scope of doped mesoporous (<10 nm) surfactant-modified alumina templated carbons for hydrogen storage applications, Int. J. Energy Res. 43 (2019) 4264–4280. doi:10.1002/er.4552.

[129] R. Muñoz, D.P. Singh, R. Kumar, A. Matsuda, Graphene oxide for drug delivery and cancer therapy, Nanostruct. Poly. Composit. Biomed. Appl. (2019). doi:10.1016/b978-0-12-816771-7.00023-5.

[130] L. Zhang, J. Xia, Q. Zhao, L. Liu, Z. Zhang, Functional graphene oxide as a nanocarrier for controlled loading and targeted delivery of mixed anticancer drugs, Small. 6 (2010) 537–544. doi:10.1002/smll.200901680.

[131] M. Hoseini-Ghahfarokhi, S. Mirkiani, N. Mozaffari, M.A. Abdolahi Sadatlu, A. Ghasemi, S. Abbaspour, M. Akbarian, F. Farjadian, M. Karimi, Applications of graphene and graphene oxide in smart drug/gene delivery: Is the world still flat? Int. J. Nanomed. 15 (2020) 9469–9496. doi:10.2147/IJN.S265876.

[132] L. Liu, Q. Ma, J. Cao, Y. Gao, S. Han, Y. Liang, T. Zhang, Y. Song, Y. Sun, Recent progress of graphene oxide-based multifunctional nanomaterials for cancer treatment, Cancer Nanotechnol. 12 (2021) 1–31. doi:10.1186/s12645-021-00087-7.

[133] H.M. Hegab, L. Zou, Graphene oxide-assisted membranes: Fabrication and potential applications in desalination and water purification, J. Memb. Sci. 484 (2015) 95–106. doi:10.1016/j.memsci.2015.03.011.

[134] S.I. Siddiqui, S.A. Chaudhry, A review on graphene oxide and its composites preparation and their use for the removal of As3+ and As5+ from water under the effect of various parameters: Application of isotherm, kinetic and thermodynamics, Process Saf. Environ. Prot. 119 (2018) 138–163. doi:10.1016/j.psep.2018.07.020.

[135] A.D. Sontakke, M.K. Purkait, Fabrication of ultrasound-mediated tunable graphene oxide nanoscrolls, Ultrason. Sonochem. 63 (2020) 104976. doi:10.1016/j.ultsonch.2020.104976.

[136] F. Alemi, R. Zarezadeh, A.R. Sadigh, H. Hamishehkar, M. Rahimi, M. Majidinia, Z. Asemi, A. Ebrahimi-Kalan, B. Yousefi, N. Rashtchizadeh, Graphene oxide and reduced graphene oxide: Efficient cargo platforms for cancer theranostics, J. Drug Deliv. Sci. Technol. 60 (2020) 101974. doi:10.1016/j.jddst.2020.101974.

[137] J. Song, X. Wang, C.-T. Chang, Preparation and characterization of graphene oxide, J. Nanomater. 2014 (2014) 1–6. doi:10.1155/2014/276143.

[138] A.D. Sontakke, P. Mondal, M.K. Purkait, Graphene oxide-based advanced nanomaterials for environmental remediation applications, in: S.J. Ikhmayies (Ed.), Advanced Nanomaterials Advanced Materials Research Technology, Springer International Publishing, Cham (2022): pp. 155–190. doi:10.1007/978-3-031-11996-5_6.

[139] B.C. Brodie, XIII. On the atomic weight of graphite, Philos. Trans. R. Soc. London. 149 (1859) 249–259. doi:10.1098/rstl.1859.0013.

[140] L. Staudenmaier, Verfahren zur darstellung der graphitsäure, Berichte Der Dtsch. Chem. Gesellschaft. 31 (1898) 1481–1487. doi:10.1002/cber.18980310237.

[141] W.S. Hummers, R.E. Offeman, Preparation of graphitic oxide, J. Am. Chem. Soc. 80 (1958) 1339. doi:10.1021/ja01539a017.

[142] D.C. Marcano, D.V. Kosynkin, J.M. Berlin, A. Sinitskii, Z. Sun, A. Slesarev, L.B. Alemany, W. Lu, J.M. Tour, Improved synthesis of graphene oxide, ACS Nano. 4 (2010) 4806–4814. doi:10.1021/nn1006368.

[143] L. Sun, B. Fugetsu, Mass production of graphene oxide from expanded graphite, Mater. Lett. 109 (2013) 207–210. doi:10.1016/j.matlet.2013.07.072.

[144] L. Peng, Z. Xu, Z. Liu, Y. Wei, H. Sun, Z. Li, X. Zhao, C. Gao, An iron-based green approach to 1-h production of single-layer graphene oxide, Nat. Commun. 6 (2015) 5716. doi:10.1038/ncomms6716.

[145] X. Pan, J. Ji, N. Zhang, M. Xing, Research progress of graphene-based nanomaterials for the environmental remediation, Chinese Chem. Lett. 31 (2020) 1462–1473. doi:10.1016/j.cclet.2019.10.002.

[146] Y. Li, L. Feng, X. Shi, X. Wang, Y. Yang, K. Yang, T. Liu, G. Yang, Z. Liu, Surface coating-dependent cytotoxicity and degradation of graphene derivatives: Towards the design of non-toxic, degradable nano-graphene, Small. 10 (2014) 1544–1554. doi:10.1002/smll.201303234.

[147] Y. Pan, N.G. Sahoo, L. Li, The application of graphene oxide in drug delivery, Expert Opin. Drug Deliv. 9 (2012) 1365–1376. doi:10.1517/17425247.2012.729575.

[148] A.D. Sontakke, R. Fopase, L.M. Pandey, M.K. Purkait, Development of graphene oxide nanoscrolls imparted nano-delivery system for the sustained release of gallic acid, Appl. Nanosci. (2022). doi:10.1007/s13204-022-02582-8.

[149] L. Li, X. Zheng, C. Pan, H. Pan, Z. Guo, B. Liu, Y. Liu, A pH-sensitive and sustained-release oral drug delivery system: The synthesis, characterization, adsorption and release of the xanthan gum-graft-poly(acrylic acid)/GO–DCFP composite hydrogel, RSC Adv. 11 (2021) 26229–26240. doi:10.1039/D1RA01012C.

[150] R.J. Nemanich, J.A. Carlisle, A. Hirata, K. Haenen, CVD diamond—research, applications, and challenges, MRS Bull. 39 (2014) 490–494. doi:10.1557/mrs.2014.97.

[151] D.J. Garrett, W. Tong, D.A. Simpson, H. Meffin, Diamond for neural interfacing: A review, Carbon N. Y. 102 (2016) 437–454. doi:10.1016/j.carbon.2016.02.059.

[152] L. Guarina, C. Calorio, D. Gavello, E. Moreva, P. Traina, A. Battiato, S.D. Tchernij, Nanodiamonds-induced effects on neuronal firing of mouse hippocampal microcircuits, Sci. Rep. (2018) 1–14. doi:10.1038/s41598-018-20528-5.

[153] H.-Y. Chan, D.M. Aslam, J.A. Wiler, B. Casey, A novel diamond microprobe for neuro-chemical and electrical recording in neural prosthesis, J. Microelectromechanical Syst. 18 (2009) 511–521. doi:10.1109/JMEMS.2009.2015493.

[154] D. Luo, L. Wu, J. Zhi, Fabrication of boron-doped diamond nanorod forest electrodes and their application in nonenzymatic amperometric glucose biosensing, ACS Nano. 3 (2009) 2121–2128. doi:10.1021/nn9003154.

[155] F. Lemaître, M. Guille Collignon, C. Amatore, Recent advances in electrochemical detection of exocytosis, Electrochim. Acta. 140 (2014) 457–466. doi:10.1016/j.electacta.2014.02.059.

[156] J.E. Field, The mechanical and strength properties of diamond, Reports Prog. Phys. 75 (2012) 126505. doi:10.1088/0034-4885/75/12/126505.

[157] M. Jelínek, K. Smetana, T. Kocourek, B. Dvořánková, J. Zemek, J. Remsa, T. Luxbacher, Biocompatibility and sp3/sp2 ratio of laser created DLC films, Mater. Sci. Eng. B. 169 (2010) 89–93. doi:10.1016/j.mseb.2010.01.010.

[158] W. Yang, O. Auciello, J.E. Butler, W. Cai, J.A. Carlisle, J.E. Gerbi, D.M. Gruen, T. Knickerbocker, T.L. Lasseter, J.N. Russell, L.M. Smith, R.J. Hamers, DNA-modified nanocrystalline diamond thin-films as stable, biologically active substrates, Nat. Mater. 1 (2002) 253–257. doi:10.1038/nmat779.

[159] A.G. Rinzler, J. Liu, H. Dai, P. Nikolaev, C.B. Huffman, F.J. Rodríguez-Macías, P.J. Boul, A.H. Lu, D. Heymann, D.T. Colbert, R.S. Lee, J.E. Fischer, A.M. Rao, P.C. Eklund, R.E. Smalley, Large-scale purification of single-wall carbon nanotubes: Process, product, and characterization, Appl. Phys. A Mater. Sci. Process. 67 (1998) 29–37. doi:10.1007/s003390050734.

[160] B.W. Smith, M. Monthioux, D.E. Luzzi, Encapsulated C60 in carbon nanotubes, Nature. 396 (1998) 323–324. doi:10.1038/24521.

[161] M. Koshino, T. Tanaka, N. Solin, K. Suenaga, H. Isobe, E. Nakamura, Imaging of single organic molecules in motion, Sci. 80, 316 (2007) 853–853. doi:10.1126/science.1138690.

[162] A. Martín, A. Escarpa, Graphene: The cutting–edge interaction between chemistry and electrochemistry, TrAC Trends Anal. Chem. 56 (2014) 13–26. doi:10.1016/j.trac.2013.12.008.

[163] X. Sun, D. Luo, J. Liu, D.G. Evans, Monodisperse chemically modified graphene obtained by density gradient ultracentrifugal rate separation, ACS Nano. 4 (2010) 3381–3389. doi:10.1021/nn1000386.

[164] Z. Sun, Z. Yan, J. Yao, E. Beitler, Y. Zhu, J.M. Tour, Growth of graphene from solid carbon sources, Nature. 468 (2010) 549–552. doi:10.1038/nature09579.

[165] J. Yu, N. Grossiord, C.E. Koning, J. Loos, Controlling the dispersion of multi-wall carbon nanotubes in aqueous surfactant solution, Carbon N. Y. 45 (2007) 618–623. doi:10.1016/j.carbon.2006.10.010.

[166] Y. Ying Wang, Z. Hua Ni, T. Yu, Z.X. Shen, H. Min Wang, Y. Hong Wu, W. Chen, A.T. Shen Wee, Raman studies of monolayer graphene: The substrate effect, J. Phys. Chem. C. 112 (2008) 10637–10640. doi:10.1021/jp8008404.

[167] A.C. Ferrari, J.C. Meyer, V. Scardaci, C. Casiraghi, M. Lazzeri, F. Mauri, S. Piscanec, D. Jiang, K.S. Novoselov, S. Roth, A.K. Geim, Raman spectrum of graphene and graphene layers, Phys. Rev. Lett. 97 (2006) 187401. doi:10.1103/PhysRevLett.97.187401.

[168] A.C. Ferrari, J. Robertson, Interpretation of Raman spectra of disordered and amorphous carbon, Phys. Rev. B. 61 (2000) 14095–14107. doi:10.1103/PhysRevB.61.14095.

[169] M.S. Dresselhaus, G. Dresselhaus, R. Saito, A. Jorio, Raman spectroscopy of carbon nanotubes, Phys. Rep. 409 (2005) 47–99. doi:10.1016/j.physrep.2004.10.006.

[170] T.M.D. Alharbi, D. Harvey, I.K. Alsulami, N. Dehbari, X. Duan, R.N. Lamb, W.D. Lawrance, C.L. Raston, Shear stress mediated scrolling of graphene oxide, Carbon N. Y. 137 (2018) 419–424. doi:10.1016/j.carbon.2018.05.040.

[171] H.-B. Zhang, W.-G. Zheng, Q. Yan, Y. Yang, J.-W. Wang, Z.-H. Lu, G.-Y. Ji, Z.-Z. Yu, Electrically conductive polyethylene terephthalate/graphene nanocomposites prepared by melt compounding, Polymer (Guildf). 51 (2010) 1191–1196. doi:10.1016/j.polymer.2010.01.027.

[172] S. Dubin, S. Gilje, K. Wang, V.C. Tung, K. Cha, A.S. Hall, J. Farrar, R. Varshneya, Y. Yang, R.B. Kaner, A one-step, solvothermal reduction method for producing reduced graphene oxide dispersions in organic solvents, ACS Nano. 4 (2010) 3845–3852. doi:10.1021/nn100511a.

[173] A. Thess, R. Lee, P. Nikolaev, H. Dai, P. Petit, J. Robert, C. Xu, Y.H. Lee, S.G. Kim, A.G. Rinzler, D.T. Colbert, G.E. Scuseria, D. Tománek, J.E. Fischer, R.E. Smalley, Crystalline ropes of metallic carbon nanotubes, Sci. 80, 273 (1996) 483–487. doi:10.1126/science.273.5274.483.

[174] S.R. Mudshinge, A.B. Deore, S. Patil, C.M. Bhalgat, Nanoparticles: Emerging carriers for drug delivery, Saudi Pharm. J. 19 (2011) 129–141. doi:10.1016/j.jsps.2011.04.001.

[175] O. Erol, I. Uyan, M. Hatip, C. Yilmaz, A.B. Tekinay, M.O. Guler, Recent advances in bioactive 1D and 2D carbon nanomaterials for biomedical applications, Nanomed. Nanotechnol. Biol. Med. 14 (2018) 2433–2454. doi:10.1016/j.nano.2017.03.021.

[176] S. Tiwari, A.D. Sontakke, K. Baruah, M.K. Purkait, Development of graphene oxide-based nano-delivery system for natural chemotherapeutic agent (Caffeic Acid), Mater. Today Proc. (2022). doi:10.1016/j.matpr.2022.11.373.

[177] B.L. Perkins, N. Naderi, Carbon nanostructures in bone tissue engineering, Open Orthop. J. 10 (2016) 877–899. doi:10.2174/1874325001610010877.

[178] A. Mahor, P.P. Singh, P. Bharadwaj, N. Sharma, S. Yadav, J.M. Rosenholm, K.K. Bansal, Carbon-based nanomaterials for delivery of biologicals and therapeutics: A cutting-edge technology, Carbon. 7 (2021) 19. doi:10.3390/c7010019.

[179] Q. Zhang, Z. Wu, N. Li, Y. Pu, B. Wang, T. Zhang, J. Tao, Advanced review of graphene-based nanomaterials in drug delivery systems: Synthesis, modification, toxicity and application, Mater. Sci. Eng. C. 77 (2017) 1363–1375. doi:10.1016/j.msec.2017.03.196.

[180] T.M. Allen, Ligand-targeted therapeutics in anticancer therapy, Nat. Rev. Cancer. 2 (2002) 750–763. doi:10.1038/nrc903.

[181] D. Yang, L. Feng, C.A. Dougherty, K.E. Luker, D. Chen, M.A. Cauble, M.M. Banaszak Holl, G.D. Luker, B.D. Ross, Z. Liu, H. Hong, In vivo targeting of metastatic breast cancer via tumor vasculature-specific nano-graphene oxide, Biomat. 104 (2016) 361–371. doi:10.1016/j.biomaterials.2016.07.029.

[182] Y. Bai, T. Xu, X. Zhang, Micromachines graphene-based biosensors for detection of biomarkers, Curr. Nanosci. (2019). doi:10.3390/mi11010060.

[183] S.M. Janib, A.S. Moses, J.A. MacKay, Imaging and drug delivery using theranostic nanoparticles, Adv. Drug Deliv. Rev. 62 (2010) 1052–1063. doi:10.1016/j.addr.2010.08.004.

[184] J. Lee, J. Kim, S. Kim, D.H. Min, Biosensors based on graphene oxide and its biomedical application, Adv. Drug Deliv. Rev. 105 (2016). doi:10.1016/j.addr.2016.06.001.

[185] H. Zhao, R. Ding, X. Zhao, Y. Li, L. Qu, H. Pei, L. Yildirimer, Z. Wu, W. Zhang, Graphene-based nanomaterials for drug and/or gene delivery, bioimaging, and tissue engineering, Drug Discov. Today. 22 (2017) 1302–1317. doi:10.1016/j.drudis.2017.04.002.

[186] H. Gu, H. Tang, P. Xiong, Z. Zhou, Biomarkers-based biosensing and bioimaging with graphene for cancer diagnosis, Nanomat. 9 (2019) 130. doi:10.3390/nano9010130.

[187] D. Chauhan, B. Nohwal, C.S. Pundir, An electrochemical CD59 targeted noninvasive immunosensor based on graphene oxide nanoparticles embodied pencil graphite for detection of lung cancer, Microchem. J. 156 (2020) 104957. doi:10.1016/j.microc.2020.104957.

[188] N.F. Chiu, T.L. Lin, C.T. Kuo, Highly sensitive carboxyl-graphene oxide-based surface plasmon resonance immunosensor for the detection of lung cancer for cytokeratin 19 biomarker in human plasma, Sens. Actuators B Chem. 265 (2018). doi:10.1016/j.snb.2018.03.070.

[189] L. Tang, Q. Xiao, Y. Mei, S. He, Z. Zhang, R. Wang, W. Wang, Insights on functionalized carbon nanotubes for cancer theranostics, J. Nanobiotechnol. 19 (2021) 423. doi:10.1186/s12951-021-01174-y.

[190] Y. Zhou, K. Vinothini, F. Dou, Y. Jing, A.A. Chuturgoon, T. Arumugam, M. Rajan, Hyper-branched multifunctional carbon nanotubes carrier for targeted liver cancer therapy, Arab. J. Chem. 15 (2022) 103649. doi:10.1016/j.arabjc.2021.103649.

[191] B. Yu, L. Tan, R. Zheng, H. Tan, L. Zheng, Targeted delivery and controlled release of Paclitaxel for the treatment of lung cancer using single-walled carbon nanotubes, Mater. Sci. Eng. C. 68 (2016) 579–584. doi:10.1016/j.msec.2016.06.025.

[192] S.M. Ghafary, M. Nikkhah, S. Hatamie, S. Hosseinkhani, Simultaneous gene delivery and tracking through preparation of photo-luminescent nanoparticles based on graphene quantum dots and chimeric peptides, Sci. Rep. 7 (2017) 1–14. doi:10.1038/s41598-017-09890-y.

[193] J. Lee, M.M. Farag, E.K. Park, J. Lim, H. Yun, A simultaneous process of 3D magnesium phosphate scaffold fabrication and bioactive substance loading for hard tissue regeneration, Mater. Sci. Eng. C. 36 (2014) 252–260. doi:10.1016/j.msec.2013.12.007.

[194] B. Huang, Carbon nanotubes and their polymeric composites: The applications in tissue engineering, Biomanufacturing Rev. 5 (2020) 1–26. doi:10.1007/s40898-020-00009-x.

[195] M. Tanaka, Y. Sato, H. Haniu, H. Nomura, S. Kobayashi, S. Takanashi, M. Okamoto, T. Takizawa, K. Aoki, Y. Usui, A. Oishi, H. Kato, N. Saito, A three-dimensional block structure consisting exclusively of carbon nanotubes serving as bone regeneration scaffold and as bone defect filler, PLoS One. 12 (2017) e0172601. doi:10.1371/journal.pone.0172601.

[196] K.P. Gopinath, D.-V.N. Vo, D. Gnana Prakash, A. Adithya Joseph, S. Viswanathan, J. Arun, Environmental applications of carbon-based materials: A review, Environ. Chem. Lett. 19 (2021) 557–582. doi:10.1007/s10311-020-01084-9.

[197] Z. Liu, Q. Ling, Y. Cai, L. Xu, J. Su, K. Yu, X. Wu, J. Xu, B. Hu, X. Wang, Synthesis of carbon-based nanomaterials and their application in pollution management, Nanoscale Adv. 4 (2022) 1246–1262. doi:10.1039/d1na00843a.

[198] J. Li, X. Wang, G. Zhao, C. Chen, Z. Chai, A. Alsaedi, T. Hayat, X. Wang, Metal–organic framework-based materials: Superior adsorbents for the capture of toxic and radioactive metal ions, Chem. Soc. Rev. 47 (2018) 2322–2356. doi:10.1039/C7CS00543A.

[199] Y. Zou, Y. Hu, Z. Shen, L. Yao, D. Tang, S. Zhang, S. Wang, B. Hu, G. Zhao, X. Wang, Application of aluminosilicate clay mineral-based composites in photocatalysis, J. Environ. Sci. 115 (2022) 190–214. doi:10.1016/j.jes.2021.07.015.

[200] M. Zarenezhad, M. Zarei, M. Ebratkhahan, Environmental technology & innovation synthesis and study of functionalized magnetic graphene oxide for Pb 2 + removal from wastewater, Environ. Technol. Innov. 22 (2021) 101384. doi:10.1016/j.eti.2021.101384.

[201] S. Pashaei-Fakhri, S. Jamaleddin, R. Foroutan, Chemosphere crystal violet dye sorption over acrylamide/graphene oxide bonded sodium alginate nanocomposite hydrogel, Chemosphere. 270 (2021) 129419. doi:10.1016/j.chemosphere.2020.129419.

[202] H. Ge, Y. Zou, J. Chen, S. Liu, A hydrophobic bio-adsorbent synthesized by nanoparticle-modified graphene oxide coated corn straw pith for dye adsorption and photocatalytic degradation-kingdom, Environ. Technol. 41 (2019) 3633–3645.

[203] S. Bhattacharya, P. Banerjee, P. Das, A. Bhowal, S.K. Majumder, P. Ghosh, Erratum: Removal of aqueous carbamazepine using graphene oxide nanoplatelets: Process modelling and optimization, Sustain. Environ. Res. 30 (17) (2020). doi:10.1186/s42834-020-00066-4.

[204] Y. Yao, H. Zhang, K. Hu, G. Nie, Y. Yang, Y. Wang, X. Duan, S. Wang, Carbon dots based photocatalysis for environmental applications, J. Environ. Chem. Eng. 10 (2022) 107336. doi:10.1016/j.jece.2022.107336.

[205] P. Duarah, A. Bhattacharjee, P. Mondal, M.K. Purkait, Green synthesized carbon and metallic nanomaterials for biofuel production: Effect of operating parameters, in: M. Srivastava, M.A. Malik, P.K. Mishra (Eds.), Green Nano Solution for Bioenergy Production Enhancement, Springer Nature, Singapore (2022): pp. 105–126. doi:10.1007/978-981-16-9356-4_5.

[206] Y. Zhou, E.M. Zahran, B.A. Quiroga, J. Perez, K.J. Mintz, Z. Peng, P.Y. Liyanage, R.R. Pandey, C.C. Chusuei, R.M. Leblanc, Size-dependent photocatalytic activity of carbon dots with surface-state determined photoluminescence, Appl. Catal. B Environ. 248 (2019) 157–166. doi:10.1016/j.apcatb.2019.02.019.

[207] K. Qi, R. Selvaraj, T. Al Fahdi, S. Al-Kindy, Y. Kim, G.C. Wang, C.W. Tai, M. Sillanpää, Enhanced photocatalytic activity of anatase-TiO 2 nanoparticles by fullerene modification: A theoretical and experimental study, Appl. Surf. Sci. 387 (2016) 750–758. doi:10.1016/j.apsusc.2016.06.134.

2 Advancement in Drug Delivery Systems

2.1 INTRODUCTION TO DRUG DELIVERY SYSTEMS

Drug delivery systems, also known as DDSs, are pharmacological formulations that assist in the targeted distribution and controlled release of therapeutics in the body. After being administered, the DDSs will release the drug's active components that will reach the point of action after crossing several biological barriers. The fundamental aim of a DDS is to safely extend, contain, and target the therapeutic at the site of disease. The need for DDSs arises as several drugs are known to exert intolerable side effects on the body parts where they are not targeted. These side effects occur from the formulation of the medicine, route of administration, and the reaction of the body, or often result from the accumulation of high blood plasma drug concentration with traditional drug administration. To ensure better patient compliance, the steps that can be taken include limiting the drug quantity and frequency so that the same effect can be derived from the treatment. It can thus be concluded that the drug's effectiveness can be significantly impacted by the way it is delivered [1,2].

It is preferable to employ a DDS to deliver any drug in the human body to obtain a controlled release (CR) rate, completely discard any side effects, and achieve the full therapeutic effect. The physicochemical properties of the therapeutic agent and the presence of bio-barriers typically influence the conditions for successful drug delivery. For the treatment of the same ailment, the properties of the drug can differ significantly depending on its size, chemical makeup, hydrophilicity, and capacity to bind a particular receptor [3]. Thus, it is essential for a delivery system to operate in the therapeutic drug window with the concentration lying between effectiveness and toxicity limits. The frequency of dose, drug clearance rates, the method of administration, and the DDS used all affect how long a drug remains in the therapeutic range. The therapeutic range must lie between the minimal effective concentration (MEC) and the minimum toxic concentration (MTC). **Figure 2.1** [1] illustrates the concept of drug delivery through the variation in the concentration of a drug with respect to time. Subsequently, few drugs have a range of optimal doses in which the most significant benefits are obtained; quantities outside or inside this range can be harmful or have no therapeutic effect. Another effective method for simulating a drug delivery is pulsed delivery, which can control the concentration profile by permitting drug discharge from the drug carrier only when prompted by an external trigger like temperature and pH conditions [1,4].

The dose forms can be liquid, semisolid, or solid. Gaseous dosage forms, like anesthetics, can also be adopted [5]. Parenteral drug delivery refers to the process of injecting or infusing medication effectively within the body. There are several distinct types of delivery, including intravenous, subcutaneous, intradermal,

DOI: 10.1201/9781003358114-2

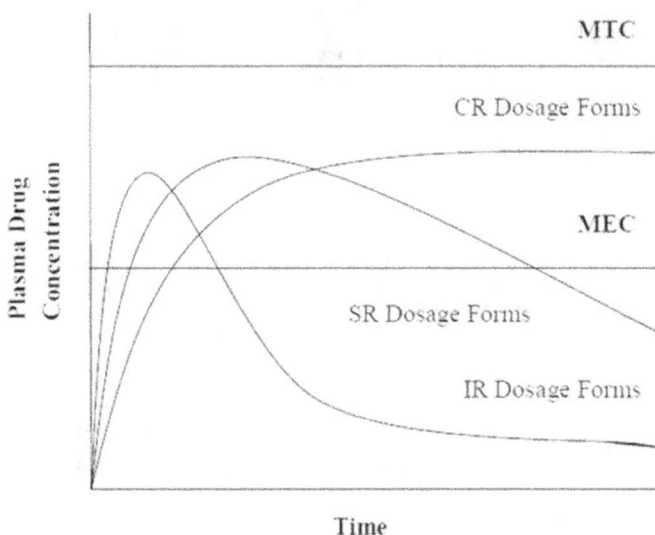

FIGURE 2.1 The Drug Plasma Levels Following a Single Oral Dose of a Drug in the Relevant Immediate Release (IR), Sustained Release (SR), and Controlled Release (CR) Forms [1].

intramuscular, and intraperitoneal, classified based on the central location of delivery. The majority of semisolid dose forms, such as creams and gels, are deposited to the skin before being ingested. Nevertheless, solid dose forms like transdermal patches as well as liquid dosage forms, like emulsions, can be employed. The dosage forms can either be modified release (MR) or instant release (IR). Similar to traditional drug delivery, IR dosage forms allow the drug to dissolve in the gastrointestinal contents without delay. Meanwhile, the drugs with delayed and extended release are both available in MR dosage formulations; the system prevents the drug release till it reaches the small intestine. Thus, these systems provide a sustained release (SR) and controlled release (CR) while consequently reducing its administration frequency [1].

The dosing frequency can be decreased by lowering the drug release rate over a longer period of time with polymer-based matrix or reservoir-controlled release mechanisms. CR DDSs, on the other hand, are intended to forecast consistent plasma drug concentrations irrespective of the biological milieu at the site of application. Hence, unlike SR systems, which control the drug's release from the pharmaceutical formulations, CR systems actively modulate the concentration of the drug within the body [6,7]. Moreover, SR systems are mostly limited to oral formulations, whereas CR systems can be supplied via a variety of methods, including transdermal, oral, and vaginal delivery. For optimal drug uptake, as well as for the drug levels in the blood and targeted site, the rate of release from the dosage type must serve as the rate-determining step. From imminent release to prolonged release dosage forms, the resultant plasma concentration versus time curves flattens down more, showing that the medication is maintained in the therapeutic range for a longer period of time following only one dosage form delivery. To overcome the problem of fluctuating drug levels associated with conventional dose forms, controlled DDSs have indeed been developed [1]. Successful formulation development depends on controlled drug releases and subsequent biodegradation.

The processes for drug release include desorption of surface-bound or adsorbed medication, migration through a polymer membrane enclosing the drug core, matrix erosion, conjunction of degradation and diffusion, and reactivity to stimuli like pH, temperature, or light. Optimizing the drug's bioavailability is the responsibility of the formulation researcher. To do this, the medicine's delivery mechanism must enable the drug to enter the systemic circulation and, more significantly, reach the targeted sites within the body, where it may be used without causing unwanted side effects. Also, the drug needs to be sustainable microbiologically and physically and chemically consistent with the excipients in the dosage forms. Designing the delivery methods in a way that can increase patient adherence is important. Instead of using parenteral medication formulations, it is possible to develop an oral solid dosage form that enables self-administration of the dose forms.

To allow repeatable medication distribution from the systems and reduce the impact on the body, such as dietary impacts on drug release, the pharmaceutical grade of the delivery systems must also be guaranteed in compliance with regulatory specifications. It is also vital to look into whether it is possible to scale up the discovered DDS beyond the laboratory to the industrial scale. The drug is not always delivered to the target organ via CR methods. To manage the bioavailability of drugs, target-specific drug delivery devices must be developed. As a result, several original ideas have been developed to specifically address the requirements of the desirable DDS. Thus, drug delivery systems have come to light, with researchers focusing on increasing bioavailability and patient compliance while lowering toxicity and adverse effects to overcome the major deficiencies of conventional drug delivery methods [3].

This chapter discusses the evolution of the DDS, including its historical aspects and classifications. The classification of the DDS based on the route of entry, release mechanism, and the recent advancement in the DDS to improve the therapeutic efficacy of the drug molecules using novel DDS approaches are also highlighted in this chapter. Furthermore, the principles of nanosized delivery systems using nanocarriers and nanoconjugates are elucidated while providing their surface characteristics and significance to the DDS. The last section briefly describes the efficacy of carbon-based nanomaterials as a drug carrier to deliver their potential in numerous biomedical applications, including drug delivery.

2.2 HISTORICAL ASPECTS OF DRUG DELIVERY SYSTEMS

Drug delivery history dates back to when humans used to intake medicines by chewing or inhaling plant and animal extracts. Over 1000 years ago, the concept of controlled drug delivery came into the picture, with a coating applied on the pills to improve their taste, which also had an effect on the drug release rate. The first-ever drug delivery products providing sustainable release were coated tablets developed in the late 1940s, where the coating and the drug were alternately stacked such that the pharmaceutical was released over time. This method not only improved the overall efficiency of the treatment but also significantly reduced the drug administration frequency while delaying the release from the stomach to the small intestine. However, this system had several limitations, like gastric emptying and low dissolution [8,9].

The commercialization of controlled drug delivery products began with the launch of Spansule® 12 hours release technology introduced by Smith, Kline & French Laboratories. This technology was used first to develop Dexedrine® and later Contac® 600 with dextroamphetamine sulfate, phenylpropanolamine hydrochloride, and chlorpheniramine maleate individually [8,10]. Since then, three historical periods have been identified in the advancement of controlled drug delivery systems, defined in three distinct generations.

The development of Spansule® marked the first generation of these drug delivery systems. The system was designed such that the patient had to take medicine only twice a day as it gave a sustained drug release for a period of 12 hours. It provides a dissolution-controlled mechanism by regulating the dissolution of the drug core through a coating barrier. Since then, various other modifications have been made to this technology to synthesize products giving better release profiles and more patient compliance [10]. The first-generation DDSs were based on oral or transdermal delivery, and the drug release mechanisms were either via dissolution, diffusion, osmosis, or ion exchange [9,10].

The second-generation DDSs were developed from 1980 to 2010 and were characterized by their zero-order release mechanism. Compared with the number of formulations synthesized, the second-generation DDSs were not as successful as the first. Based on the assumption that maintaining a consistent drug concentration was better, all research efforts were concentrated on composing a constant rate of release (zero-order DDSs). After ten years of extensive research, it was announced that zero-order release kinetics is not strictly necessary for a DDS to be classified as a sustained release DDS and following this discovery, significant advancements were made in this field. The second-generation DDSs utilized smart polymers and hydrogels that were sensitive to external factors. Tumor-targeting nanoparticle-based drug delivery systems were also designed with time; however, all these DDSs had a shortcoming with their inability to cross biological barriers [9,10].

The third-generation DDSs are currently being constructed to overcome the challenges offered to the second-generation DDSs by biological barriers and characteristics of the drug and the delivery system. Researchers have been focusing on reducing the side effects, working on the drug's poor solubility and high molecular weights, and having better control of the release kinetics. Low water solubility can lead to problems, including decreased bioavailability and higher drug product costs. For instance, medicines with low water solubility have reduced uptake in the gastrointestinal system when taken orally. Low solubility, on the other hand, might lead to drug precipitation and agglomeration, which can result in some hazardous consequences. As a result, tremendous endeavors have been undertaken to increase drug solubility [11].

Proteins and polypeptides are examples of bioactive molecules that have a role in regulating the body's performance and are thus important for sustaining health. These drugs must be administered in specified amounts, at the appropriate times, and to specific body sites [12]. These complex molecular drugs are often administered parenterally; however, due to their large size, the digestive tract is unable to absorb them. As a result, novel delivery techniques such as pulmonary, nasal, and transdermal systems have been employed [9].

As previously stated, drug delivery is defined as a mechanism designed to release a drug at a preset duration and rate. Organizing the carrier to target a certain location and discharge at a specified pace are two obstacles that one may encounter while developing an effective carrier. Developing an ideal drug delivery system is a considerable challenge since the drug must be directed to a specific site and released continuously over time with zero negative impact on the body. With the advancement in science and technology, various interdisciplinary types of research are being conducted to develop the most efficient and perfectly biocompatible DDSs [10,13].

2.3 CLASSIFICATIONS OF DRUG DELIVERY SYSTEMS

2.3.1 CONVENTIONAL DRUG DELIVERY SYSTEMS

Traditional drug delivery systems, also known as conventional DDSs, are classical methods for administering drugs into the body. These methods include simple oral, inhaled, or intravenous drug administration. Some advantages of these DDSs include the convenience of administration, accurate measurement of dose, higher shelf life, dose adjustment, and low cost. They are typically utilized when the objective is to achieve rapid drug absorption, subsequently facilitating a quick drug release. However, the traditional delivery methods fail to maintain a fixed and constant drug concentration over time. They do not provide a target-specific release and are often associated with the premature metabolism of drugs and excretion from the body. One way to address the issue of drug concentration instability is by administering multiple doses at regular intervals, but this approach has some limitations. Drug concentration in the blood plasma tends to fluctuate irregularly, and patients may forget to take the prescribed dose at the correct time. Given these issues, the need for new and innovative drug delivery systems has become increasingly apparent [2,14,15].

2.3.2 NOVEL DRUG DELIVERY SYSTEMS

Novel drug delivery systems can solve several drawbacks of traditional drug delivery methods. They are also referred to as controlled drug delivery systems as they can improve the efficiency of any treatment by enhancing drug potency, improving drug safety, and enabling the targeted delivery of drugs to specific tissues or cells in the body. The definition of "controlled release" extends beyond sustainable drug release but must also exhibit two essential characteristics: predictability and reproducibility. The advantages of controlled DDSs include drug release at a specific rate, direct delivery to a particular site, extended residence period, protection from metabolism, and enhanced bioavailability. Controlled drug delivery systems can be categorized into four types. The first type is rate-programmed DDSs, where the system design is modified to alter the diffusion rate of drug molecules, which further varies the release rate. The activation-modulated DDSs, a second type of novel DDS, work with external simulations like physical and chemical processes, which then control the drug release process. The third type of controlled DDSs is feedback-regulated DDS. With this type of DDS, sensors on the devices measure the concentration of certain biochemical substances, and this concentration controls the drug release. Finally, site-targeted DDSs are often used for treating diseases like cancer. They deliver a specific drug dose to a particular site in the body for a set period. Such types of DDS assist in eliminating side effects of drugs while providing high biocompatibility, improved drug absorption, distribution, and metabolism, maintaining consistent drug concentration in blood, and cutting down dose frequency and cost [2,15,16].

The rate-programmed DDSs are further classified into polymer-matrix diffusion-controlled, membrane permeation-controlled, hybrid type, and micro-reservoir partition-controlled DDS. The activation-modulated DDSs can be established through external and internal stimuli, including physical, chemical, and biological stimuli. The physical stimuli comprise temperature, pressure, magnetic and electric fields, along with ultrasound and light waves. At the same time, chemical stimuli include pH, hydrolysis, and reactive oxygen species (ROS). In addition, the biological stimuli mainly comprise proteins, enzymes, and aptamers. A feedback-regulated DDS comprises bio-erosion, bio-responsive and self-modulated DDS, wherein the drug release is mostly modulated or controlled via biological substances. The targeted DDS mainly primarily works on two mechanisms, namely, the passive and active targeting mechanisms through systemic targeting and intracellular targeting. In the case of passive targeting, macromolecules get aggregated selectively over the targeted tissues due to the enhanced permeability and retention characteristics. In contrast, the active targeting mechanism occurs as a result of precise interactions between the target cell's receptors and nanocarrier [15,17].

2.3.3 BASED ON THE ROUTE OF ADMINISTRATION

2.3.3.1 Oral Administration

Oral drug intake is the most common and conventional method of administration. It comprises tablets, capsules, and syrup that are taken orally and pass through the digestive system. It has several advantages, such as the convenience of administration, its noninvasive nature, and its low cost. However, in oral DDSs, there is almost no control over the drug release, leading to a fluctuating concentration in the plasma, which results in side effects. Besides that, additional drug absorption from standard formulations may vary significantly based on the physicochemical characteristics of the drug and its carrier type, as well as a number of physiological variables like the absence or presence of food, pH, gastrointestinal tract motility, etc. Thus, it is essential to design the carrier in a way that it provides controlled release [15,18].

2.3.3.2 Rectal Delivery

The rectal delivery system is inserted through the rectum, which dissolves at body temperature to release the drug. As it doesn't involve first-pass metabolism, it can be helpful in cases like an unconscious patient. Though this delivery route can be a good substitute for oral administration, it often leads to patient discomfort. Moreover, it can be beneficial in cases with poorly absorbed drugs in the upper gastrointestinal tract as the medication can bypass the liver, leading to higher bioavailability.

Subsequently, the protection provided to these drugs from enzymatic degradation can lead to better efficacy. For a drug that requires a high dose, developing an oral dosage form may be difficult because of problems like low solubility or instability; thus, rectal administration may be a practical substitute [19].

2.3.3.3 Intravenous Delivery

Intravenous administration is the fastest and most bioavailable method of delivering a drug into the body's systemic circulation. It has several advantages, like allowing the medication to infuse straight into the bloodstream, leading to rapid delivery in the body; helping control drug levels in the body by enabling precise dosing; providing immediate effect and quick onset of drug action; suitable for drugs containing irritants; and easy access to the bloodstream for blood sampling and monitoring of drug levels. However, it has some disadvantages, like infection and tissue damage, and requires trained personnel for its application [20].

2.3.3.4 Subcutaneous Delivery

In this delivery method, the drug is delivered in subcutaneous tissue in a liquid form. One of the most significant advantages of this delivery method is that the drug can be self-administered by the patient, leading to improved compliance and reduced expenditure. This delivery method is also less painful than intravenous and intramuscular administration and has fewer chances of infection caused by the treatment. However, this delivery method is limited to small volumes of the drug, making it unsuitable for treatments that require high doses. Also, some medications may retain or degrade at the injection site, causing low treatment efficiency [21].

2.3.3.5 Intramuscular Delivery

In intramuscular delivery, a liquid medication is injected via an injector into the muscle tissue. Since the drug is injected directly into the muscle, which can be absorbed into the bloodstream, this administration technique is appropriate for medications that are not readily soluble or absorbed through other methods. Additionally, in contrast to the subcutaneous (SC) approach, which can only administer smaller amounts of the drug due to the constrained space between the skin and underlying tissues, intramuscular administration enables the administration of a larger volume of the drug [4,15].

2.3.4 BASED ON THE RELEASE MECHANISM

2.3.4.1 Dissolution

The process of dissolution refers to the transfer of molecules of a solute into a solvent vehicle. In the case of an active agent, this involves moving drug molecules or ions from a solid phase into the surrounding medium. Examining the rate at which the drug dissolves from its solid form can predict the drug release rate from a therapeutic system. When no chemical reaction is involved, a higher level of solubility leads to a more rapid dissolution rate. When the solvating medium surrounding a solid drug particle is not saturated, dissolution can occur. The process is influenced by several factors, including the solvating medium, the surface area of the solid, the thickness of the boundary layer, the diffusion coefficient, agitation of the medium, and temperature, which can regulate the dissolution process of the drug particle [14,22].

2.3.4.2 Partitioning

The monitoring of drug release is significantly influenced by the way the drug partitions in the media. Drug delivery systems can be composed of materials that may display varying affinities and polarities toward different mediums; this nature can control drug delivery. When a drug molecule encounters interfaces between different materials or phases, its movement between these phases depends on their concentrations, chemical potentials, and affinity for each phase. This affinity can be quantified with the partition coefficient, which is the ratio of drug solubility in two phases. Suppose a polymeric DDS designed with micelles possessing hydrophilic coronas and hydrophobic cores is dissolved in an aqueous environment; the hydrophilic drugs will be retained in the coronas for a short period, while hydrophobic drugs will be released for longer durations due to their partitioning in the cores [17,22,23].

2.3.4.3 Diffusion

Diffusion-controlled drug delivery systems utilize inert water-insoluble polymeric membrane matrices to load drugs and release them via diffusion. The release rate of drugs is regulated by Fick's laws of diffusion, and the diffusion of the drug is the rate-limiting step here. Fick's first law of diffusion states that the molar flux is directly proportional to the concentration gradient. On the other hand, Fick's second law of diffusion states that a solution's rate of concentration change at a specific point in space is proportional to the second derivative of the concentration gradient with space. This law deals with variations in the concentration gradient with time at any distance [2,14,17].

These systems can be classified into membrane control reservoir systems and monolithic or matrix systems. Membrane-controlled systems hold the drug as a reservoir in the core, surrounded by a thin polymeric membrane. This membrane can either be porous or nonporous. The release of drugs occurs via diffusion through the membrane; its thickness and porosity, along with the drug's physicochemical properties, determine the release rate. Monolithic or matrix-controlled delivery systems involve either the homogeneous dissolution or dispersion of the drug throughout the polymer matrix. Here the release occurs via diffusion when the outer layer dissolves, allowing the drug to diffuse out of the matrix. If the drug is dissolved and loaded below the solubility limit in monolithic systems, the drug release decreases as the matrix's size decreases. The release follows a nonzero order, meaning that the absorption rate is not equal to the elimination rate. On the other hand, in systems where the drug is dispersed in the polymer matrix, it is loaded above the solubility limit [2,14].

2.3.4.4 Osmosis

Comprehensive treatment depends on selecting the proper medication and dose over time. The ability of rate-controlled release systems to preserve the active drug levels in the body at the ideal level lowers the risk of adverse effects and subpar therapeutic effectiveness.

Osmosis, among the most elementary biological concepts, has been used in a technological device for the past 50 years to facilitate the modulation of the drug release rate. Osmosis-based drug delivery devices have been suggested as a practical way to regulate the release rate. These are dependable, well-proven systems that permit a variety of uses, from implanted devices that effectively regulate the dissolution of the active ingredient over time spans of months, years, or longer to oral dosage forms that deliver the active ingredient in less than 24 hours. The osmosis concept can also be used with other techniques to regulate the rate of drug release [2].

Osmotic drug delivery is a method that employs osmotic pressure to achieve controlled drug delivery. Osmosis describes the process of solvent movement from an area of lower to higher solute concentration via a semipermeable membrane. Osmotic pressure is generated by the movement of water through a semipermeable membrane that separates two solutions with different solute concentrations. The system includes a drug, which can act as an osmogene, a semipermeable membrane with high wet strength, water permeability, and biocompatibility to withstand the pressure inside. An outer coating material permeable to water but impermeable to solute can also be used here. This DDS commonly employs polymers like cellulose acetate, cellulose triacetate, and ethyl cellulose [2,14].

2.3.4.5 Swelling

Many materials swell when they come into contact with water due to their hydrophilic nature. Such materials are utilized to prepare swelling-based drug delivery systems. Polymers are primarily used to prepare controlled release systems because their chain can be organized three-dimensionally. When this polymer is exposed to water, its internal network expands, creating bonds, and the slow dissolution of the polymer into water begins. Subsequently, the system's volume increases along with the emergence of spaces between the polymeric chains. This system expansion is utilized to regulate the drug release from the polymeric systems. The drug here is dissolved or dispersed in the polymer system and released when the polymer is dissolved in water [2,14].

In actuality, the shape of the matrices or membranes may be used to macroscopically examine the importance of the swelling. The water that is absorbed by a polymer system enhances its thickness and volume during the initial phase of drug delivery. Such growth in thickness is countered by the subsequent unilateral withdrawal of polymeric chains and the dissolving of the drug or fillers utilized, resulting in a reduction in the matrix's volume. Ultimately, once the complete polymer is inflated, the matrix dissipates. It would be more appropriate to refer to this kind of system as a "swellable-soluble matrix." In this instance, swelling frequently occurs before polymer disintegration. However, occasionally, the substance just partially swells, and the matrix persists. Such phenomena can happen if water and the polymer aren't compatible enough, if the polymer chain is long enough, or if cross-links are added to produce a polymer matrix [2,17].

2.3.4.6 Erosion

The polymers utilized in diffusion-controlled DDS serve a mostly passive function. They operate as carriers and slow down the distribution of the active drug to the intended target. A few polymeric carriers have been developed to participate more actively in the drug delivery procedure. Some polymer-based drug carriers have the property of eroding when they undergo a chemical reaction. In biodegradable or erodible systems, these polymeric materials are utilized that immobilize and contain the active substance, which is then released once the net has eroded. The most significant advantage of an erodible system is that it dissolves and degrades when it enters the body; thus, it requires no separate removal procedure. However, the carrier system must be nontoxic and erodible; either bulk or surface erosion governs the erosion process. In bulk erosion, the entire polymer disintegrates to release the drug trapped in the system, while surface erosion occurs when water slowly invades the system dissolving only the surface. The erosion process depends on the chemical structure and composition, configuration, and molecular weight of the polymer used [2,14].

2.4   PRINCIPLES OF NANOSIZED DELIVERY SYSTEMS

Nanoscience appraises materials at the molecular, macromolecular, and atomic levels; at these scales, physical material characteristics differ dramatically from those at higher scales. For many purposes, nanotechnologies can modify the size and forms of these materials at the nanoscale. Drug authorities determine that a nanoscale product is one that has, at a minimum, one dimension that falls within the range of 1–100 nm [24,25]. Also, if a substance or finished product exhibits size-related characteristics or phenomena up to 1 μm (1000 nm), the US FDA deems it to comprise nanomaterials [24]. Nanomaterials are defined by the International Organization for Standardization (ISO) as materials with any external dimension or internal or surface attributes that lie on the nanoscale [26]. Drug nanosystems provide a number of advantages. For instance, they may be employed to enhance absorption profiles for targeted and controlled drug delivery, to offer optimum therapeutic action with minimal adverse reactions, to reduce the delivery frequency for high metabolic stability, or to preserve and sustain the drug material against spontaneous degradation all through storage and *in-vivo*. Moreover, it has been demonstrated that cells may absorb nanoparticles as such [27].

The toxicity concerns associated with nanosized materials might vary significantly according to the substance and structure of the nanosystems; however, regardless of the nanosystems, the possible exposures and toxicology of the nanosystems must be meticulously evaluated [28,29]. Regarding nanoscale materials, it is important to pay attention to both the material's toxicity and the tiny-size nanotoxicity [30,31].

Nanomaterials have the ability to cause *in-vivo* oxidative stress, inflammatory responses, cytotoxicity, and genotoxicity [30]. Particular attention must be paid to the sustainability of nonbiodegradable and gradually disintegrating nanosystems [28,32]. Several nanosized DDSs have been demonstrated for pharmaceutical and medical applications using a range of delivery methods, since they can transport a lot of drugs and do not require a high-dose carrier to attain the therapeutic concentrations due to the higher surface area of the nanomaterials [33]. Depending on the kind of carrier used, greater drug-loading nanomedicine could be categorized into four groups: 1. inert carriers, where the drug is mounted on inorganic carriers like mesoporous nanoparticles of silica or mesoporous carbon nanoparticles; 2. the drug appears to be part of a carrier like linear or branched polymer-drug conjugates; 3. the drug as a carrier like drug nanoclusters; and 4. amphoteric drug-drug conjugates. Many studies have been conducted on polymeric drug nanoparticles since the 1970s [34].

Subsequently, there has been a lot of investigation into nanosized systems, including solid lipid nanoparticles, liposomes, dendrimers, and carbon-based nanomaterials [35]. Such nanosized drug delivery methods were invented to strengthen the drug's solubility and dissolution rate, which frequently results in enhanced pharmacokinetic/pharmacodynamic characteristics and better *in-vivo* effectiveness [36]. The bioavailability and safety of nano drugs can be further increased by functionalizing them or incorporating targeted functionalities [37].

While analyzing the entire market position of nano drugs in US dollars in 2017, drug nanostructures and polymeric nanoparticles accounted for around 80% of the market [35]. The number of drug items utilizing nanomaterials that are submitted to the US FDA each year has exhibited rising trends [38,39]. There are several varieties of nano-drug systems. In some instances, the drug is entrapped within a sheer drug substance that is only enclosed with a few active ingredients (drug nanocrystals). However, in the majority of applications, the drug is contained inside some sort of nanocarrier. The nanocarriers generally employed for drug delivery applications include polymeric nanoparticles, micelles, mesoporous nanostructures, hydrogels, dendrimers, liposomes, and carbon-based nanomaterials (**Figure 2.2**) [40]. The characteristics of some of these nanocarriers are briefly discussed as follows.

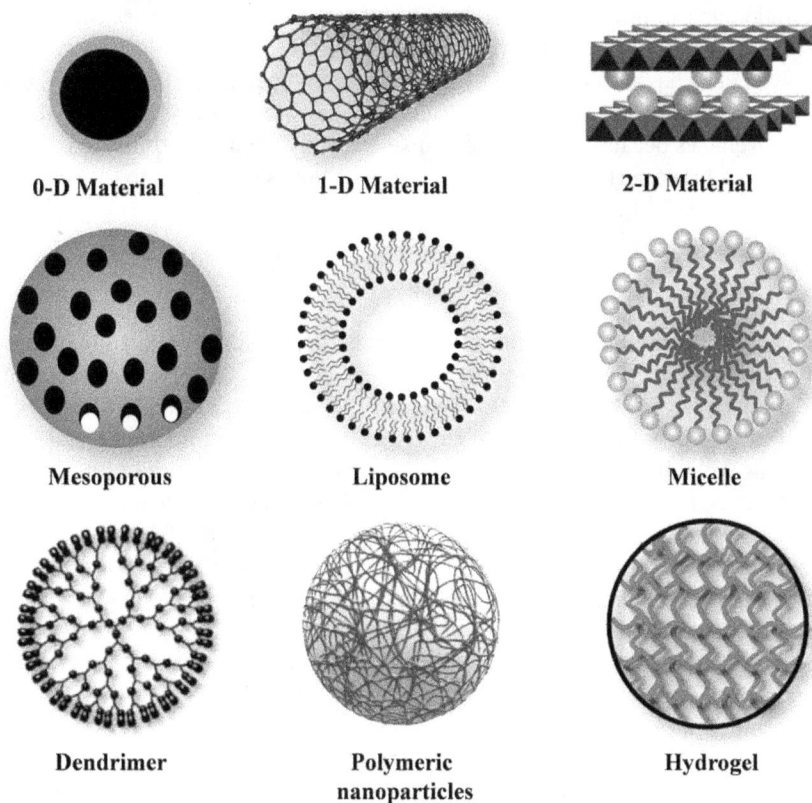

0-D Material **1-D Material** **2-D Material**

Mesoporous **Liposome** **Micelle**

Dendrimer **Polymeric nanoparticles** **Hydrogel**

FIGURE 2.2 Types of Nanocarriers Used as a Controlled Drug Delivery Vehicle [40].

2.4.1 POLYMERIC NANOPARTICLES

Polymeric nanostructures are made from solid, often spherical polymers that might be either organic or synthetic. Drug delivery is among the most significant biological applications of polymeric nanoparticles. Numerous methods of delivery have been attempted with these nanoparticles to administer a variety of medications, including tiny hydrophilic as well as hydrophobic pharmaceutical drugs, peptides, vaccines, and biomolecules [41]. The most effective biodegradable polymers for exploring polymeric nanoparticles are various types of poly(lactide-co-glycolide) and poly(lactide) copolymers [42]. Polymeric nanoparticles offer significant benefits such as facilitating controlled drug release to the targeted region, stabilizing malleable molecules (such as proteins), and allowing surface modification with receptors for covert and targeted drug administration [43].

2.4.2 LIPOSOMES

One of the most researched nano-delivery technologies for use in the cosmetics and pharmaceutical industries is the liposome. These are spherical vesicles that typically range in size from 50 to 450 nm and are made up of phospholipid bilayers, particularly phosphatidylcholines, that surround an aqueous core. To decrease liposome penetration and improve *in-vivo* and *in-vitro* endurance of the bilayer frameworks, cholesterol is introduced to the bilayer membrane of liposomes. Both hydrophilic (dissolved in an aqueous core) and hydrophobic (entrapped in the lipid bilayer) drugs can be delivered using this type of structure. They are regarded as effective drug delivery vehicles because of their biocompatibility and biodegradability and the fact that the membrane surrounding the active ingredients is equivalent to the cell membranes *in-vivo* [35,44].

2.4.3 LIPIDS

The two types of lipid nanoparticles involve solid lipid nanoparticles and lipid carriers with the nanostructure. The former has several qualities, including simple production at a cheap cost, the avoidance of organic solvent, and characteristics like photo-, moisture-, and chemical sensitivity. Nevertheless, due to the precise crystal lattice that forms while in storage, its crystal structure restricts the capacity of drugs it can hold. Moreover, the drug release profile, as well as some other characteristics, may change while the material is being stored. Lipid carriers in the form of nanostructures have been developed to address the aforementioned problems. The defect of the structure may be maintained and increased using a wide variety of lipid molecules. The defect increases their ability to load drugs [45].

Solid lipid nanoparticles (SLNs) are made up of 0.1%-30% (w/w) solid fat floating in an aqueous medium. The lipid particles are solid at both the body and room temperature. Surfactants (0.5%–5% (w/w)) or the functionalization of the surfaces utilizing certain hydrophilic components both lower the free energy of the hydrophobic surfaces. Controlling particle size, drug loading, release behavior, and shelf life may be accomplished by choosing the appropriate lipids and surfactants [46]. SLNs are frequently made using lipids such as fatty acids, waxes, steroids, and glycerides.

2.4.4 DENDRIMERS

Dendrimers are macromolecules made of polymers. They have a precisely articulated structure with one atom or molecule at the center, followed by multiple repeating branches that emerge proportionately from the core, often acquiring a spherical three-dimensional globular shape [47,48]. Functional groups on the molecular surface are primarily responsible for dendrimer characteristics. Polyamidoamine and poly(propyleneimine) dendrimers are extensively researched dendrimers for biological purposes. Since dendrimers include amine groups, their therapeutic uses are constrained. Dendrimers are often modified to lessen or completely remove the toxicity problems caused by these positively charged or cationic groups. Simple encapsulation, electrostatic interactions, or other functionalization methods can all be used to load drugs into dendrimers [35].

2.4.5 INORGANIC NANOPARTICLES

Silver, gold, silicon, iron oxide, and silica are among the materials that make up inorganic nanoparticles (NPs). In contrast to other nanocarriers like liposomes and dendrimers, gold and silver NPs have specific uses in surface plasmon resonance (SPR) investigation. Such nanomaterials exhibit high biocompatibility and adaptability after surface modification. Drugs can be physically bonded to the surface of gold NPs by electrostatic or covalent bonding and physical absorption, with the distribution and release to the target location being regulated by biological or environmental stimuli [49]. Silver NPs have antibacterial properties, but there haven't been many investigations on how well they carry drugs [50].

The scientific and medical communities are paying more and more attention to porous silicon and silica NPs. It has been effectively shown that nanocrystalline porous silicon has prospective uses in drug delivery, diagnosis, and therapeutics. Several researchers are looking into the potential of such NPs for oral, transdermal, and parenteral administration of pharmaceutical agents due to their outstanding *in-vivo* biocompatibility as well as biodegradability [50].

2.4.6 CARBON-BASED NANOMATERIALS

Carbon is one of the most flexible elements in the periodic table, owing to its vast, diversified array of various types and degrees of bonds that may form with it or with countless other elements [51,52]. Additionally, the ability for carbon orbitals to combine in the sp, sp^2, and sp^3 orientations opens up the possibility of a variety of allotropic forms. The three most common allotropes of carbon that are found naturally are graphite, diamond, and amorphous carbon. Up until now, these three allotropes have been augmented by synthetically produced graphene and its derivatives, fullerenes, carbon nanotubes (CNTs), quantum dots (QDs), and nanodiamonds [52,53]. Since the introduction of fullerenes in 1985 and the subsequent appearances of CNTs and graphene in 1991 and 2004, the main emphasis on carbon-based nano-materials (CBNs) has substantially increased. These CBNs are widely used in a broad spectrum of disciplines, including material science [54], energy generation and storage [55], environmental research [56], and biomedical [57,58], as a result of their special attributes.

Because of their extraordinary mechanical robustness, thermal and electrical conductivity, and optical properties, two major compounds of the CBN family—graphene and CNTs—have received the most attention and have been the focus of extensive investigations. The ability of CBNs to deliver therapeutic drug molecules and enable imaging of cells and tissues feasible, both of which are crucial for iden-tifying and treating unhealthy and damaged tissues, has had a considerable impact on the biomedical field recently. Drug and gene delivery, photothermal and photo-dynamic therapy, bioimaging, biosensing, fluorescent cell labeling, and regenerative medicine are some of the possible biological applications of CBNs [58,59]. CBNs can be used to sequence and diagnose cells and tissues since they contain intrinsic fluorescence, a restricted emission spectrum that may be adjusted, and great photo-stability. Its surfaces can also be altered using a range of functional groups to enhance their properties. Because of their large surface areas and exceptional opto-electronic and electromechanical properties, CBNs are among the most popular and effective choices for drug delivery applications [60].

Graphene oxide (GO), a hydrophilic derivative of graphene, has been intensively employed for numerous biomedical applications, especially drug delivery. In con-trast to graphene, GO nanosheets are enriched with oxygenated functional groups such as epoxy, hydroxyl, and carboxyl groups, which offer suitable hydrophilicity, aqueous stability, and biocompatibility with GO. These functional groups further provide functionalization ability to GO with numerous biomolecules, targeting ligands, polymers, and other functional groups through covalent and non-covalent interactions, which further enhances their colloidal stability, compatibility, drug loading capacity, and targetability [58,61]. Similarly, CBNs, including graphene, quantum dots (QDs), CNTs, fullerene, rGO, graphene oxide nanoscrolls (GONS), and graphene nanorods have been utilized for drug delivery-related applications [58,61,62]. The characteristics and efficacy of CBNs are highlighted in the subse-quent section.

2.5 EFFICACY OF CARBON-BASED MATERIALS AS DRUG CARRIERS

The human race today has access to a wide range of nano-enabled products or nanosystems that are employed for a wide range of biomedical applications. Such nano-constructs and interactions with drugs, enzymes, nucleic acids, viruses, pro-teins, cellular lipid bilayers, cellular receptor sites, and antigens (essential for immu-notherapy) are included in the category of nanostructures that are multidimensional [63]. CBNs are a class of nanosystems that have been thoroughly researched with potential for drug delivery and other medicinal applications. Lately, they have proven successful in a variety of industries, notably for theranostics, cancer treatment, and regenerative medicine [58] (**Figure 2.3**) [64].

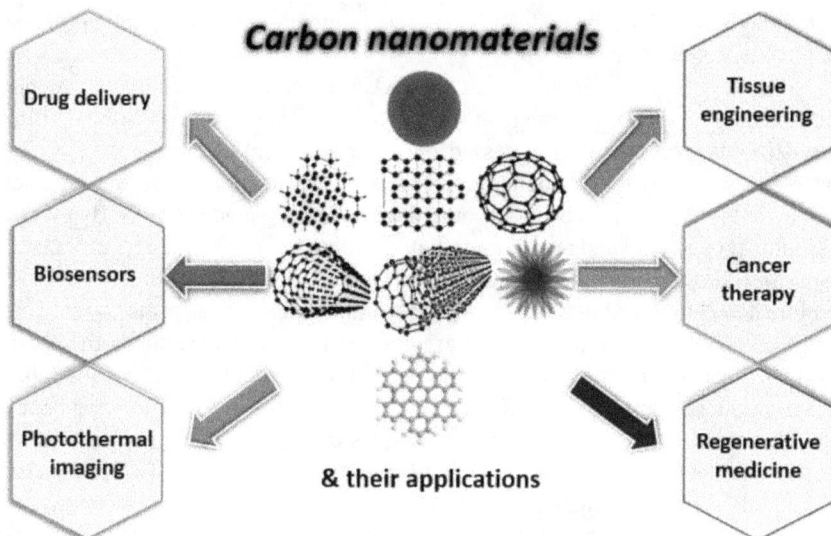

FIGURE 2.3 The Biomedical Applications of Carbon-Based Nanomaterials. [Replicated with permission from *Mahor et al. (2021)*] [64].

Carbon nanoparticles are especially well suited for use in the diagnostic and therapeutic fields due to their exceptional electrical and mechanical properties and large surface areas. In the areas of medicines and diagnostics, the following are the main benefits of utilizing CBNs:

1. They may absorb a significant amount of drug due to their supramolecular "π–π stacking" characteristic.
2. CBNs can be used as novel therapeutic components due to their distinct optical properties and easy fusion with illuminating components.
3. CBNs have outstanding NIR heat conversion competence that makes them a good choice for photothermal treatment (PTT).
4. Therapeutic agents can be released under regulated conditions using tunable surface chemistry.

The colloidal stability of CBNs in organic or aqueous environments impedes their use in biomedical applications [65]. All the same, this might be overcome by activating the CBNs' surfaces by functionalization utilizing both covalent and non-covalent methods. The functionalization of CBNs is one such unavoidable stage that modifies the surface by integrating various functional entities. Covalent functionalization can be accomplished in a variety of ways, including oxidation, plasma treatments, dehydrogenation, etc. [64]. They have been widely utilized in the delivery of drugs in great portions because of the surface modification of CBNs, which enables them to, for example, permeate biological membranes. By functionalizing CBNs with specific targeting ligands like aptamers and folic acid (FA), which also minimizes their cytotoxicity toward healthy cells, it is possible to increase the therapeutic efficiency of CBN-assisted DDSs.

Modest targeting molecules, such as FA [66], which targets folate receptors espoused on the exterior of a range of robust cancerous cells, ligands with an affinity for a particular receptor overexpressed on a particular malignant tumor [58,67], a monoclonal antibody that recognizes tumor-associated antigens [68], and magnetic nanoparticles [69], can also be incorporated with the drug-loaded CBNs. By using an external magnetic field and receptor-mediated endocytosis or drug aggregation at the target site, these approaches enable targeted drug delivery. Functionalized CBNs have therefore been employed in the transport of biomolecules such as proteins, enzymes, nucleic acids, and metabolites. CBNs have been utilized to deliver chemotherapeutic agents, fluorescent tumor detection markers, PTT, and other therapeutics [64,69].

The graphene quantum dots (GQDs) are the tiniest derivatives of graphene in the CBN family. Due to their small size, GQDs can transport nucleic acids to cell cytosols and nuclei by crossing the blood-brain barrier (BBB). GQDs are an excellent candidate for gene carriers due to their low toxicity, excellent solubility, and luminous attributes that make it simple to monitor drug release. Due to their fascinating physicochemical and biological properties, GQDs have received a lot of attention for applications in drug delivery. On the margins of GQDs, several functional groups provide strong binding sites for treatments, drugs, and targeted ligands. Moreover, the presence of sp^2 carbon in the GQDs structure makes it possible for aromatic ring-containing chemotherapeutic drug molecules to adhere to the surface of GQDs for increasing drug loading efficiency [70,71]. Moreover, chemotherapeutic medications like doxorubicin (DOX) and methotrexate (MTX) cannot be adequately delivered to a specific tissue in the body due to their limited water solubility. A hydrophilic carrier with a greater surface-to-volume ratio, like GQDs, can carry such chemotherapeutic drugs effectively. By π-π stacking onto the basal plane, GQDs offer many binding sites to the liking of pharmacological molecules.

Graphene oxide, a hydrophilic derivative of graphene, has shown tremendous promise in biological applications. As shown in **Figure 2.4** [58], GO was successfully tested for several biomedical applications. The oxygen-rich functional groups on GO surfaces are crucial to the properties and bio-application of these surfaces. In addition, the controlled oxidation of GO enables the adjustment of its mechanical, electrical, and optical characteristics. The versatility of GO made it a more accessible precursor for wide-ranging applications by providing several options to bind various molecules to nanosheets.

Targeted DDSs have advanced as a result of breakthroughs in nanotechnology and nanocarriers. Because of the nanostructures' ideal drug loading and release behavior and target-specificity, the DDSs ensure that the drug is distributed properly throughout the patient's body [72]. Because of their outstanding physicochemical properties, graphene and GO have attracted scholarly attention for potential biological uses. GO-based nanocarriers have several advantageous traits, including biocompatibility, large surface area and aspect ratio, colloidal stability, pH sensitivity, and photothermal characteristics [73]. Drugs may be mounted on the hydrophobic tails of GO by means of electrostatic interactions and π-π staking because of its amphiphilic properties [74]; for example, drug molecules can interact electrostatically owing to the

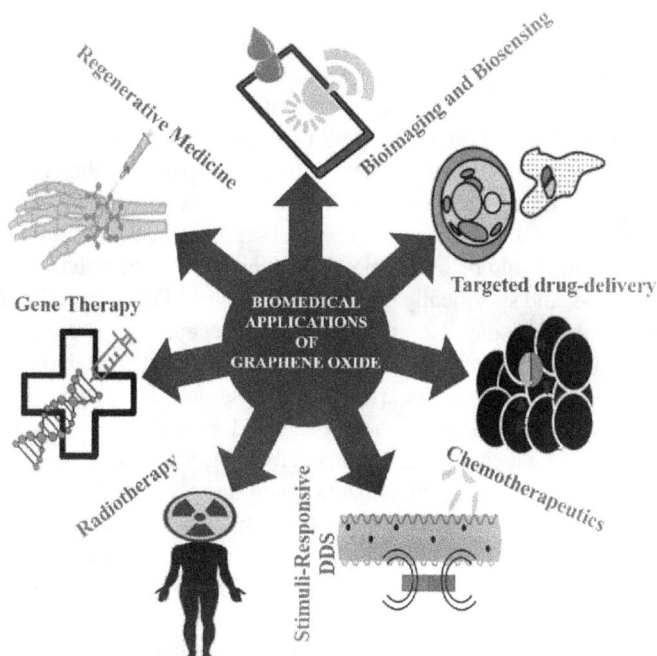

FIGURE 2.4 Biomedical Applications of GO-Based Nanocarriers. [Reprinted with permission from *Sontakke et al. (2023)*] [58].

ionizable carboxylic acid group on the edges of GO nanosheets [75]. GO may interact with cross-linking agents via covalent and non-covalent alterations to improve its stability and offer multimodal detection [76]. Moreover, graphene oxide is most stable at pH 7 or 8, and since the tissues at cancer locations have low pH, this causes the drug release by weakening the hydrogen bonds among drug molecules and GO [74].

CBNs have demonstrated tremendous potential for tissue engineering applications owing to their outstanding mechanical and chemical characteristics. The discovery of drugs for bone, cardiac, and neurological regeneration made good use of CNTs. The bone may repair and reconstruct itself after minor injuries or fractures. Nevertheless, if the defects are larger than a threshold size (5 mm) in pathogenic injuries, acute bone attrition, or core tumor excision, the bone is no longer able to repair itself [77,78]. In this example, many therapies, including xenografts, allografts, and autografts, were used. However, these procedures have significant drawbacks, including restricted availability and donor site morbidity for autografts, a chance of infection and resistance transfer for allografts, and a poor clinical prognosis and the likelihood of immunogenicity for xenografts [78]. As a result, a novel and extremely promising method known as tissue-engineered synthetic bone scaffolds has received a huge amount of attention and offers the support necessary for cell adhesion, growth, and transformation.

Overall, it was discovered that the CBNs, including graphene, GO, rGO, CNTs, and quantum dots, have demonstrated suitable efficacy and great potential to address most of the challenges related to drug delivery application.

2.6 SUMMARY

In this chapter, we have highlighted the evolution of DDS with its classification, historical aspects, and the principles behind the utilization of nanosized materials for drug delivery-related applications. The DDS was classified into conventional and novel methodologies based on their advancements in release patterns, the concentration of drugs in plasma, and other aspects to improve therapeutic efficacy and reduce the side effects in numerous therapeutics. It was observed that the shortcomings of the conventional systems could be overcome via rate-programmed, activation-modulated, feedback-regulated, and specifically by site-targeted novel DDS. The DDS was further classified based on the route of entry and release mechanism. The aspects of these types of DDS have delivered a detailed understanding of the mechanism and challenges for their utilization in nanocarrier-based drug delivery. It was concluded that the release profiles of the drug through the nanocarriers must be adjusted based on the type of disease, and nanocarriers offer those advantages to modify their structure as per the requirement through functionalization and morphological modifications. The major concern over the toxicity and targetability of nanocarriers may also be addressed through their functionalization. This chapter has also highlighted the attributes of several types of nanocarriers used in the advanced DDS. The CBNs, including graphene, GO, quantum dots, and CNTs, have demonstrated suitable therapeutic efficacy toward drug delivery for different therapeutics, including chemotherapy and tissue engineering. However, except for quantum dots with their tiny size, the toxicity of other CBNs is still a matter of concern, which must be addressed in the future. Meanwhile, GO has provided acceptable solutions to these challenges through its structural, functional, and morphological modification into GONS and GO quantum dots. Nevertheless, detailed *in-vivo* toxicity assessments are obligatory for their future applications.

REFERENCES

[1] S. Maiti, K.K. Sen, Introductory chapter: Drug delivery concepts, in: S. Maiti, K.K. Sen (Eds.), Advances Technology Delivered Theraphy, InTech, Rijeka (2017): Ch. 1. doi:10.5772/65245.

[2] S. Adepu, S. Ramakrishna, Controlled drug delivery systems: Current status and future directions, Mol. 26 (2021) 5905. doi:10.3390/molecules26195905.

[3] F. Laffleur, V. Keckeis, Advances in drug delivery systems: Work in progress still needed? Int. J. Pharm. 590 (2020) 119912. doi:10.1016/j.ijpharm.2020.119912.

[4] P. Trucillo, Drug carriers: Classification, administration, release profiles, and industrial approach, Processes. 9 (2021) 470. doi:10.3390/pr9030470.

[5] T. Perrie, R. Yvonne, Pharmaceutics - Drug Delivery and Targeting, 2nd ed., Pharmaceutical Press (2012). https://www.pharmpress.com/product/9780857110596/fasttrack-pharmaceutics-drug-delivery-and-targeting.

[6] J. V. Bondi, D.G. Pope, Drug Delivery Systems, Humana Press, Totowa, NJ (1987): pp. 291–325. doi:10.1007/978-1-4612-4828-6_11.

[7] P. Prajapat, D. Agrawal, G. Bhaduka, A brief overview of sustained released drug delivery system, J. Appl. Pharm. Res. 10 (2022) 5–11. doi:10.18231/j.joapr.2022.10.3.5.11.

[8] H. Park, A. Otte, K. Park, Evolution of drug delivery systems: From 1950 to 2020 and beyond, J. Control. Release. 342 (2022) 53–65. doi:10.1016/j.jconrel.2021.12.030.

[9] Y.H. Yun, B.K. Lee, K. Park, Controlled drug delivery: Historical perspective for the next generation, J. Control. Release. 219 (2015) 2–7. doi:10.1016/j.jconrel.2015.10.005.

[10] H. Reza Rezaie, M. Esnaashary, A. Aref Arjmand, A. Öchsner, The history of drug delivery systems, in: A Review of Biomaterials and Their Applications in Drug Delivery, Springer Singapore (2018): pp. 1–8. doi:10.1007/978-981-10-0503-9_1.

[11] C.-X. He, Z.-G. He, J.-Q. Gao, Microemulsions as drug delivery systems to improve the solubility and the bioavailability of poorly water-soluble drugs, Expert Opin. Drug Deliv. 7 (2010) 445–460. doi:10.1517/17425241003596337.

[12] M. Rawat, D. Singh, S. Saraf, S. Saraf, Lipid carriers: A versatile delivery vehicle for proteins and peptides, Yakugaku Zasshi. 128 (2008) 269–280. doi:10.1248/yakushi.128.269.

[13] W. Zhang, Q. Zhao, J. Deng, Y. Hu, Y. Wang, D. Ouyang, Big data analysis of global advances in pharmaceutics and drug delivery 1980–2014, Drug Discov. Today. 22 (2017) 1201–1208. doi:10.1016/j.drudis.2017.05.012.

[14] M.L. Bruschi, Main mechanisms to control the drug release, in: Strategy to Modify Drug Release from Pharm System, Elsevier, Cambridge (2015): pp. 37–62. doi:10.1016/B978-0-08-100092-2.00004-7.

[15] H. Reza Rezaie, M. Esnaashary, A. Aref arjmand, A. Öchsner, Classification of drug delivery systems, A Rev. Biomater. Their Appl. Drug Deliv. (2018) 9–25. doi:10.1007/978-981-10-0503-9_2.

[16] A. Bhattacharjee, M.K. Purkait, S. Gumma, Loading and release of doxorubicin hydrochloride from iron(iii) trimesate MOF and zinc oxide nanoparticle composites, Dalt. Trans. 49 (2020) 8755–8763. doi:10.1039/d0dt01730b.

[17] R.A. Siegel, M.J. Rathbone, Overview of controlled release mechanisms, in: J. Siepmann, R.A. Siegel, M.J. Rathbone (Eds.), Fundamental Applied Controlled Release Drug Delivery, Springer, Boston, MA (2012): pp. 19–43. doi:10.1007/978-1-4614-0881-9_2.

[18] R.K. Verma, B. Mishra, S. Garg, Osmotically controlled oral drug delivery*, Drug Dev. Ind. Pharm. 26 (2000) 695–708. doi:10.1081/DDC-100101287.

[19] V. Jannin, G. Lemagnen, P. Gueroult, D. Larrouture, C. Tuleu, Rectal route in the 21st Century to treat children, Adv. Drug Deliv. Rev. 73 (2014) 34–49. doi:10.1016/j.addr.2014.05.012.

[20] S.H. Yalkowsky, J.F. Krzyzaniak, G.H. Ward, Formulation-related problems associated with intravenous drug delivery, J. Pharm. Sci. 87 (1998) 787–796. doi:10.1021/js980051i.

[21] S.S. Dychter, D.A. Gold, M.F. Haller, Subcutaneous drug delivery, J. Infus. Nurs. 35 (2012) 154–160. doi:10.1097/NAN.0b013e31824d2271.

[22] A.T. Florence, D. Attwood, Physicochemical Principles of Pharmacy, in Manufacture, Formulation and Clinical Use, Pharmaceutical Press, Basingstoke (2015).

[23] A. Bhattacharjee, M.K. Purkait, S. Gumma, Doxorubicin loading capacity of MIL-100(Fe): Effect of synthesis conditions, J. Inorg. Organomet. Polym. Mater. 30 (2020) 2366–2375. doi:10.1007/s10904-020-01456-2.

[24] FDA, Guidance for industry considering whether an FDA-regulated product involves the application of nanotechnology, Biotechnol. Law Rep. 30 (2011) 613–616. doi:10.1089/blr.2011.9814.

[25] EU-Commission, Commission Recommendation of 18 October 2011 on the Definition of Nanomaterial Text with EEA Relevance, EU-Commission, Brussels (2011): p. 2.

[26] L. Peltonen, M. Singhal, J. Hirvonen, Principles of Nanosized Drug Delivery Systems, Elsevier, Cambridge (2020): pp. 3–25. doi:10.1016/B978-0-08-102985-5.00001-2.

[27] N. Darville, J. Saarinen, A. Isomäki, L. Khriachtchev, D. Cleeren, P. Sterkens, M. van Heerden, P. Annaert, L. Peltonen, H.A. Santos, C.J. Strachan, G. Van den Mooter, Multimodal non-linear optical imaging for the investigation of drug nano-/microcrystal–cell interactions, Eur. J. Pharm. Biopharm. 96 (2015) 338–348. doi:10.1016/j.ejpb.2015.09.003.

[28] R.H. Müller, S. Gohla, C.M. Keck, State of the art of nanocrystals—special features, production, nanotoxicology aspects and intracellular delivery, Eur. J. Pharm. Biopharm. 78 (2011) 1–9. doi:10.1016/j.ejpb.2011.01.007.

[29] D. Haldar, P. Duarah, M.K. Purkait, Progress in the Synthesis and Applications of Polymeric Nanomaterials Derived from Waste Lignocellulosic Biomass, Elsevier, Cambridge (2022): pp. 419–433. doi:10.1016/B978-0-323-90485-8.00006-0.

[30] P. Khanna, C. Ong, B. Bay, G. Baeg, Nanotoxicity: An interplay of oxidative stress, inflammation and cell death, Nanomat. 5 (2015) 1163–1180. doi:10.3390/nano5031163.

[31] Y. Wang, A. Santos, A. Evdokiou, D. Losic, An overview of nanotoxicity and nanomedicine research: Principles, progress and implications for cancer therapy, J. Mater. Chem. B. 3 (2015) 7153–7172. doi:10.1039/C5TB00956A.

[32] C.M. Keck, R.H. Müller, Nanotoxicological classification system (NCS)—a guide for the risk-benefit assessment of nanoparticulate drug delivery systems, Eur. J. Pharm. Biopharm. 84 (2013) 445–448. doi:10.1016/j.ejpb.2013.01.001.

[33] A.M. Alkilany, L.B. Thompson, S.P. Boulos, P.N. Sisco, C.J. Murphy, Gold nanorods: Their potential for photothermal therapeutics and drug delivery, tempered by the complexity of their biological interactions, Adv. Drug Deliv. Rev. 64 (2012) 190–199. doi:10.1016/j.addr.2011.03.005.

[34] J.P. Rao, K.E. Geckeler, Polymer nanoparticles: Preparation techniques and size-control parameters, Prog. Polym. Sci. 36 (2011) 887–913. doi:10.1016/j.progpolymsci.2011.01.001.

[35] H. Reza Rezaie, M. Esnaashary, A. Aref Arjmand, A. Öchsner, A Review of Biomaterials and Their Applications in Drug Delivery, Springer, Singapore (2018). doi:10.1007/978-981-10-0503-9.

[36] S.-Y. Chuang, C.-H. Lin, T.-H. Huang, J.-Y. Fang, Lipid-based nanoparticles as a potential delivery approach in the treatment of rheumatoid arthritis, Nanomat. 8 (2018) 42. doi:10.3390/nano8010042.

[37] Z. Zhao, A. Ukidve, V. Krishnan, S. Mitragotri, Effect of physicochemical and surface properties on in vivo fate of drug nanocarriers, Adv. Drug Deliv. Rev. 143 (2019) 3–21. doi:10.1016/j.addr.2019.01.002.

[38] S.R. D'Mello, C.N. Cruz, M.-L. Chen, M. Kapoor, S.L. Lee, K.M. Tyner, The evolving landscape of drug products containing nanomaterials in the United States, Nat. Nanotechnol. 12 (2017) 523–529. doi:10.1038/nnano.2017.67.

[39] M. Kapoor, S.L. Lee, K.M. Tyner, Liposomal drug product development and quality: Current US experience and perspective, AAPS J. 19 (2017) 632–641. doi:10.1208/s12248-017-0049-9.

[40] S. Senapati, A.K. Mahanta, S. Kumar, P. Maiti, Controlled drug delivery vehicles for cancer treatment and their performance, Signal Transduct. Target. Ther. 3 (2018) 7. doi:10.1038/s41392-017-0004-3.

[41] M. Hans, A. Lowman, Biodegradable nanoparticles for drug delivery and targeting, Curr. Opin. Solid State Mater. Sci. 6 (2002) 319–327. doi:10.1016/S1359-0286(02)00117-1.

[42] B.L. Banik, P. Fattahi, J.L. Brown, Polymeric nanoparticles: The future of nanomedicine, WIREs Nanomed. Nanobiotechnol. 8 (2016) 271–299. doi:10.1002/wnan.1364.

[43] G. Bao, S. Mitragotri, S. Tong, Multifunctional nanoparticles for drug delivery and molecular imaging, Annu. Rev. Biomed. Eng. 15 (2013) 253–282. doi:10.1146/annurev-bioeng-071812-152409.

[44] G. Bozzuto, A. Molinari, Liposomes as nanomedical devices, Int. J. Nanomed. 10 (2015) 975. doi:10.2147/IJN.S68861.

[45] S. Das, A. Chaudhury, Recent advances in lipid nanoparticle formulations with solid matrix for oral drug delivery, AAPS PharmSciTech. 12 (2011) 62–76. doi:10.1208/s12249-010-9563-0.

[46] N. Naseri, H. Valizadeh, P. Zakeri-Milani, Solid lipid nanoparticles and nanostructured lipid carriers: Structure, preparation and application, Adv. Pharm. Bull. 5 (2015) 305–313. doi:10.15171/apb.2015.043.

[47] K. Madaan, S. Kumar, N. Poonia, V. Lather, D. Pandita, Dendrimers in drug delivery and targeting: Drug-dendrimer interactions and toxicity issues, J. Pharm. Bioallied Sci. 6 (2014) 139. doi:10.4103/0975-7406.130965.

[48] P. Kesharwani, L. Xie, S. Banerjee, G. Mao, S. Padhye, F.H. Sarkar, A.K. Iyer, Hyaluronic acid-conjugated polyamidoamine dendrimers for targeted delivery of 3,4-difluoroben-zylidene curcumin to CD44 overexpressing pancreatic cancer cells, Colloids Surf. B Biointerfaces. 136 (2015) 413–423. doi:10.1016/j.colsurfb.2015.09.043.

[49] F.-Y. Kong, J.-W. Zhang, R.-F. Li, Z.-X. Wang, W.-J. Wang, W. Wang, Unique roles of gold nanoparticles in drug delivery, targeting and imaging applications, Mol. 22 (2017) 1445. doi:10.3390/molecules22091445.

[50] H.A. Santos, E. Mäkilä, A.J. Airaksinen, L.M. Bimbo, J. Hirvonen, Porous silicon nanoparticles for nanomedicine: Preparation and biomedical applications, Nanomed. 9 (2014) 535–554. doi:10.2217/nnm.13.223.

[51] G.A. Silva, Nanotechnology approaches to crossing the blood-brain barrier and drug delivery to the CNS, Curr. Res. Pharm. Technol. 4 (2011) 81–84. doi:10.1201/b13128-27.

[52] R. Rauti, M. Musto, S. Bosi, M. Prato, L. Ballerini, Properties and behavior of carbon nanomaterials when interfacing neuronal cells: How far have we come? Carbon N. Y. 143 (2019) 430–446. doi:10.1016/j.carbon.2018.11.026.

[53] D. Pantarotto, J.P. Briand, M. Prato, A. Bianco, Translocation of bioactive peptides across cell membranes by carbon nanotubes, Chem. Commun. 4 (2004) 16–17. doi:10.1039/b311254c.

[54] Q. Li, J. Song, F. Besenbacher, M. Dong, Two-dimensional material confined water, Acc. Chem. Res. 48 (2015) 119–127. doi:10.1021/ar500306w.

[55] D. Yu, K. Goh, H. Wang, L. Wei, W. Jiang, Q. Zhang, L. Dai, Y. Chen, Scalable synthesis of hierarchically structured carbon nanotube–graphene fibres for capacitive energy storage, Nat. Nanotechnol. 9 (2014) 555–562. doi:10.1038/nnano.2014.93.

[56] Q. Xue, H. Chen, Q. Li, K. Yan, F. Besenbacher, M. Dong, Room-temperature high-sensitivity detection of ammonia gas using the capacitance of carbon/silicon heterojunctions, Energy Environ. Sci. 3 (2010) 288. doi:10.1039/b925172n.

[57] C. Lee, X. Wei, J.W. Kysar, J. Hone, Measurement of the elastic properties and intrinsic strength of monolayer graphene, Sci. 80, 321 (2008) 385–388. doi:10.1126/science.1157996.

[58] A.D. Sontakke, S. Tiwari, M.K. Purkait, A comprehensive review on graphene oxide-based nanocarriers: Synthesis, functionalization and biomedical applications, FlatChem. 38 (2023) 100484. doi:10.1016/j.flatc.2023.100484.

[59] K.D. Patel, R.K. Singh, H.W. Kim, Carbon-based nanomaterials as an emerging platform for theranostics, Mater. Horizons. 6 (2019) 434–469. doi:10.1039/c8mh00966j.

[60] W. Tao, D. Ni, G. Liu, P. Huang, X. Mou, K. Yang, D. Maiti, X. Tong, Carbon-based nanomaterials for biomedical applications: A recent study, Front. Pharmacol. (2019). doi:10.3389/fphar.2018.01401.

[61] S. Tiwari, A.D. Sontakke, K. Baruah, M.K. Purkait, Development of graphene oxide-based nano-delivery system for natural chemotherapeutic agent (Caffeic Acid), Mater. Today Proc. (2022). doi:10.1016/j.matpr.2022.11.373.

[62] A.D. Sontakke, R. Fopase, L.M. Pandey, M.K. Purkait, Development of graphene oxide nanoscrolls imparted nano-delivery system for the sustained release of gallic acid, Appl. Nanosci. 12 (2022) 2733–2751. doi:10.1007/s13204-022-02582-8.

[63] S.R. Mudshinge, A.B. Deore, S. Patil, C.M. Bhalgat, Nanoparticles: Emerging carriers for drug delivery, Saudi Pharm. J. 19 (2011) 129–141. doi:10.1016/j.jsps.2011.04.001.

[64] A. Mahor, P.P. Singh, P. Bharadwaj, N. Sharma, S. Yadav, J.M. Rosenholm, K.K. Bansal, Carbon-based nanomaterials for delivery of biologicals and therapeutics: A cutting-edge technology, Carbon. 7 (2021) 19. doi:10.3390/c7010019.

[65] D. Konios, M.M. Stylianakis, E. Stratakis, E. Kymakis, Dispersion behaviour of graphene oxide and reduced graphene oxide, J. Colloid Interface Sci. 430 (2014) 108–112. doi:10.1016/j.jcis.2014.05.033.

[66] Q. Zhang, Z. Wu, N. Li, Y. Pu, B. Wang, T. Zhang, J. Tao, Advanced review of graphene-based nanomaterials in drug delivery systems: Synthesis, modification, toxicity and application, Mater. Sci. Eng. C. 77 (2017) 1363–1375. doi:10.1016/j.msec.2017.03.196.

[67] T.M. Allen, Ligand-targeted therapeutics in anticancer therapy, Nat. Rev. Cancer. 2 (2002) 750–763. doi:10.1038/nrc903.

[68] D. Yang, L. Feng, C.A. Dougherty, K.E. Luker, D. Chen, M.A. Cauble, M.M. Banaszak Holl, G.D. Luker, B.D. Ross, Z. Liu, H. Hong, In vivo targeting of metastatic breast cancer via tumor vasculature-specific nano-graphene oxide, Biomaterials. 104 (2016) 361–371. doi:10.1016/j.biomaterials.2016.07.029.

[69] A.D. Sontakke, M.K. Purkait, A brief review on graphene oxide Nanoscrolls: Structure, Synthesis, characterization and scope of applications, Chem. Eng. J. 420 (2021) 129914. doi:10.1016/j.cej.2021.129914.

[70] S. Tiwari, A.D. Sontakke, K. Baruah, M.K. Purkait, Development of graphene oxide-based nano-delivery system for natural chemotherapeutic agent (caffeic acid), Mater. Today Proc. (2022). doi:10.1016/j.matpr.2022.11.373.

[71] S. Kumbhar, M. De, Carbon quantum dots modified Bi2WO6 nanosheets for photo-oxidation of glycerol to value-added product, Mater. Today Proc. (2022). doi:10.1016/j.matpr.2022.11.230.

[72] A. Shah, S. Aftab, J. Nisar, M.N. Ashiq, F.J. Iftikhar, Nanocarriers for targeted drug delivery, J. Drug Deliv. Sci. Technol. 62 (2021). doi:10.1016/j.jddst.2021.102426.

[73] K. Muazim, Z. Hussain, Graphene oxide—a platform towards theranostics, Mater. Sci. Eng. C. 76 (2017). doi:10.1016/j.msec.2017.02.121.

[74] Y. Qu, F. He, C. Yu, X. Liang, D. Liang, L. Ma, Q. Zhang, J. Lv, J. Wu, Advances on graphene-based nanomaterials for biomedical applications, Mater. Sci. Eng. C. 90 (2018) 764–780. doi:10.1016/j.msec.2018.05.018.

[75] G. Shim, M.G. Kim, J.Y. Park, Y.K. Oh, Graphene-based nanosheets for delivery of chemotherapeutics and biological drugs, Adv. Drug Deliv. Rev. 105 (2016). doi:10.1016/j.addr.2016.04.004.

[76] S. Song, H. Shen, Y. Wang, X. Chu, J. Xie, N. Zhou, J. Shen, Biomedical application of graphene: From drug delivery, tumor therapy, to theranostics, Colloids Surf. B Biointerfaces. 185 (2020) 110596. doi:10.1016/j.colsurfb.2019.110596.

[77] J. Lee, M.M. Farag, E.K. Park, J. Lim, H. Yun, A simultaneous process of 3D magnesium phosphate scaffold fabrication and bioactive substance loading for hard tissue regeneration, Mater. Sci. Eng. C. 36 (2014) 252–260. doi:10.1016/j.msec.2013.12.007.

[78] B. Huang, Carbon nanotubes and their polymeric composites: The applications in tissue engineering, Biomanufacturing Rev. 5 (2020) 1–26. doi:10.1007/s40898-020-00009-x.

3 Graphene-Based Nanocarriers as Drug Delivery System

3.1 INTRODUCTION TO GRAPHENE-BASED NANOCARRIERS

Carbon is named after the Latin word *carbo*, which denotes charcoal. Due to the peculiar electronic structure of carbon, it can be hybridized to establish sp^3, sp^2, and sp networks, leading to the formation of more well-known stable allotropes unlike any other component. Graphite is a ubiquitous natural mineral with a long history of being the most predominant allotropic form of carbon. Graphite is made up of sp^2-hybridized carbon atomic layers held together by weak van der Waals interactions. Graphene is a single layer of carbon atoms that are closely packed into a two-dimensional (2D) honeycomb crystal structure. The prefix "graph" for graphite and the ending "-ene" for the C-C double bond make up the word "graphene." In 1994, Boehm, Setton, and Stumpp proposed the use of this term [1,2]. Graphene's structure is akin to several joined benzene rings with hydrogen atoms substituted by carbon atoms (**Figure 3.1a**), and it is regarded as hydrophobic due to the unavailability of oxygen-containing groups [3]. It is likewise an allotrope of carbon with sp^2-linked atoms arranged in a plane and a molecular bond length of 0.142 nm. Graphite is developed by stacking graphene layers with an interlayer spacing of 0.335 nm [4]. Graphite has a three-dimensional structure as a result of such stacking, whereas graphene is a 2D, one-atom-thick substance [5].

Graphene has one π orbital and three σ bonds that are perpendicular to the plane. The robust in-plane σ-bonds serve as the hexagonal rigid backbone chain, whereas the out-of-plane π bonds regulate the interactions between graphene layers. In almost any event, alterations in graphitic layers are mostly caused by the lack of one or more sp^2 carbon atoms or even the inclusion of one or more additional atoms with sp^3 hybridization [5]. Due to their outstanding mechanical, thermal, electrical, and foldable characteristics, single sp^2-bonded carbon atom allotropes lie in zero to three dimensionalities, including fullerene, graphene, nanotube, and graphite, which have been incorporated into distinct polymeric composites throughout the last decades [6]. It has a tensile strength of ~125 GPa and an elastic modulus of ~1.1 TPa, rendering graphene 100 times stronger than steel [7]. In comparison to copper, which has a thermal conductivity of 401 W/mK, graphene has a thermal conductivity of ~5000 W/mK. With a conductance of 10^6 S/m and an impedance of 31 Ω/sq, graphene's electrons may move with ultra-high mobility of (2×10^5 cm^2/V. s), which itself is 140 times greater than silicon's. The sp^2 hybridization, whereby it provides an additional

DOI: 10.1201/9781003358114-3

electron to the π bond and results in strong conductivity at ambient temperature, is the cause of this exceptionally high mobility [8].

Additionally, graphene is a naturally occurring semiconducting material that has a benzene ring-like electronic structure composed of six π-orbitals, three of which are occupied for bonding and three of which are vacant for antibonding, isolated by an energy band gap. Due to a small amount of valence and conduction band overlap caused by the fusing among these benzene rings, electrons from the top valence band can go to the bottom conduction band without generating heat **(Figure 3.1b)** [9,10]. The surface area of graphene is presided by the accumulation of its layers. When pristine graphene is modified with additional compounds, the agglomeration can be reduced, and the effective surface area will be increased [11]. The nanoparticles' biological responsiveness strongly depends on their surface area due to the surface phenomena, including physisorption and catalytic chemical reaction. Monolayer graphene has the greatest surface area among sp^2-hybridized carbon sheets (2600 m^2/g), which is significantly higher than that of pure single-walled carbon nanotubes (SWCNTs) (1300 m^2/g). This is because each carbon atom in monolayer graphene is accessible to the extracellular environment on both sides. Additionally, dependent on the number of layers, the surface area and biological molecule adsorption competency drastically decline with increasing layer numbers [12].

Graphene represents the most significant component of a larger group of graphene-based nanomaterials (GBNs), which also includes few-layer graphene (FLG), graphene oxide (GO), reduced GO (rGO), and nano GO (NGO). We often refer to a monolayer nanosheet as graphene, but FLG is made up of two to ten stacked layers of graphene and was first produced as a by-product of the synthesis of graphene [13]. Graphene, in its oxidized state, is called GO, which is made of a monolayer graphene nanosheet and oxygenated functional groups such as hydroxyl, carboxyl, and epoxide groups all over its edges and surface. The reduction of GO by chemical and thermal processing in reducing environments results in rGO, which has a lower oxygen

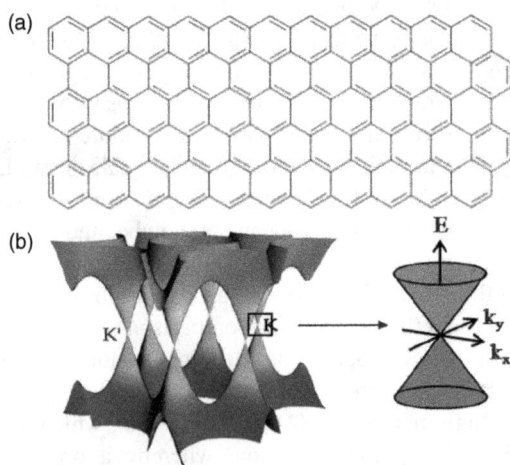

FIGURE 3.1 (a) Structure of Graphene Nanosheet, (b) Electronic Band Structure of Graphene. [Reprinted with permission from *Rao et al. (2009)*] [10].

concentration. GO with a lateral dimension of less than 100 nm is called NGO and is occasionally referred to as graphene nanosheets.

The distinctive physicochemical characteristics of graphene have sparked an unprecedented surge in its interest among scientists since it was discovered in 2004 [13,14]. Graphene applications in nanoelectronics, material science, and engineering have recently been extensively researched and demonstrated [15,16]. However, the enormous aptitude of graphene with its oxidized form, graphene oxide (GO), in biomedical sectors has been unveiled recently. Despite this new interest, graphene and GBN have already explored their wide range of applications in the biomedical sector, such as drug delivery, tissue engineering, biosensing, disease diagnostics, cancer targeting, and photothermal treatment (PTT) [12,17]. The characteristics of graphene, including its large specific surface area due to the 2D flat structure of the nanosheets and the configurable surface and morphological modifications resulting in their improved biocompatibility, led to its fast dissemination. This is a significant value addition since it enables the attachment or adsorption of biomolecules or functional groups to both sides of the graphene surface, enabling substantial functionalization and drug-loading efficiencies. Considering all these characteristics, graphene nanoparticles are much more promising than CNTs. Although the significant surface characteristic and superior drug loading capacity of GBNs make them suitable for novel drug delivery systems (DDSs), the poor aqueous stability, biocompatibility, biodistribution, and toxicity of GBNs are the major constraints over their applicability in the biomedical application [18].

The great propensity of exfoliated graphene nanosheets to persistently agglomerate or even rearrange, establishing additional multilayers and resembling graphite, is one of the major disadvantages of graphene [19]. This characteristic is caused by substantial π–π stacking interactions between individual nanosheets of graphene and van der Waals forces. Since graphene persists hydrophobic nature, functionalization is required to make it more processable and dispersible in aqueous and organic solutions [19,20]. A graphene surface may also be functionalized chemically or physically to incorporate biological moieties to combine the remarkable characteristics of graphene with biological activity [21]. To improve the characteristics of graphene, both covalent and non-covalent functionalization have already been extensively adopted [22,23]. Combining covalent and non-covalent functionalization has also been demonstrated to be a successful strategy. Covalent functionalization typically involves chemically derived forms of GO or rGO developed by cross-linking hydrophilic polymers or nucleic acids (NAs), coupling amines to carboxylic groups, or sulfonating processes. However, the non-covalent alterations use hydrophobic forces or π–π interactions on a graphene surface or rely on the stabilizing ability of surfactants that adhere to the surface to produce colloidal dispersions of graphene nanosheets [24].

Considering the significance of graphene and GBN for various biomedical applications, including drug and gene delivery, this chapter elucidates the recent developments in their application for cancer therapeutics, tissue engineering, and neurodegenerative diseases. The present chapter also highlights the details of the synthesis of graphene through both the "Top-down" and "Bottom-up" approaches. Furthermore, the functionalization strategies utilized to improve the surface characteristics of graphene are also described in detail. Recommendations are made to overcome the challenges involved in the synthesis and functionalization of graphene-based nanocarriers to enhance their compliance with modern therapeutics. This chapter also highlights the recent advances in the structural and functional modifications of graphene for enhancing its therapeutic efficacy in cancer and other infirmities therapy. The last section reviews the results of application-driven research on graphene-based nanocarriers related to cancer treatment, gene therapy, neurodegenerative diseases, and tissue engineering, offering exhaustive knowledge about its efficiency in drug delivery-related applications.

3.2   SYNTHESIS OF GRAPHENE

Following the discovery of graphene in 2004, a number of techniques have been employed to synthesize graphene. According to the intended purity of graphene, these fabrication processes are referred to for extracting graphene from the carbon source [25]. The synthesis methods of graphene are primarily divided into "Top-down" and "Bottom-up" methods. The top-down approach works by exfoliating graphite, which is employed as the starting material. The top-down processes divide exfoliation into four categories: mechanical, chemical, electrochemical, and laser ablation. It is quite simple to use the top-down method for industrial-scale graphene fabrication. However, a traditional top-down technique, such as Hummer graphite oxidation, demands a regulated reaction and invariably results in a large number of structural flaws that impede its electrical conductivity. On the other hand, "Bottom-up" methods are described as strategies for the imposition of a starting material that is conducted out of under-regulated parameters by modulating the parameters such as flow rate, pressure, and temperature [26]. The high-quality graphene with certain structural flaws and strong electrical characteristics could be fabricated using the bottom-up approach. Unfortunately, because it is synthesized in such tiny amounts, it can only be applied in a limited domain. Additionally, it is conceivable to develop a defect-free graphene structure with tailored layers for subsequent integration in specialized applications. The typical bottom-up approaches for synthesizing graphene include CVD, pyrolysis, and epitaxial growth. The details of these fabrication processes employed for synthesizing graphene are provided subsequently.

3.2.1   MECHANICAL CLEAVAGE FROM NATURAL GRAPHITE

Mechanical cleavage or exfoliation is often referred to as the peel-off process or the Scotch tape method. Novoselov and Geim employed this technique for the first time to fabricate graphene, forcing the graphene nanosheets to separate by an adhesive tape [25,27]. This technique leaves numerous graphene layers on the tape once it has been peeled off, although subsequent peeling enables it to be divided up into a few graphene flakes. The tape is applied to a specific substrate for the detachment of graphene layers, and then further peeling is performed using brand-new tape to produce flakes that are varied in dimensions, which are certainly visible on SiO2/Si surfaces with a light microscope [28]. Due to the sluggishness and ambiguity of this process, the obtained graphene is most frequently utilized for investigating its characteristics instead of being employed for practical purposes [27]. Additionally, this procedure may be carried out utilizing other components, including an electric field [29], epoxy resin [30], and transfer printing technology [5]. Although this procedure is easy, its primary drawback is that it results in a tiny amount of graphene with certain structural flaws.

3.2.2 CHEMICAL AND ELECTROCHEMICAL EXFOLIATION

Chemical exfoliation is also termed liquid phase exfoliation (LPE). LPE is a new top-down technique that consists solely of sonication or high-shear mixing to exfoliate natural graphite [31,32]. The exfoliation process of graphite through LPE is illustrated in **Figure 3.2a** [31]. Until recently, two separate graphite flaying procedures have been used with LPE: cavitation during sonication and high-shear mixing. Since the LPE operates under extremely benign circumstances, neither a vacuum nor a high-temperature system is necessary. The sonification-aided LPE method is less advised for industrial-scale applications than that of the high-shear mixing or microfluidizer approach [33]. This is because the LPE sonication approach produces less graphene and necessitates a significant amount of energy. Furthermore, high-shear mixing methods exfoliate graphite more effectively than those of LPE sonication. Large volumes of graphene can be produced efficiently via chemical exfoliation. However, this approach has several drawbacks, including the requirement for precise chemical reactions and the tendency to yield poor conductive graphene nanosheets. However, electrochemical-assisted exfoliation techniques alleviate these hurdles to some extent.

Electrochemical graphite exfoliation has recently developed into a simplistic yet productive approach for the industrial-scale synthesis of graphene [34]. This technique uses many types of graphite, including graphite foils, sheets, cylinders, and powder, as electrodes in an aqueous or non-aqueous electrolyte, together with an electrical charge to induce electrode expansions. Anode, cathode, electrolyte, and power supply are the specified number of key components required for the electrochemical process. Since the anode is a carbon source, graphene will be produced by oxidizing and exfoliating it. The cathode material can be altered by utilizing graphite or platinum.

A standard experimental setup of the electrochemical exfoliation process is illustrated in **Figure 3.2**b [31]. The electrodes, that is, cathode and anode, are submerged in the electrolyte at different depths. According to the targeted exfoliation mechanism, either a negative or positive voltage is supplied to the anode [35]. The electrochemical operation depends critically on the type of electrodes and electrolyte employed since it can impact the amount of graphene that is produced at the end.

Pencil graphite was employed as the source of graphite by Liu et al. (2013), which ultimately adopted it as the cathode and anode for the synthesis of graphene via the electrochemical exfoliation system. A voltage within +7 V and -7 V is supplied, and the electrodes are submerged in 1 M H_3PO_4 solution, which was employed as an electrolyte. The resulting graphene was not uniform, and there was a considerable variation in thickness and dimension [36]. In another study by Parvez et al. (2013), graphite was employed as an anode, whereas the cathode was supplemented by a platinum (Pt) electrode. These electrodes were submerged in the electrolyte solution of sulfuric acid,

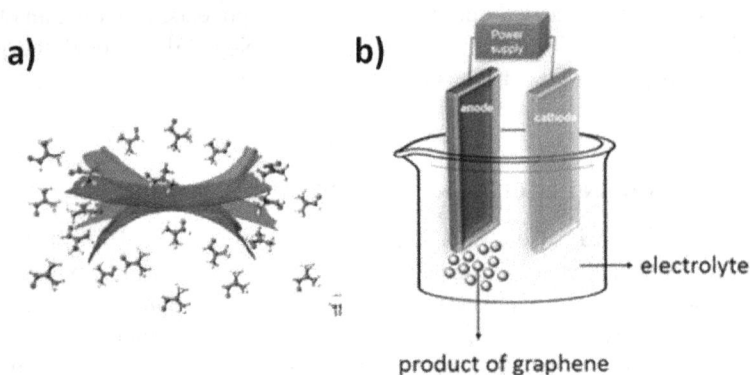

FIGURE 3.2 Schematic Representation for the Synthesis of Graphene by (a) Liquid-Phase Exfoliation (LPE) and (b) A Typical Experimental Setup of the Electrochemical Exfoliation Process for the Synthesis of Graphene [31].

and the electrochemical exfoliation of graphite was tested at 10 V for 10 min. This technique successfully fabricated graphene nanosheets with one to three layers and a yield of roughly 60% [37]. According to the findings of the aforementioned studies, sulfuric acid is considered a competent electrolyte for the electrochemical deposition of graphene and exfoliation of graphite. The electrolyte process may be encouraged by the sulfate ions' size of 0.46 nm, which is comparable to the graphite interlayer spacing of 0.335 nm. Additionally, gases like SO_2, O_2, and H_2 are released during the electrolysis of sulfate ions and co-intercalated water [38]. Graphite was flaked throughout the complexation process due to the use of an acid electrolyte. However, in contrast to what was anticipated, this technique produces multiple layers of graphene. Furthermore, Parvez et al. (2014) suggested a detailed mechanism for the electrochemical exfoliation of graphite in an ammonium sulfate solution, as presented in **Figure 3.3**. In this process, the voltage output was adjusted to 10 V, and graphite electrodes were submerged in an electrolyte solution. During the electrolysis, water reduction at the cathode results in the formation of hydroxyl (OH^-) ions, which are effective nucleophiles. The corners and borders of the graphite grains are attacked by nucleophiles, which further promotes the oxidation processes and the physical adsorption of sulfate ions in the graphite layer. The expansion and depolarization of the graphite layer are driven by oxidation reactions. Throughout this reaction, water molecules co-intercalate with SO_4^{2-} ions. Gas molecules, namely, SO_2 and O_2, were produced as a result of SO_4^{2-} ion reduction and oxidation of water molecules. The energy available to gas species allows them to detach the graphite layer and develop multilayer graphene. The process of exfoliating graphite is also influenced by the concentration of electrolytes at the applied voltage. To obtain 5 wt.% graphenes, the minimum electrolyte concentration for the graphite electrolysis reaction was < 0.01 M. It was suggested that the yield of graphene-containing products might improve over 75 wt.% provided the concentration was raised to a 0.01 to 1.0 M limit. The overall mechanism of graphite exfoliation by electrochemistry in inorganic salts is supported by this event [37,39].

Similarly, the hybrid method comprising sonication and an electrochemical oxidation process was also employed for the synthesis of graphene. Such combined

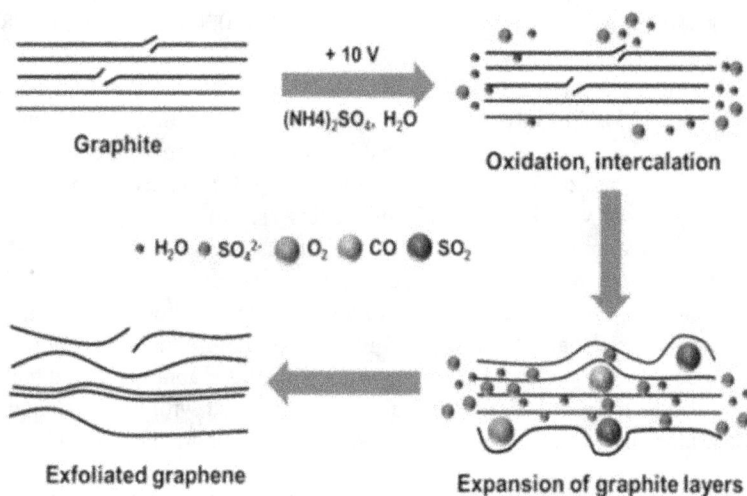

FIGURE 3.3 Proposed Mechanism for the Electrochemical Exfoliation of Graphite in an Ammonium Sulfate Solution. [Reprinted with permission from *Parvez et al. (2014)*] [39].

techniques can mitigate the requirement for rigorous operation stages, elevated temperatures, and excessive pressures in the synthesis method [31].

3.2.3 LASER ABLATION

A novel technique for synthesizing nanomaterials, particularly graphene, is laser ablation. This approach offers a number of potential benefits, such as environmental friendliness, simple experimental modes, long-term stability of nanoparticles, the absence of toxic synthesis reagents, and undesirable contaminants in nanoparticle compositions [40,41]. Cappelli et al. (2015) produced graphene using laser ablation. Their study was carried out utilizing a near-IR Nd: YAG laser ($\lambda = 523$ nm, frequency = 10 Hz, pulse width (τ) = 7 ns, and deposition period = 15 min) on silicon (Si) wafers with variable surface temperatures (from ambient temperature to 900 °C) [42]. The development process is then carried out under a range of configurations to produce high-quality graphene [43].

Solid carbon source is essential in laser ablation methodologies to enable the laser source for carbon eradication and synthesize graphene [44,45]. Throughout the fabrication of graphene, a number of laser parameters need to be regulated [46]. The quality of the final product may change depending on the way these parameters are set up for the laser ablation device. The laser's physical characteristics, such as its fluence, wavelength, frequency (repetition rate), and pulse duration, should be regulated as the initial parameter. The next controllable variables are the substrate's temperature, distance, ambient pressure, and gas conditions. The product is also influenced by substrate choice. In a study employing the laser ablation technique, Koh et al. (2012) examined the viability of different metals as a substrate for the production of graphene. Nickel (Ni), cobalt (Co), copper (Cu), and iron (Fe) were the metals that were examined. According to the findings, graphene made from Ni, Co, Cu, and Fe frameworks does have a lattice constant of 0.357, 0.361, 0.352, 0.251, and 0.287 nm, correspondingly [45].

A high-grade bilayer graphene was produced utilizing a Ni/SiO_2 substrate by Hemani et al. (2013). This information was supported by Raman spectroscopy, which demonstrated findings that were 60% better than those obtained with other substrates [44]. Pechlivani et al. (2017) evaluated the impact of pulses on diverse substrates. To achieve the required wavelengths and pulse energies, ultra-short pulse lasers were deployed. The outcomes of this investigation demonstrated that the development of ultra-short pulse laser technology has the potential to promote micro-graphene as an effective material in the manufacturing industry [47]. De Bonis et al. (2015) also used ultra-short laser ablation, which resulted in exceptional graphene production [48]. **Figure 3.4** describes the general configurations of the laser ablation-based technique for the synthesis of graphene, wherein direct laser contact with the carbon/graphite solid causes it to lose some of its frameworks and yielding graphene [31].

3.2.4   CHEMICAL VAPOR DEPOSITION (CVD)

Chemical vapor deposition (CVD) is one of the bottom-up synthesis processes utilized on a larger scale to synthesize high-grade graphene [49]. In this procedure, a surface substrate and gas molecules are combined inside a reactor vessel while the reaction environment is controlled through temperature, gas flow rate, and pressure [50]. A conventional CVD instrument consists of a quartz reactor, a mass flow controller, thermocouples for temperature monitoring, a pump, gas distribution lines, a power system, a vacuum system, and a computer for auto-control. For the CVD process that produces graphene films, a variety of substrates are employed, including nickel (Ni), iron (Fe), and copper (Cu). Typically, carbon sources include hydrocarbon gases like methane (CH_4) and acetylene (C_2H_2). The carbon source is stimulated using two CVD techniques: thermal CVD and plasma-enhanced CVD (PECVD) [51].

To synthesize graphene, thermal CVD employs a vacuum tube, furnace, pressure gauges, vacuum pump, and mass flow regulator to regulate the amount of hydrocarbon

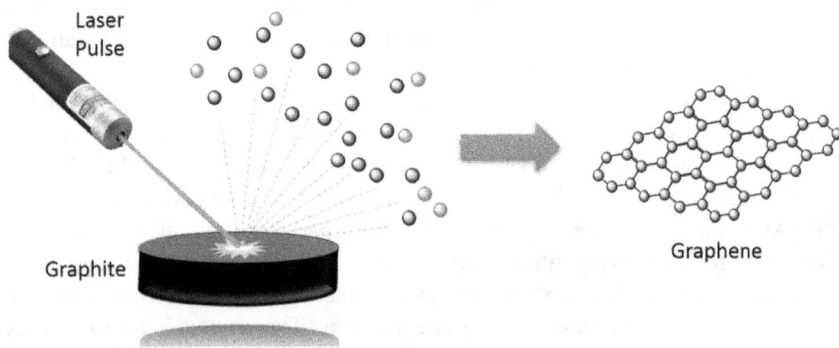

FIGURE 3.4 A General Configuration of the Laser Ablation-Based Technique for the Synthesis of Graphene [31].

and career gas. In PECVD, plasma prompts the gas source to break down before reacting with the metal substrate to trigger the development of graphene filaments [52]. Plasma has been developed using many power sources, including radio frequency (RF), microwave, and direct current (DC) [53]. The ability of graphene growth methodology to proceed at low pressure and temperatures is a major benefit of PECVD over thermal CVD [54]. High temperature causes the decomposition of carbon sources into carbon and hydrogen atoms.

In this CVD technique, the undesirable compounds on the metallic surface of the catalyst are eliminated and cleaned using H_2 and Ar gas as carrier gases. Graphene has traditionally been grown via CVD on transitional metallic substrates like Cu and Ni [55]. There are two primary phases in this growing process: 1. thermal decomposition of the gas reactant to produce carbon, and 2. exploitation of segmented carbon on the surface of the metallic catalyst to produce the carbon framework of graphene [56]. One method is to first anneal nickel in an H_2 environment at the required temperature of 900–1000 °C with grain size in order to produce graphene using polycrystalline nickel [5]. In this case, CH_4 is employed as the carbon source, and the substrate is subject to a combination of H_2 and CH_4. The carbon atom dissolves in the Ni substrate during the hydrocarbon's breakdown and yields the solid solution. Because Ni has the ability to dissolve at high temperatures, it may be solidified and condensed in argon gas to yield a precipitate of Ni-C that can scratch graphene (**Figure 3.5**) [5]. Ni is an excellent substrate toward the synthesis of graphene;

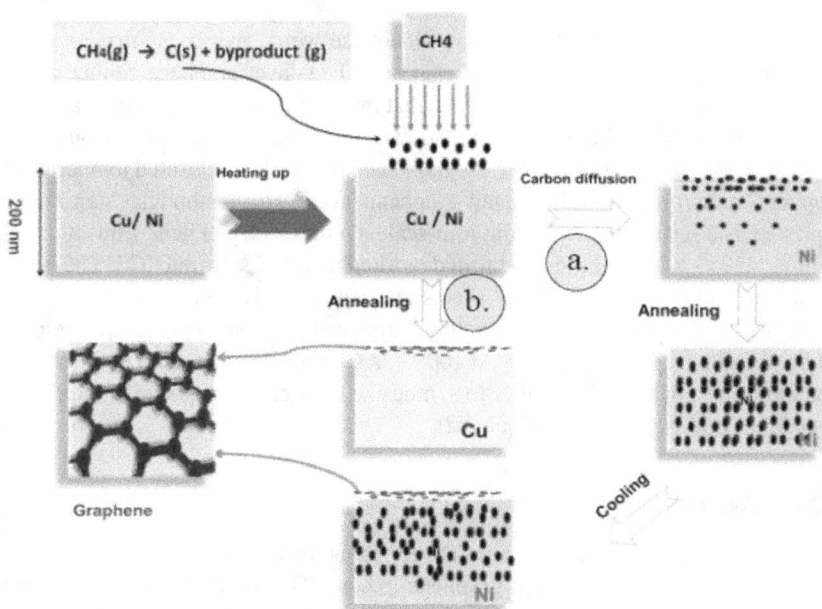

FIGURE 3.5 Growth Mechanism of Graphene on Cu/Ni Substrate Through Chemical Vapor Deposition (CVD)(a) Graphene Growth by Dissolution-Precipitation Mechanism and (b) Graphene Growth Direct by Deposition Mechanism. [Adapted with permission from *Mbayachi et al. (2021)*] [5].

however, the dimension and proportion of monolayer graphene might vary depending on the purity of the Ni film. The thickness and purity of graphene are influenced by the cooling rate, and the structure of Ni may also have an impact on the morphology of obtained graphene [57].

To determine the relative significance and relevance of the factors, Papon et al. (2017) used a technique called "designs of experiments." The interplay of a number of independent variables in the fabrication of graphene on a Cu substrate was explained by this design. The outcome demonstrated a considerable effect of substrate temperature, duration, heating rate, and pre-annealing time on the final purity of the graphene produced. The time frame of the graphene development process and the rates at which the temperature of the source of carbon is rising are the two major factors that specifically influence the size of the graphene outcome [58]. It signifies that the researchers only need to tweak these elements to affect the size substantially. Additionally, Liu and Liu (2017) highlighted that strong control over the reaction conditions could result in the production of large-area, high-grade graphene with distinct structures and layers [59].

In general, the CVD technique continues to be one of the most effective ways to produce significant amounts of graphene. Comparing the CVD process to other techniques like Scotch tape, thermal breakdown, reduction of GO, LPE, and even other bottom-up methods, the graphene obtained approximately 1.5 times better.

3.2.5 PYROLYSIS

The Greek *pyro* and *lysis* elements are where the word "pyrolysis" first appeared. Pyro denotes fire, and lysis indicates separation. Few-layer graphene can be synthesized via a simplistic process of pyrolysis that involves synthesizing carbon atoms on a metal surface [60]. The thermal breakdown of silicon carbide (SiC) is one of the frequently used methods of producing graphene. Si desorbs at elevated temperatures, keeping C remaining to produce a few graphene layers. This method has significantly improved as a result of the ongoing mm-scale synthesis of graphene films at a temperature of 750 °C on a thin nickel film deposited on a SiC substrate [61]. The benefit of this technique is that graphene sheets are continuously produced all across the whole SiC-coated surface. Unfortunately, large-scale production of graphene could not be possible using this process. At 1000 k, a similar system is used in the thermal breakdown of ethylene. The ability to synthesize high-grade graphene monolayers is a benefit of this synthesis technique [62].

3.2.6 ARC DISCHARGE

The arc discharge is indeed a comparatively economical and ecologically responsible technique for manufacturing graphene [63,64]. The arc discharge process may synthesize graphene in the presence of H_2, He, or N_2 [65]. To fabricate few-layered graphene underneath a combination of He and carbon dioxide (CO_2), Wu et al. (2010) designed the arc discharge technique [66]. The outcome demonstrates that the acquired graphene has fewer flaws than graphene made using chemical processes. For further applicability, the produced graphene may also be readily dispersed in organic solvents. Excellent graphene for constructing electrodes with different devices may be produced under suitable He and CO_2 environments within the arc discharge technique. The graphene made by this process also has the benefit of being an excellent option for an electrical charger utilized for conducting composites. A repeatable and sustainable aqueous arc discharge technique that yields excellent-grade dual and triple-layer graphene was described by Kim et al. (2016) [67]. Meanwhile, it is necessary to design a purification technique since they discovered contaminants while utilizing this approach.

Cheng et al. (2017) executed a study on the exploration of the arc discharge technique to make graphene through combining a vacuum arc discharge with the CVD process. Graphene is fabricated on a copper foil with the aid of a furnace operating at an elevated temperature and a vacuum arc discharge. This fusion technique may form a single sheet of graphene at high temperatures [68]. To fabricate graphene nanosheets on a mass scale, Wu et al. (2016) revealed the mechanics of the arc discharge approach. In their study, an activated carbon (AC) was employed as the anode and the cathode in the arc discharge process beneath the mixed gases (H_2 and N_2). Due to the concurrent reaction and evaporation caused by the alternating current used throughout the process, sediments at the cathode are not formed. By doing this, the temperature is raised, which is necessary to speed up the dispersion of carbon atoms and clusters. As the diffusing rate increases, both the carbon atoms and gas molecules might interact with one another. Because H_2 gas has an extremely rapid cooling rate, graphene products may be easily developed. To achieve these circumstances and produce graphene with acceptable quality, they have blended H_2 gas with an inert gas like N_2, which possesses a lower thermal conductivity [69].

3.3 FUNCTIONALIZATION OF GRAPHENE

Despite the enormous potential for applications, it is imperative to perceive that the graphene itself is hydrophobic and exhibits zero band gap, instability in aqueous conditions, and inertness to reactions, which weaken its potential to compete in the biomedical industry. This is among the factors contributing to the enormous rise in research initiatives focused on the functionalization of graphene, encompassing interactions between graphene (and its derivatives) and inorganic and organic molecules, chemical alteration of the large graphene surface, as well as a comprehensive description of numerous covalent and non-covalent interactions with graphene [3,70,71]. Functionalization with oxygenated functional groups through the formation of GO has multiplied the adaptability of graphene in drug delivery, cancer therapeutics, and other biomedical applications. Furthermore, the widening of the graphene band gap induced by doping and intercalation might aid in the development of effective nanoelectronics components. The graphene-based nanomaterials potentially provide a gateway to new domains of biotechnology unless they were biofunctionalized with certain biomolecules such as proteins, nucleic acids, enzymes, and peptides [72]. In addition, due to its aptitude to quench a variety of chemical dyes, quantum dots (QDs), and rapid DNA sequencing, graphene has recently been recognized as a viable element in the design of fluorescence resonance energy transfer (FRET) biosensors [73]. Graphene can be functionalized via covalent and non-covalent interactions through numerous value-added functional entities, which further improves the surface characteristics of graphene; the details are provided subsequently.

3.3.1 Covalent Functionalization

The covalent functionalization of graphene has been the subject of several studies, with the primary goals being to offer graphene with improved aqueous solubility, ease of processing, reduced toxicity, and biocompatibility [3,12]. After molecules are bonded covalently to graphene, the sp^2 carbon atoms of the π-network undergo rehybridization into an sp^3 orientation. This results in a partial or complete breakdown of the π–π conjugation and impairments to the inherent chemical and physical characteristics of graphene.

Graphene may be functionalized either at the basal surface or at the edges, albeit it demands a variable amount of energy. As a result of their rehybridization to the sp^3 tetrahedral configuration, the dangling terminal bonds actually respond with reduced energy barriers since it does not put excessive strain on the innermost carbon elements. The covalent functionalization of graphene can occur in either two ways: 1. through the development of covalent cross-linking between reactive species like dienophiles and free radicals and the C=C bonds of pure graphene; or 2. through the development of covalent links between organic functionalities and the oxygen groups of GO. The latter approach is most frequently used to attach solubilizing and biologically active compounds to graphene. In fact, GO is a preferable contender for biomedical application than pure graphene due to its oxygen-rich functional groups, such as the carboxyl, epoxy, and hydroxyl groups, which offer improved dispersibility, biocompatibility, and the potential for their subsequent surface modification [12,74].

Previously, numerous covalent functionalization strategies were adopted for the surface modification of graphene through organic compounds. The functionalization of graphene with organic compounds has significantly improved its dispersibility and, ultimately, colloidal stability as well as biocompatibility. The cycloaddition reaction, free radical addition, and nucleophilic addition reactions drove organic group functionalization.

3.3.1.1 Cycloaddition

The cycloaddition can be distinctively carried away through zwitterionic intermediate, the 1,3-dipolar cycloaddition of azomethine ylide, Diels–Alder cycloaddition, and other organic intermediates such as nitrene, carbene, and aryne. The combination of 4-dimethylamino pyridine with an acetylene dicarboxylate produces a zwitterionic intermediate, which reacts with an acetylene dicarboxylate to yield a five-membered ring. According to the substituted functional groups, the functionalized nanoparticles of graphene can be dispersed in organic solvents like DMF, $CHCl_3$, or water [75].

Nitrenes are active compounds formed only after the photochemical or thermal ablation of an N_2 molecule from the organic azides. They effortlessly combine with the graphene C=C double bonds to establish three-membered aziridine rings that link the organic azide component to the surface of graphene nanosheets. Graphene nanosheets are ultimately adorned with aromatic compounds [76], polymers [77], or aliphatic chains that may then be supplemented with functional

groups like carboxyl or hydroxyl groups depending upon the organic component [74,78]. These functional units may help to post-functionalize the obtained
graphene. For instance, carboxyl groups preferentially absorb gold nanoparticles
(NPs) distributed in a solution of carboxy-alkyl aziridine functionalized graphene,
enabling the gold NPs to be immobilized on the functionalized graphene. Graphene
that has undergone chemical modification is simple to dissolve in organic solvents.
A significant expansion in the sp^3/sp^2 ratio of graphene's carbon atoms occurs concurrently with the development of aziridine rings, and this increase is seen as a rise
in the I_D/I_G ratio of functionalized graphene. When graphene combines with a sur-
plus of the alkyl azides by a factor of 10, the I_D/I_G ratio is demonstrated to enhance
even more. This finding demonstrates a clear correlation across the reagent ratio
and the extent of graphene's surface modification. In other terms, the proportion of
the reagents might influence the extent of graphene functionalization [78]. Nitrene
addition might potentially be employed in polymer grafting on graphene nanosheets
[76]. Numerous azide groups must be present in the polymeric chains of these polymers. By adding nitrene, it is possible to covalently attach polyacetylene containing
alkyne azide groups on its side chain onto a surface of graphene. Because of the
chemical affinities of the obtained polymeric matrix, the functionalized polyacetylene exhibit improved dispersibility in conventional organic solvents. Previously,
a similar method was employed to functionalize graphene with phenylalanine. The
reaction occurs once N-protected azido phenylalanine is combined with exfoliating
graphene nanosheets distributed in o-dichlorobenzene **(Figure 3.6)** [74,79].

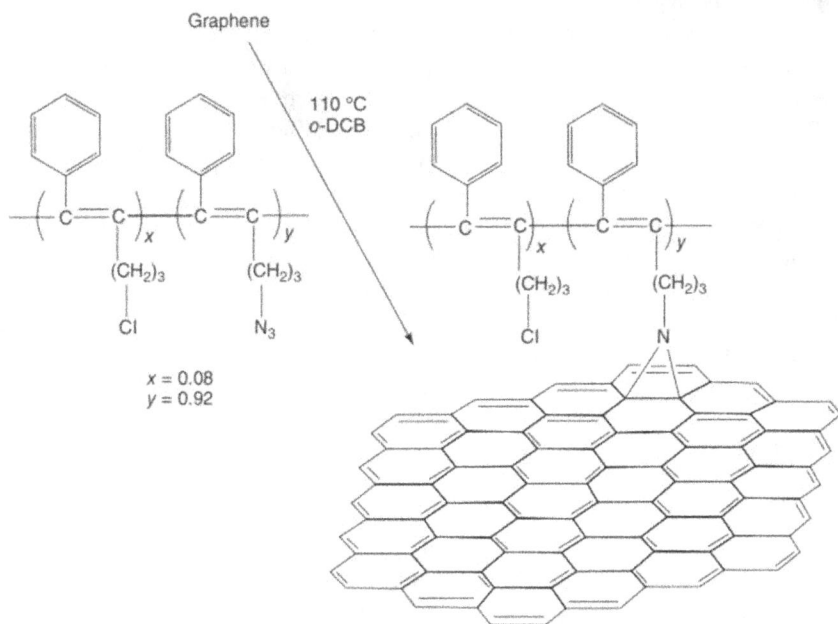

FIGURE 3.6 Formation of a Polyacetylene/Graphene Composite through an Aziridine Ring
Linker. [Reproduced with permission from *V. Georgakilas (2014)*] [74].

Similar to nitrene, carbenes are extremely reactive organic precursors with low electron density, which can target C-H bonds with sp^3 carbon atoms in place of hydrogen or C=C bonds in a [1+2] cycloaddition process. Due to the abundance of C=C and C-H bonds at the edges and defective sites of graphene, the interactions of graphene with carbenes results in the surface modification of graphene via both possible mechanisms. Despite sufficient information from the early functionalization of CNTs, and fullerenes employing carbene derivatives, the interaction of graphene and carbene is still not fully utilized [74]. In the [1+2] reactions, dichlorocarbene synthesized from chloroform that has been treated with sodium hydroxide (NaOH) is introduced to graphene nanoplatelets to formulate three-membered rings [3,74].

Ismaili et al. (2011) demonstrated the encapsulation of gold NPs on the surface of graphene through organic linkers, which resulted in a much more complex graphene functionalization via carbene [80]. Carbene was synthesized by photochemically treating a 3-aryl-3(trifluoromethyl)-diazirine derivative that had gold NPs coupled at the side of the molecule by an Au-S interaction. Carbenes were also formed through the breakdown of diazirines and the separation of nitrogen atoms as N_2, which may be accomplished via heating or incinerating diazirine compounds. The benefit of not offering potential intramolecular recombination routes for the associated carbenes, which results in by-products and lowers the productivity of a carbene addition process, makes 3-Aryl-3(trifluoromethyl)-diazirine compounds a common choice for carbene synthesis. In this case, gold NPs encapsulated with alkane thiol chains were partially functionalized by 3-aryl-3-(trifluoromethyl)-diazirine molecules via a thiol-alkyloxy linker in which thiol is linked to gold and oxygen onto the aryl ring [3].

As previously mentioned, arynes are another group of very reactive organic intermediates that are synthesized from phenyl derivatives by removing two ortho heteroatoms. As a result of their reactivity, arynes may easily undergo [2+2] or [4+2] cycloadditions with dienes or C=C bonds. Zhong et al. (2010) employed 2-(trimethylsilyl) aryl triate as a precursor for the synthesis of the aryne intermediate under the novel framework in which graphene nanosheets were functionalized by aryne cycloaddition. The dissolution rate of the functionalized graphene was significantly improved in an organic and polar solvent like DMF, o-DCB (1,2-dichlorobenzene), ethanol, chloroform, and water while succeeding the interaction of the modified arene to graphene by a four-membered ring. Similarly, various distinct functional groups can supersede the arenes [81].

3.3.1.2   Free radical addition

Free radicals are extremely reactive organic mediators that engage sp^2 carbon atoms and establish covalent bonds. They are often synthesized from organic compounds by meticulously removing an easily leaving component that dissociates a covalent bonding. A common method for producing free radicals is to heat the diazonium salt of an organic molecule. Meanwhile, the radicals are formed by eliminating an N_2 molecule. The hybridization of the reacting carbon atoms shifts from sp^2 to sp^3 when an organic radical is introduced to the surface of graphene. Such alteration disrupts the aromatic structure, resulting in a significant impact on the electrical characteristics of graphene [74]. According to Tour et al. (2010), the graphene conductivity decreases as a consequence of the time of the radical addition reaction, which may be regulated effectively [82].

In contrast, functionalizing graphene results in the introduction of a band gap that can be specified, enabling graphene with remarkable semiconducting characteristics [83]. This process has also been used to place aryl diazonium salts on graphene surfaces, demonstrating its significant adaptability. These functional groups include carboxy, chlorine, bromine, nitro, iodine, and cyano. Herein, the thermally or chemically reduced graphene that has been made into nanostructures is the primary component. A surfactant is then employed to make the reduced graphene disperse. The functionalized graphene compounds could be dissolved in polar aprotic solvents [84]. Numerous types of graphene, including epitaxial graphene [85] and graphene obtained through mechanical cleavage [86], have indeed been subjected to diazonium salt interactions.

To examine the antibacterial properties of the synthesized graphene compound, chlorophenyl groups have also been introduced to graphene nanosheets by the diazonium salt reactions. The extensive bactericidal potential of chlorine is a significant characteristic of chlorophenyl-functionalized graphene [86]. Sun et al. (2010) attempted to effectively functionalize the edges of graphene nanosheets while keeping the graphitic surface unaltered and further employed the diazonium salt reaction to accomplish this goal. It was not feasible to regulate the addition of free radicals to the reacting graphene region upon full exfoliation of the monolayers since the edges, and the remained surface are both equally exposed to the radical species. This is not the case for expanded graphite, in which the edges are fully exposed, whereas the major graphene surface is shielded against large 4-bromophenyl radicals with a relatively tiny space between graphene nanosheets. As a result, the edges of the graphene nanosheets were efficiently functionalized with bromophenyl groups due to the interaction between the 4-bromophenyl diazonium salt and thermally expanded graphite. Following the process, the edge-functionalized graphene nanosheets dispersed readily in DMF [87].

The incorporation of free radicals is also evident in polymer grafting on graphene processes. A number of well-known free radical polymerization techniques, including atom transfer radical polymerization (ATRP) and reversible addition-fragmentation chain transfer (RAFT), have indeed been implemented to formulate polymer nanocomposites comprising polymeric chains deposited on the surface of graphene [3,88]. Previously, a polystyrene-polyacrylamide copolymer was grafted onto the graphene sheet via in-situ free radical polymerization of the monomers in the vicinity of distributed graphene nanosheets. Through adjusting the monomer ratio, the amphiphilic characteristics of the graphene/copolymer composite may be modulated. Since the acrylamide monomer is hydrophilic as well as the styrene monomer is organophilic, they may both be dispersed in water and xylene, respectively [88].

3.3.2 Non-covalent Functionalization

Non-covalent functionalization is a potent technique frequently used for inducing desirable characteristics in graphene nanosheets while preventing desired loss of its parent properties. To establish non-covalent bonding, graphene delivers accessible π-electrons. The non-covalent interactions are crucial for comprehending biomolecular structures, molecular clusters, supramolecular assembly, ionophores, and nanomaterial engineering [3,74]. Since pure graphene nanosheets are hydrophobic and cannot disperse in polar liquids, conversely, graphene nanosheets may be functionalized to make them dispersible and perhaps soluble in an aqueous medium and organic solvent [89]. As it is vital to prevent stacking, the non-covalent functionalization with organic molecules via π-interactions would be greatly desired, as demonstrated by water-soluble fullerenes [90]. In this context, developing new nanomaterials for designing unique nanodevices depends on the antagonism and collaboration among individual interactions. Configurations and molecular characteristics of the nanosystems may change significantly as a result of even slight variations in the electronic structure of π-electron molecular structures. The non-covalent interactions mainly comprise π–π, and electrostatic interactions, in addition to hydrogen bonding and van der Waals interactions.

An understanding of the aromatic complexes is greatly aided by the non-covalent π–π interactions. There are two notably distinct scenarios with these systems. In the first scenario, the electron density configurations of the two aromatic moieties are extremely close or identical. Negative and strongly delocalized π-electron clouds distinguish aromatic systems. Chemical understanding dictates that such molecular structures should interact adversely. Nonetheless, since the proportion of electrostatic energy is much inferior to that of dispersion energy, π–π - interactions are still not governed via electrostatic interaction yet rather by dispersion forces. To develop novel nanostructures and nanomaterials, a comprehensive investigation of the energy constituents in π–π interactions is beneficial. Until the H-π interaction is significant, aromatic compounds interact with graphene through the π–π interaction [91]. The bonding among graphene and the immobilized molecule is frequently strengthened by the electrostatic interactions induced by charge transfer. Charge transport is also responsible for shifting the Dirac cone and doping graphene. Nucleobases on graphene have gained significant interest due to their potential usage in DNA sequencing [3,92]. The non-covalent interaction of graphene with aromatic molecules, polymers, and biomolecules is discussed subsequently.

3.3.2.1 Aromatic molecules

The aromaticity provided by the π-conjugation of graphene made it significant for the non-covalent functionalization of graphene through aromatic molecules. These molecules subsequently position themselves all along graphene's basal surface and engage in interactions via π–π stacking. The significant affinity of pyrene for graphite's basal plane might be used to improve the properties of a graphite surface. As a consequence, several research teams have begun to investigate the complexation of graphene utilizing pyrene derivatives [93,94]. In addition to numerous other characteristics, these functionalizations have yielded graphene that is water-soluble [3,95], with improved solar cell power transmission [96], and also doped with n/p types [97].

It is possible to make graphene/reduced graphene oxide (rGO) water soluble [74,98]. This aqueous stability can be achieved by sonicating graphite/or rGO in the vicinity of the pyrene stabilizer. It is interesting to note that even when destabilized by extremely low pH levels or freeze drying, these kinds of materials have been demonstrated not to agglomerate [99]. This action is supposed to be induced by the residual pyrene stabilizer groups on the surface, thereby preventing the material from aggregating.

Utilizing aromatic macrocycles like phthalocyanines and porphyrins, graphene may also be functionalized through non-covalent interactions [3,100]. Non-covalently functionalizing with water-soluble porphyrins makes it possible to provide desired water solubility to graphene. Using a vacuum filtering procedure coupled with thermal annealing, those solutions are then employed to generate extremely conductive and transparent graphene sheets. Through functionalizing graphene sheets with porphyrin or phthalocyanine, it is possible to develop light-harvesting sheets that may be utilized to analyze a variety of proteins [101]. The synthesis of a hemin-graphene hybrid composite via π–π interactions may be accomplished with a conventional wet-chemical method [102]. This novel nanomaterial was employed to distinguish between single-stranded (ss) and double-stranded (ds) DNA due to its peroxidase-like activity, good solubility, as well as stability in aqueous media. Based on this understanding, an assay for precise visual assessment of single-nucleotide polymorphisms at room temperature was designed. It was estimated that once the hemin-graphene compound was complexed with streptavidin and paired with a biotinylated molecular beacon, DNA could be electrochemically detected at the molar level [74]. A highly precise and selective electrochemical detector for dopamine was developed using an analogous wet-chemistry method [103]. The ascorbic acid and uric acid inhibition typically accompanied with dopamine detection could not be recognized using a glassy carbon electrode covered with the graphene/meso-tetra (4-carboxyphenyl) porphyrin composite. This is supposed to result from preferred π–π interactions between negatively charged porphyrin and positively charged dopamine. The non-covalent coupling of meso-tetrakis(4-methoxyl-3-sulfonate phenyl) porphyrin with graphene resulted in a robust and efficient label-free adenosine triphosphate sensing platform [104]. With a limit of detection of 0.7 nM for photosensitizers, this substance might be utilized to distinguish among adenosine triphosphate and cytidine/guanosine/uridine triphosphate nucleosides [100].

3.3.2.2 Polymers

Graphene may be functionalized with polymers through non-covalent interactions to provide materials for electronics, biomedical, green chemistry, capacitors, and other applications. Due to the π–π interactions between the aromatic framework of sulfonated polyaniline and the graphene basal plane, it was possible to make graphene water stable by utilizing these substances [105]. These substances also demonstrated significant electrocatalytic activity, conductance, and stability. A polystyrene/graphene nanocomposite may be developed by in situ stripping of graphite nanoplates in the vicinity of a polystyrene solution [106]. Due to the equal distribution of graphene throughout the matrix, the resulting composites were demonstrated to be conductive; surprisingly, the polystyrene segments prevented the graphene nanoplates from aggregation due to significant π–π interactions.

These significant non-covalent interactions among both the graphene carboxylic as well as the polyimide substrate prevent emulsification throughout thermal imidization, resulting in a clear polyimide/graphene polymer composite with superior mechanical strength [107]. It is considered that the 2D configuration of the graphene nanosheets transverse to the polyimide films and the uniform distribution of graphene all across the polymer matrices are the sources of the specimens' improved mechanical resilience. The inclusion of graphene increased the shape memory of the polyimide/graphene composite well beyond the glass transition temperature (GT) (250 °C). It is possible to develop pH-dependent soluble composites such as rGO/chitosan through the reduction of GO with a natural polymer, chitosan [108]. This substance exhibited pH-dependent solubility in water, which is likely to be mediated by electrostatic interaction and h-bonding between functional entities of chitosan and graphene. It was demonstrated in a subsequent investigation that this compound might function as a pH sensor due to its reversible pH switching across dispersion and agglomeration [109]. Similar methods exist for stabilizing graphene in the aqueous phase, including the use of biopolymers like cellulose and lignin compounds [110].

Through the straightforward process of sonication of the substrates, a thermoresponsive graphene/poly-(N-isopropyl acrylamide) composite can be developed. The compound was demonstrated to have a reduced critical solution temperature of 24 °C, under which it would be distributed in an aqueous system. Graphene was successfully dispersed in water using the $\pi-\pi$ stacking phenomenon that occurred among poly-(2,5-bis(3-sulfonatopropoxy)-1,4-ethynyl-phenylene-alt-1,4-ethynyl phenylene) sodium salt (PPE-SO$_3$Na$^+$) and graphene [111]. The (PPE-SO$_3$) sodium salt offers the substance with extra negative charges, which presents a unique technique to functionalize the graphene-based substance effectively. Utilizing poly oxy-ethylene sorbitan laurate, graphene may be stabilized in an aqueous system [112]. This approach allowed for the synthesis of a film that demonstrated resilience in water and biocompatibility to mammalian cell lines, making it suitable for use in biological applications such as tissue engineering, wherein excellent mechanical strength is required.

It is also conceivable to develop amphiphilic graphene compounds parallel to the water-soluble varieties. The rGO can be made soluble in a wide range of polar and nonpolar organic media by functionalizing it with polyethylene glycol (PEG) and polyethylene oxide (OPE) triblock copolymer. By functionalizing graphene with ionic liquid molecules, it is possible to induce phase transition between immiscible liquids [113].

3.3.2.3 Biomolecules

Graphene nanostructure can eventually be functionalized non-covalently with the biomolecules like peptides, enzymes, and nucleic acids for their application in drug and gene delivery. Liu et al. (2010) demonstrated the non-covalent functionalization of graphene through thiolated DNA **(Figure 3.7)**. The gold NPs that are subsequently attached to such water-soluble DNA/graphene combination may enable the application of these compounds in systems for bio-detection, catalysis, and field effects [114]. Graphene oxide/DNA material may be employed through a self-assembly procedure to produce a 3D hydrogel [115]. The process of self-assembly is initiated by putting the material in solution at 90 °C, which causes the DNA segments to unfold and enable a connection of distinct GO sheets as ss-DNA. This substance was demonstrated to have a high dye-adsorption capacity, self-healing properties after heating, chemical stability, and strong mechanical properties. Additionally, < 2 nm Pt nanostructures have been uniformly grown on the graphene surface under the direct influence of DNA-functionalized graphene [116]. In addition, this

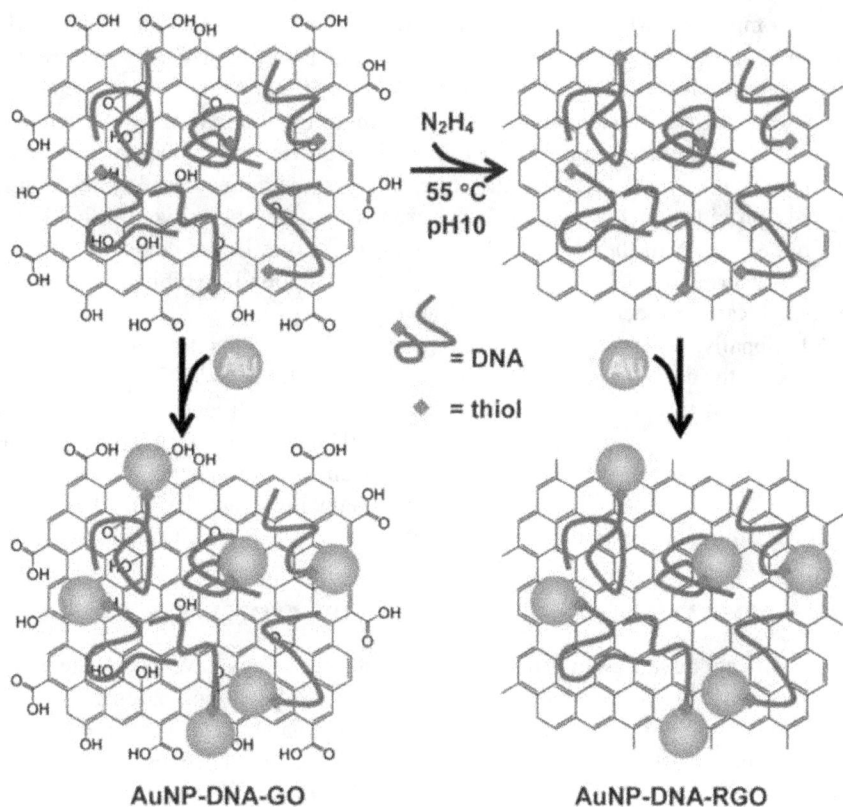

FIGURE 3.7 Non-covalent Functionalization of GO and rGO through Thiolated DNA and Gold NPs. [Reproduced with permission from *Liu et al. (2010)*] [114].

approach provides an electrochemically active surface area that is multiple times larger than that of Pt-graphene without DNA functionalization. It was discovered that when this substance was used in the oxygen reduction reaction (ORR), it displayed greater ORR half-wave current and potential as compared to the Pt-graphene and standard Pt/C catalyst.

The non-covalent interactions among a graphene nanosheet and a lipids backbone make it simple to form a monolayer of phospholipids over it, forming a distinct planar mimic of the biological membranes. Through reactivating the fluorescence of a fluorescein-labeled phospholipid that has been incorporated into the monolayer, a potential biosensor can be developed to monitor the functioning of the phospholipase D-enzyme. Enzymes may also be immobilized on graphene covered with a lipid monolayer, and this kind of substance can potentially be employed as a biosensor [74]. Encapsulated in the lipid/graphene framework, the enzyme Microperoxidase-11 demonstrated exceptional sensitivity and reproducibility for hydrogen peroxide detection with a limit of detection of 7.2×10^{-7} M. The advantage of adopting these particular lipid/graphene compounds is that they are biocompatible, which results in the development of an ideal situation for the immobilization of enzymes that are proficient in preserving their structure and bioavailability. Additionally, enzymes may directly functionalize graphene mono-layers. Lu et al. (2012) demonstrated in their investigation that pH-dependent and water-soluble graphene could be obtained through the non-covalent functional-ization of rGO with β-lactoglobulin. Surprisingly, the connected β-lactoglobulin not only provides anchoring sulfhydryl groups that may be utilized to hold gold NPs but also aids in the reduction of GO. Furthermore, it was demonstrated that the Au-functionalized-lactoglobulin/graphene compound exhibited a surface-enhanced Raman spectroscopic effect [117].

Additionally, a graphene surface was functionalized by the anticoagulant hepa-rin, making the compound more biocompatible and water-soluble. Compared to pure herapin, which utilized 85.6 IU mL^{-1} of anticoagulant anti-factor Xa activity, the herapin/graphene composite consumed just 29.6 IU mL^{-1}. Given that the herapin can maintain its reactivity even after being functionalized to graphene, this is encour-aging for biological applications. Herapin is a reducing agent that may be used to functionalize graphene by reducing the substrates composed of GO [118].

3.4 APPLICATION OF GRAPHENE IN DRUG DELIVERY

The significant advancements in the field of nanotechnology have driven the recent advancements for its application in numerous biomedical applications. Nanoma-terials, with their distinct characteristics like a smaller size, higher reactivity, larger surface area, and controllable surface chemistry, have provided signifi-cant advantages for their application in cancer diagnosis and therapeutics as well as in DDS and tissue engineering. The application of nanomaterial-based DDS potentially leads to 1. extended systemic circulation [119], 2. regulated administra-tion of chemotherapy drugs to the target cells/tissue, and, therefore, 3. enhanced pharmacokinetic and pharmacodynamic profiles [120]. Nanoscale-targeted DDSs have the potential to concentrate in the tumor microenvironment using a "passive-targeting" mechanism based on the enhanced permeability and retention (EPR) effect and to target cancerous cells using an "active-targeting" approach that involves expressing oncomarkers [121]. Furthermore, smart stimuli-responsive nanocarriers could react to physicochemical and biological disturbances in the tumor microenvironment, such as low pH, elevated temp, reduced oxygen level, and highly expressed proteases [122].

In addition to other nanomaterials, graphene-based nanocarriers have received prodigious attention in the DDS field since they are known to be excellent drug carriers for a plethora of drugs, such as chemotherapeutic agents, genes, and small interfering RNAs (siRNAs) [123]. The unique physicochemical features of graphene and its oxidized derivative, GO, have been extensively employed for numerous bio-medical applications (**Figure 3.8**) [124]. Graphene derivatives like GO and rGO have been widely employed as effective photosensitizing agents in photodynamic (PDT) and photothermal (PTT) treatment due to inherent optical absorption in the NIR range. The applications of graphene-based nanocarriers in drug delivery for cancer therapeutics and tissue engineering are presented subsequently.

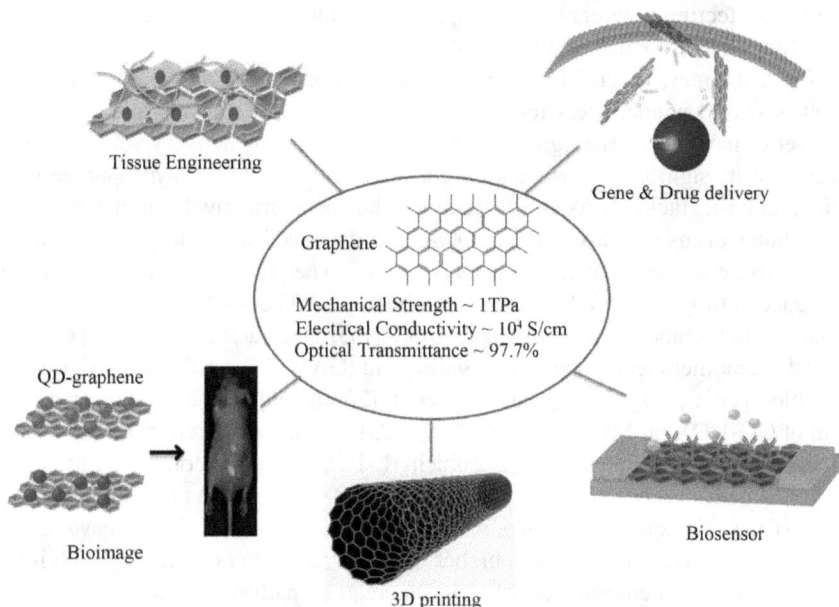

FIGURE 3.8 Biomedical Applications of Graphene-Based Nanomaterials. [Reprinted with permission from *Shin et al. (2016)*] [124].

3.4.1 CHEMOTHERAPY

Graphene, with its high degree of hydrophobicity and absence of an oxygen-containing functional group, exhibits poor aqueous stability and dispersion. However, it provides suitable functionalization ability through covalent and non-covalent interactions for improving its physicochemical characteristics. As a result, GO can be readily synthesized using graphene functionalization, a covalent functionalization technique wherein the oxygenated groups such as epoxy, hydroxyl, and carboxyl can be impregnated on the edges and basal planes of the graphene nanosheets to augment its water solubility [125,126]. However, GO has the propensity to agglomerate in physiological solutions in the vicinity of salts and proteins due to electrostatic charge shielding and the establishment of nonspecific interaction with proteins [127]. Furthermore, two major techniques, comprising covalent and non-covalent alterations by various modifiers, have been used to improve the physiological stability, cellular absorption, and transfection effectiveness of graphene-based nanocarriers [128]. Covalent functionalization techniques were employed when the modified graphene must have stability and superior mechanical characteristics, whereas non-covalent functionalization is favored when the graphene's dielectric properties and wide surface area are required. Both techniques of modification can provide higher drug loading capacity and DNA/RNA condensation, making them favorable for drug delivery and intracellular gene delivery applications [17]. The aqueous stability of graphene-based nanocarriers also leads to biocompatibility-related issues for their application in DDS. It was observed that the conjugation and modification with the protecting polymers might improve their biocompatibility as well as circulation time in the bloodstream [129].

In recent times, several investigations have been conducted on the aptitude of graphene-based nanocarriers for the delivery of anticancer agents and genes. The discoveries have established graphene as a prospective drug delivery vehicle, largely because of its significant surface area, tiny size, electrostatic or hydrophobic interaction, and π-π stacking. As an illustration, it has been effectively employed to load hydrophobic drugs like doxorubicin (DOX) and docetaxel with a targeting ligand for the selective eradication of cancer cells [130–132]. The graphene-based nanocarriers were successfully employed for the chemotherapy application by delivering conventional chemotherapeutic drugs such as DOX [133] and Paclitaxel (PTX) [134] and natural chemotherapeutic agents like gallic acid (GA) [135], caffeic acid (CA) [136], and chlorogenic acid [137]. Quagliarini et al. (2020) studied the anticancer mechanism of GO-DOX on MCF-7 and MDA-MB 231 (breast cancer cells) and compared its performance with liposomal-doxorubicin (L-DOX), another commonly used drug for breast cancer. They reported that the GO-DOX complex had higher efficiency than L-DOX. Encapsulating drugs with nanocarriers increases their bioavailability and cellular uptake. GO provides higher cell internalization by binding with integrins at the plasma membrane of cells, which creates a pathway for conjugated drugs. Thus, GO-DOX exhibits superior performance as it delivers DOX by attaching it to the cell membrane and destroying the DNA [138]. Recently, Guo et al. (2021) established a drug delivery system with PEG-modified and oxidized sodium alginate functionalized GO nanosheets to deliver PTX and treat gastric cancer. PTX@ GO-PEG-OSA was designed to overwhelm the drug resistance faced by PTX in gastric cancer cells due to P-glycoprotein (P-gp). When exposed to NIR radiations, the PTX@GO-PEG-OSA NSs exhibit a photo-thermal effect that generates ROS, limits mitochondrial respiratory chain complex enzyme activity, and diminishes ATP supplement to P-gp. Thus, this nanocarrier system provides better efficiency than free PTX [139].

Gu et al. (2018) reported that GA exerts an anticancer effect by inhibiting mitochondrial respiration in cancer cells [140]. Zhang (2019) studied the effect of GA on NSCLC A549 cells with and without cisplatin, another chemotherapeutic. The findings showed that GA controlled the proliferation and persuaded apoptosis of cancerous cells. Also, GA enhanced the effect of cisplatin [141]. Recently, Sontakke et al. (2022) developed a novel GO nanoscrolls (GONS)-based nano delivery system for the sustained release of GA. The nanoscrolls were fabricated via the low-frequency ultrasonication method and further loaded with GA. The loading capacity for the presented nanocarrier was ~30%. The GONS-GA nanocomposite demonstrated suitable anticancer efficacy against A549 lung cancer cells (IC$_{50}$ = 60.7 µg/mL) [142]. Dorniani et al. (2016) loaded GA on GO nanocarriers. The application of the GO/GA system was studied on normal fibroblast and liver cancer cells at different concentrations. It was conveyed that the complex hindered the growth of cancer cells and had no side effects on normal cells [135].

Meanwhile, traditional drug delivery methods have some drawbacks, such as the release of the drug before reaching the targeted site, low efficiency, low drug retention, poor solubility in the physiological medium, and side effects on healthy cells

[143]. The advantages of smart drug systems, as summarized by Shah et al. (2021), are improved utilization of the drug and lowered administration frequency, drug protection from degradation, and reduced side effects [144]. The advances in nanotechnology have led to the advancement in nanocarrier-based targeted DDS. The DDSs, which are target-specific, lead to the proper distribution of the drug in the patient's body as the nano-structures have the required size and display excellent drug loading and release behavior [144]. Graphene and graphene oxide (GO) have exceptional physicochemical qualities, which have sparked interest in research for its biomedical applications. Meanwhile, the targetability of the GO-based nanocarriers can be enhanced by its functionalization with the targeting ligands such as folic acid, aptamers, and lactoferrin. As the cancer cells are overexpressed to folate receptors, the FA functionalized nanocarriers loaded drug conjugates accumulate over the tumor cell, henceforth increasing their local concentration and enhancing the therapeutic efficiency in chemotherapy.

Fong et al. (2017) recently developed a folic acid (FA) conjugated GO nanocarrier (GO-FA) for the targeted delivery of DOX. For intratumoral drug administration, the drug-loaded nanocomposite (GO-FA-DOX) was encapsulated with the injectable and thermosensitive hyaluronic acid-chitosan-g-poly(N-isopropyl acrylamide) (HACPN) hydrogel. The breakdown duration of HACPN hydrogel may be modulated, potentially resulting in a controlled distribution of DOX from the GO-FA nanocarrier. Furthermore, biopsies of major organs and blood analysis indicated no adverse effects of the medication, confirming its safety [145]. Pourjavadi et al. (2020) designed a GO-based DDS for the loading and controlled release of both hydrophobic and hydrophilic anticancer drugs [146]. The hydrophobic drug (curcumin) was loaded by π-π interaction and hydrophilic (DOX) by covalent bonding. Also, GO was modified with oxygen-rich polymers to enhance its aqueous solubility. The system displayed pH-triggered release behavior, and dual-loading resulted in better drug internalization. Zhou et al. (2014) developed nanocarriers based on GO and polyelectrolytes that showed charge-reversal and pH-responsive behavior [147]. The system could release the loaded DOX under an acidic environment. The surface charge alternated when GO-Abs/PEI/PAH-Cit/DOX entered the cell resulting in the release of the drug, which reached the cytoplasm and then the nucleus of cancer cells.

For developing the GO-based electrically controlled DDS, Weaver et al. (2014) incorporated GO nanosheets into a conducting polymer. The poly(pyrrole) (PPy)/ GO composite was developed to deliver dexamethasone, and the system could be simulated electrically [148]. The nanocomposite demonstrated a linear release profile that was stable for a large number of simulations. Wang et al. (2017) designed a magnetically controlled drug delivery system, Fe_3O_4/GO nanocarriers, to deliver 5-fluorouracil [149]. The composite had combined properties of GO and Fe_3O_4 and could release the drug under externally applied magnetism. They also concluded that the drug loading of Fe_3O_4/GO was higher than Fe_3O_4 and it had good dispersity in water. Recently, Liang et al. (2019) have employed a modified Hummers's method to synthesize targeted NCGO-FA nanocomplexes effectively. The carboxyl functional groups of the nanoscale GO were activated to obtain NCGO prior to its functionalization with FA. The resultant nanocomplex was further loaded with the photosensitizer MB dyes and anticancer agent DOX via non-covalent interactions to develop a dual responsive, namely, thermal and pH-responsive NCGO@ DOX-FA and NCGO@MB-FA nanoplatform for combined chemo-photothermal therapy. The NCGO-FA nanocomplexes demonstrate outstanding photothermal conversion efficiency and photo-stability in addition to a significant drug loading capacity and dual-responsive drug release properties to temperature and pH. More significantly, compared to separately administered photothermal treatment or chemotherapy, the photothermal-photodynamic or photothermal-chemo simultaneous therapies using the NCGO@DOX-FA or NCGO@MB-FA nanoplatform demonstrated an exceptional synergistic impact, resulting in a distinct anticancer efficiency [150].

Imani et al. (2022) recently investigated the prospect of siRNA-based gene delivery using a PEG/R8/FA multifunctionalized GO loaded via chloroquine (CQ). By using physical and chemical step-by-step conjugation, the FA was effectively attached to the GO-PEG-R8 (GPP) nanocarrier, and the efficiency of FA encapsulation was improved. The rate of MCF-7 cellular internalization through receptor-mediated endocytosis was substantially increased by incorporating FA into the R8/PEG-functionalized nanocarrier. Due to CQ's lysosomotropic action, incorporating CQ at an optimum concentration of 10 μM through π-π interactions allowed the GPPF nanocarrier to discharge from the lysosomal partition. Additionally, compared to free CQ therapy, the pH-dependent release of CQ through nanocarriers (95.3% at pH 4.5) was safer and more effective. In addition, the antimalarial drug CQ was unanimously implemented as an anticancer agent. It is a lysosomotropic substance that predominantly deposits in lysosomal regions. As a result, it has frequently been employed to improve the efficiency of gene delivery. The presented study also delivers its significance for combined gene-chemo therapy [151,152]. Similarly, Chen et al. (2022) have designed a GO-PEI-DTX-anti-miRNA21-based DDS for combined chemo-gene-photothermal therapy [153].

The fundamental problem in treating cancer, like other solid tumors, is the development of drug resistance. One of the largest contributors to drug resistance in cancer therapy continues to be the upregulation of multidrug transport machinery, although gene therapy may offer a promising strategy to combat inherent or developed drug resistance. In this regard, certain genes like pro-apoptotic, carcinogenic transporter genes could be modulated by genetic materials (such as oligonucleotide antisense, siRNA, etc.) [154,155]. It has been demonstrated that functionalized graphene-based NSs may effectively transfer nucleic acids into cancer cells while also having the ability to impose PTT/PDT effects [156,157]. For instance, Zeng et al. (2017) demonstrated FA-conjugated high molecular weight branching PEI-modified PEGylated nanographene (PPG-FA) as a dual carrier for the targeted administration of both siRNA and DOX to suppress the development of efflux transporter, P-glycoprotein (P-gp). The PPG-FA carrier was loaded with DOX and siRNA via electrostatic interaction and π-π stacking. The platform displayed significant DOX and siRNA loading, and it was discovered that heat and pH were requisite for their release. Moreover, it was applied as a combination treatment depending on the photothermal impact of GO under NIR illumination and the anticancer activity of DOX [158].

3.4.2 Tissue Engineering

Tissue engineering is an interdisciplinary area that leverages skills in biology, physiology, medicine, and engineering to design biomimetic tissue structures for regenerative medicine in addition to therapeutic and diagnostic investigations [159,160]. Biomaterials are essential elements in tissue engineering since they can drive cellular proliferation, promote certain biological activities, and regulate cell-cell interactions [161]. Furthermore, the biomechanical, electrical, or physical characteristics of various body tissues differ. As solitary materials may not imitate the biological and physical characteristics of native tissue, hybrid composites comprising multiple elements that may accommodate the diverse requirements are commonly employed to build artificial tissues. Researchers have been inspired to employ graphene-based nanomaterials in tissue engineering and regenerative medicine because of their exceptional electrical and mechanical attributes [162–164]. It has been discovered that graphene may efficiently adsorb nucleobases through the π–π interaction and shield nucleotides from enzymatic breakage [165]. In tissue regeneration, gene therapy has lately gained prominence as a treatment for disorders. Protecting DNA from deterioration and delivering high transfection effectiveness are two fundamental needs of a gene delivery vector [166]. Additionally, both viral and nonviral vectors have attended immense attention in the field of gene delivery science [167]. In light of this, graphene nanosheets would be a good choice for a vector since cells could readily absorb them. For example, Chen et al. (2011) demonstrated that PEI-GO could augment transfection efficiency through a proton-sponge effect by transfecting plasmid DNA into HeLa cells using a poly(ethylenimine)-GO (PEI-GO) carrier [168].

To develop 2D or 3D graphene-based frameworks, several researchers have used a range of techniques, including coating, hydrogel mixing, wet/dry spinning operations, and 3D printing. For tissue regeneration applications, graphene and its derivatives may be coupled with additional biomaterials to improve their biomechanical, electrical, and physical characteristics. Recently, Purohit et al. (2020) used freeze-drying to develop gelatin-alginate (GA)-based 3D polymeric scaffolds using graphene oxide-nanohydroxyapatite (GO-nHAp) nanocomposites as reinforcing agents. The main physicochemical characteristics of this scaffold and the synergistic effects of all its constituent parts were established for application in tissue regeneration. Additionally, it demonstrated swelling behavior in water, demonstrating its hydrophilic character and suitability for practice in tissue engineering. The presence of GO-nHAp in this scaffold increased its compressive strength to 14.72 MPa while lowering its rate of biodegradation. These characteristics, along with the scaffold's biocompatibility, considerably increase its suitability for bone tissue engineering [169].

Similarly, for bone regeneration, Sharma et al. (2022) developed a polydopamine-rGO doped 3D printable PLA scaffold with significant functionalities, including antioxidant, pro-angiogenic, anti-biofilm, and osteoinduction. Development of tissues like bone, which confronts a plethora of biological and physiological constraints leading to declining performance and ultimate rejection of grafts, significantly requires the assimilation of multifunctionality in a single tailored scaffold. The presented approach offered an easy way to develop a multifunctional bone scaffold that may confront issues like biofilm formation brought on by infection, reduced oxidative stress caused by ROS, encourages assimilation with the native tissue due to proangiogenic potential, and endorses bone formation via its osseointegration effect and superior *in-vivo* compatibility and adequacy [170].

Meanwhile, as a component of mammalian tissue that offers cells structural support, the extracellular matrix (ECM) plays a crucial function in tissue development. Additionally, ECM functions as a regional repository for developmental factors that regulate cell development and phenotype. In this aspect, a scaffold that closely resembles the structure of the ECM is essential for the development of the healing of wounds. In a recent study, Ryu et al. (2022) established enzyme-mediated GO cross-linked gelatin-based hydrogels exhibiting excellent mechanical properties to simulate ECM and successfully adhere to the adjacent tissue with significant adhesive potential. In comparison to gelatine-based hydrogels and fibrin glue as a reference, the tissue adhesive potential of GO/gelatine-based hydrogel was three times and eight times greater, respectively. The hydrogels demonstrated biodegradability as well as encouraged cell proliferation in an *in-vitro* proteolytic disintegration characteristic and human dermal fibroblast proliferation investigation [171].

In addition, graphene-based nanostructures can also be applied for neural and cardiac tissue engineering. Injecting exogenous neural stem/precursor cells (NSCs) into animal models has been utilized extensively to treat neuronal disorders [124]. For instance, Dibajnia et al. (2013) increased rehabilitation from brain ischemia by injecting NSCs effectively into the lateral ventricle [172]. The initial investigation into the basic impacts of materials based on graphene on the activities of human NSCs (hNSCs) was conducted by Park et al. (2011). The hNSCs showed a superior proliferation rate in comparison to the control group when they were cultivated in a medium with growth factors and a 2D graphene sheet. A neuronal-specific marker (TUJ1) was also produced by cells in the absence of growth hormones, and differentiated neurons showed outstanding neuronal functioning on the graphene surface [173]. It was discovered that graphene and embryonic stem cells (ESCs) function well together because they provide a stimulating environment for pluripotent cells to transform into neurons [174]. Yang et al. (2014) evaluated the capacity of ESCs to differentiate into neurons on graphene and GO. In an investigation using ESCs grown on GO substrates, they discovered that dopaminergic neuronal development was twice as high as it was on graphene. Furthermore, they verified that the concentration of GO might control the development of dopaminergic neurons in ESCs. Particularly, the maximum tested concentration of GO (100 g/mL) resulted in a threefold rise in the number of differentiated dopaminergic neurons compared to the smallest dosage (1 g/mL) [175].

3.5 SUMMARY

The fabrication of materials based on graphene has progressed significantly during the past ten years. Graphene-based nanomaterials have been discovered to offer a wide range of applications in the disciplines of chemotherapy and tissue engineering due to their superior physicochemical and biological characteristics. Graphene has demonstrated significant adsorbing capacity to chemotherapeutic agents for their application in DDSs due to its unique atomic structures. Furthermore, the exceptional electrical conductance of graphene and its derivatives is projected to boost the activity and growth of electrical-responsive cells, including cardiomyocytes and neurons, as well as improve the memory of cellular signals. Also, the coupling of graphene and its derivatives with additional composites that have characteristics like wettability or flexibility makes them attractive alternatives to developing multifunctional smart materials.

In this chapter, we discussed the prospective uses of graphene and graphene-based nanocarriers for therapeutic drug delivery in chemotherapy, neurological, and tissue engineering applications. Based on all the preceding investigations, it was highlighted that graphene has unique properties and enormous potential for use in tissue and neurovascular tissue engineering, cancer diagnostics, and therapy. The present chapter describes the structure and properties of graphene as well as recent developments in graphene synthesis using both the top-down and bottom-up methods. Several functionalization methodologies have been examined to improve the surface and physicochemical characteristics of graphene. It was observed that the non-covalent functionalization of graphene-based nanocarriers through numerous biomolecules and polymers had delivered substantial improvement in the aqueous stability and biocompatibility of these composites. Among the fabrication methods, CVD and laser ablation methods provided promising results considering the amount, homogeneity, and characteristics of obtained graphene. Meanwhile, the cost of the production process for the synthesis of graphene is a major challenge faced by the research community, in addition to the toxicity of graphene for biomedical applications. The emergence of green synthesis approaches has provided a timely solution to these challenges, which must be explored in the future. Also, it is obligatory to explore the detailed *in-vivo* and *in-vitro* toxicological aspects of graphene and related materials for their application in DDSs.

REFERENCES

[1] H.P. Boehm, R. Setton, E. Stumpp, International union of pure and applied chemistry inorganic chemistry division commission on high temperature and solid state chemistry* nomenclature and terminology of graphite intercalation compounds, Pure Appl. Chem. 66 (1994) 1893–1901. doi:10.1351/pac199466091893.

[2] S. Baig, M. Ahmed, A. Batool, A. Bashir, S. Mumtaz, M. Ikram, M. Saeed, K. Shahzad, M. Umer Farooq, A. Maqsood, M. Ikram, Introductory Chapter: Brief Scientific Description to Carbon Allotropes - Technological Perspective, in: Graphene - Recent Advances and Future Perspective, IntechOpen, Cambridge (2022): pp. 225–240. doi:10.5772/intechopen.107940.

[3] V. Georgakilas, M. Otyepka, A.B. Bourlinos, V. Chandra, N. Kim, K.C. Kemp, P. Hobza, R. Zboril, K.S. Kim, Functionalization of graphene: Covalent and noncvalent approaches, derivatives and applications, Chem. Rev. 112 (2012) 6156–6214. doi:10.1021/cr3000412.

[4] R. Mmaduka Obodo, I. Ahmad, F. Ifeanyichukwu Ezema, Introductory chapter: graphene and its applications, in: Graphene - Recent Advances and Future Perspective, IntechOpen, Cambridge (2019): p. 13. doi:10.5772/intechopen.86023.

[5] V.B. Mbayachi, E. Ndayiragije, T. Sammani, S. Taj, E.R. Mbuta, A. Ullah Khan, Graphene synthesis, characterization and its applications: A review, Results Chem. 3 (2021) 100163. doi:10.1016/j.rechem.2021.100163.

[6] G. Yang, L. Li, W.B. Lee, M.C. Ng, Structure of graphene and its disorders: A review, Sci. Technol. Adv. Mater. 19 (2018) 613–648. doi:10.1080/14686996.2018.1494493.

[7] A.D. Sontakke, S. Tiwari, M.K. Purkait, A comprehensive review on graphene oxide-based nanocarriers: Synthesis, functionalization and biomedical applications, FlatChem. 38 (2023) 100484. doi:10.1016/j.flatc.2023.100484.

[8] K.I. Bolotin, K.J. Sikes, Z. Jiang, M. Klima, G. Fudenberg, J. Hone, P. Kim, H.L. Stormer, Ultrahigh electron mobility in suspended graphene, Solid State Commun. 146 (2008) 351–355. doi:10.1016/j.ssc.2008.02.024.

[9] Z. Zhen, H. Zhu, Structure and properties of graphene, in: H. Zhu, Z. Xu, D. Xie, Y.B.T.-G. Fang (Eds.), Graphene, Elsevier, Cambridge (2018): pp. 1–12. doi:10.1016/B978-0-12-812651-6.00001-X.

[10] C.N.R. Rao, K. Biswas, K.S. Subrahmanyam, A. Govindaraj, Graphene, the new nano-carbon, J. Mater. Chem. 19 (2009) 2457. doi:10.1039/b815239j.

[11] K. Lü, G. Zhao, X. Wang, A brief review of graphene-based material synthesis and its application in environmental pollution management, Chinese Sci. Bull. 57 (2012) 1223–1234. doi:10.1007/s11434-012-4986-5.

[12] C. Spinato, C. Ménard-Moyon, A. Bianco, Chemical functionalization of graphene for biomedical applications, Funct. Graphene. 9783527335 (2014) 95–138. doi:10.1002/9783527672790.ch4.

[13] K.S. Novoselov, A.K. Geim, S.V. Morozov, D. Jiang, Y. Zhang, S.V. Dubonos, I.V. Grigorieva, A.A. Firsov, Electric field effect in atomically thin carbon films, Sci. 306 (2004) 666–669. doi:10.1126/science.1102896.

[14] A.K. Geim, Graphene: Status and prospects, Sci. 324 (2009) 1530–1534. doi:10.1126/science.1158877.

[15] X. Huang, Z. Yin, S. Wu, X. Qi, Q. He, Q. Zhang, Q. Yan, F. Boey, H. Zhang, Graphene-based materials: Synthesis, characterization, properties, and applications, Small. 7 (2011) 1876–1902. doi:10.1002/smll.201002009.

[16] L. Dai, Functionalization of graphene for efficient energy conversion and storage, Acc. Chem. Res. 46 (2013) 31–42. doi:10.1021/ar300122m.

[17] M. Teimouri, A.H. Nia, K. Abnous, H. Eshghi, M. Ramezani, Graphene oxide–cationic polymer conjugates: Synthesis and application as gene delivery vectors, Plasmid. 84–85 (2016) 51–60. doi:10.1016/j.plasmid.2016.03.002.

[18] T.P. Dasari Shareena, D. McShan, A.K. Dasmahapatra, P.B. Tchounwou, A review on graphene-based nanomaterials in biomedical applications and risks in environment and health, Nano-Micro Lett. 10 (2018) 1–34. doi:10.1007/s40820-018-0206-4.

[19] D. Li, M.B. Müller, S. Gilje, R.B. Kaner, G.G. Wallace, Processable aqueous dispersions of graphene nanosheets, Nat. Nanotechnol. 3 (2008) 101–105. doi:10.1038/nnano.2007.451.

[20] Y. Si, E.T. Samulski, Synthesis of water soluble graphene, Nano Lett. 8 (2008) 1679–1682. doi:10.1021/nl080604h.

[21] C. Shan, H. Yang, D. Han, Q. Zhang, A. Ivaska, L. Niu, Water-soluble graphene covalently functionalized by biocompatible poly-l-lysine, Langmuir. 25 (2009) 12030–12033. doi:10.1021/la903265p.

[22] C.-T. Hsieh, W.-Y. Chen, Water/oil repellency and work of adhesion of liquid droplets on graphene oxide and graphene surfaces, Surf. Coatings Technol. 205 (2011) 4554–4561. doi:10.1016/j.surfcoat.2011.03.128.

[23] J. Park, M. Yan, Covalent functionalization of graphene with reactive intermediates, Acc. Chem. Res. 46 (2013) 181–189. doi:10.1021/ar300172h.

[24] N. Mohanty, V. Berry, Graphene-based single-bacterium resolution biodevice and DNA transistor: Interfacing graphene derivatives with nanoscale and microscale biocomponents, Nano Lett. 8 (2008) 4469–4476. doi:10.1021/nl802412n.

[25] K.S. Novoselov, D. Jiang, F. Schedin, T.J. Booth, V. V Khotkevich, S.V. Morozov, A.K. Geim, Two-dimensional atomic crystals, Proc. Natl. Acad. Sci. 102 (2005) 10451–10453. doi:10.1073/pnas.0502848102.

[26] J.Y. Lim, N.M. Mubarak, E.C. Abdullah, S. Nizamuddin, M. Khalid, Inamuddin, Recent trends in the synthesis of graphene and graphene oxide based nanomaterials for removal of heavy metals—a review, J. Ind. Eng. Chem. 66 (2018) 29–44. doi:10.1016/j.jiec.2018.05.028.

[27] R.S. Edwards, K.S. Coleman, Graphene synthesis: Relationship to applications, Nanoscale. 5 (2013) 38–51. doi:10.1039/c2nr32629a.

[28] C. Casiraghi, A. Hartschuh, E. Lidorikis, H. Qian, H. Harutyunyan, T. Gokus, K.S. Novoselov, A.C. Ferrari, Rayleigh imaging of graphene and graphene layers, Nano Lett. 7 (2007) 2711–2717. doi:10.1021/nl071168m.

[29] X. Liang, A.S.P. Chang, Y. Zhang, B.D. Harteneck, H. Choo, D.L. Olynick, S. Cabrini, Electrostatic force assisted exfoliation of prepatterned few-layer graphenes into device sites, Nano Lett. 9 (2009) 467–472. doi:10.1021/nl803512z.

[30] H. Prakash, N. Chandra, R. Prakash, Shivani, Effect of decoherence on fidelity in teleportation using entangled coherent states, J. Phys. B At. Mol. Opt. Phys. 40 (2007) 1613. doi:10.1088/0953-4075/40/8/012.

[31] K.A. Madurani, S. Suprapto, N.I. Machrita, S.L. Bahar, W. Illiya, F. Kurniawan, Progress in graphene synthesis and its application: History, challenge and the future outlook for research and industry, ECS J. Solid State Sci. Technol. 9 (2020) 093013. doi:10.1149/2162-8777/abbb6f.

[32] J. Phiri, P. Gane, T.C. Maloney, General overview of graphene: Production, properties and application in polymer composites, Mater. Sci. Eng. B. 215 (2017) 9–28. doi:10.1016/j.mseb.2016.10.004.

[33] X. Zhang, B.R.S. Rajaraman, H. Liu, S. Ramakrishna, Graphene's potential in materials science and engineering, RSC Adv. 4 (2014) 28987–29011. doi:10.1039/c4ra02817a.

[34] C.-Y. Su, A.-Y. Lu, Y. Xu, F.-R. Chen, A.N. Khlobystov, L.-J. Li, High-quality thin graphene films from fast electrochemical exfoliation, ACS Nano. 5 (2011) 2332–2339. doi:10.1021/nn200025p.

[35] A. Öztürk, M. Alanyalıoğlu, Electrochemical fabrication and amperometric sensor application of graphene sheets, Superlattices Microstruct. 95 (2016) 56–64. doi:10.1016/j.spmi.2016.04.039.

[36] J. Liu, H. Yang, S.G. Zhen, C.K. Poh, A. Chaurasia, J. Luo, X. Wu, E.K.L. Yeow, N.G. Sahoo, J. Lin, Z. Shen, A green approach to the synthesis of high-quality graphene oxide flakes via electrochemical exfoliation of pencil core, RSC Adv. 3 (2013) 11745–11750. doi:10.1039/c3ra41366g.

[37] K. Parvez, R. Li, S.R. Puniredd, Y. Hernandez, F. Hinkel, S. Wang, X. Feng, K. Müllen, Electrochemically exfoliated graphene as solution-processable, highly conductive electrodes for organic electronics, ACS Nano. 7 (2013) 3598–3606. doi:10.1021/nn400576v.

[38] S. Yang, M.R. Lohe, K. Müllen, X. Feng, New-generation graphene from electrochemical approaches: Production and applications, Adv. Mater. 28 (2016) 6213–6221. doi:10.1002/adma.201505326.

[39] K. Parvez, Z.S. Wu, R. Li, X. Liu, R. Graf, X. Feng, K. Müllen, Exfoliation of graphite into graphene in aqueous solutions of inorganic salts, J. Am. Chem. Soc. 136 (2014) 6083–6091. doi:10.1021/ja5017156.

[40] S. Barcikowski, G. Compagnini, Advanced nanoparticle generation and excitation by lasers in liquids, Phys. Chem. Chem. Phys. 15 (2013) 3022–3026. doi:10.1039/C2CP90132C.

[41] M. Dell'Aglio, R. Gaudiuso, O. De Pascale, A. De Giacomo, Mechanisms and processes of pulsed laser ablation in liquids during nanoparticle production, Appl. Surf. Sci. 348 (2015) 4–9. doi:10.1016/j.apsusc.2015.01.082.

[42] E. Cappelli, S. Orlando, M. Servidori, C. Scilletta, Nano-graphene structures deposited by N-IR pulsed laser ablation of graphite on Si, Appl. Surf. Sci. 254 (2007) 1273–1278. doi:10.1016/j.apsusc.2007.09.098.

[43] F. Kazemizadeh, R. Malekfar, One step synthesis of porous graphene by laser abla-
     tion: A new and facile approach, Phys. B Condens. Matter. 530 (2018) 236–241.
     doi:10.1016/j.physb.2017.11.052.

[44] G.K. Hemani, W.G. Vandenberghe, B. Brennan, Y.J. Chabal, A.V. Walker, R.M. Wallace,
     M. Quevedo-Lopez, M.V. Fischetti, Interfacial graphene growth in the Ni/SiO2 system
     using pulsed laser deposition, Appl. Phys. Lett. 103 (2013). doi:10.1063/1.4821944.

[45] A.T.T. Koh, Y.M. Foong, D.H.C. Chua, Comparison of the mechanism of low defect
     few-layer graphene fabricated on different metals by pulsed laser deposition, Diam.
     Relat. Mater. 25 (2012) 98–102. doi:10.1016/j.diamond.2012.02.014.

[46] K. Wang, Laser based fabrication of graphene, Adv. Graphene Sci. 5772 (2013) 55821.

[47] E.M. Pechlivani, D. Papas, E. Mekeridis, A. Laskarakis, G. Nomikos, S. Logothetidis,
     Ultra-short pulse laser for patterning high quality graphene electrodes, Mater. Today
     Proc. 4 (2017) 5074–5081. doi:10.1016/j.matpr.2017.04.116.

[48] A. De Bonis, M. Curcio, A. Santagata, J.V. Rau, A. Galasso, R. Teghil, Fullerene-
     reduced graphene oxide composites obtained by ultrashort laser ablation of fullerite in
     water, Appl. Surf. Sci. 336 (2015) 67–72. doi:10.1016/j.apsusc.2014.09.141.

[49] D.A.C. Brownson, C.E. Banks, The electrochemistry of CVD graphene: Progress and
     prospects, Phys. Chem. Chem. Phys. 14 (2012) 8264–8281. doi:10.1039/c2cp40225d.

[50] D.A.C. Brownson, C.E. Banks, CVD graphene electrochemistry: The role of graphitic
     islands, Phys. Chem. Chem. Phys. 13 (2011) 15825–15828. doi:10.1039/c1cp21978b.

[51] L. Cheng, K. Yun, A. Lucero, J. Huang, X. Meng, G. Lian, H.S. Nam, R.M. Wallace,
     M. Kim, A. Venugopal, L. Colombo, J. Kim, Low temperature synthesis of graphite on
     Ni films using inductively coupled plasma enhanced CVD, J. Mater. Chem. C. 3 (2015)
     5192–5198. doi:10.1039/c5tc00635j.

[52] M. Li, D. Liu, D. Wei, X. Song, D. Wei, A.T.S. Wee, Controllable synthesis of graphene
     by plasma-enhanced chemical vapor deposition and its related applications, Adv. Sci. 3
     (2016) 1–23. doi:10.1002/advs.201600003.

[53] N. Woehrl, O. Ochedowski, S. Gottlieb, K. Shibasaki, S. Schulz, Plasma-enhanced
     chemical vapor deposition of graphene on copper substrates, AIP Adv. 4 (2014).
     doi:10.1063/1.4873157.

[54] Y. Okigawa, R. Kato, T. Yamada, M. Ishihara, M. Hasegawa, Electrical properties and
     domain sizes of graphene films synthesized by microwave plasma treatment under a low
     carbon concentration, Carbon N. Y. 82 (2015) 60–66. doi:10.1016/j.carbon.2014.10.029.

[55] S. Xu, L. Zhang, B. Wang, R.S. Ruoff, Chemical vapor deposition of graphene on thin-
     metal films, Cell Rep. Phys. Sci. 2 (2021) 100372. doi:10.1016/j.xcrp.2021.100372.

[56] T. Mahmoudi, Y. Wang, Y.-B. Hahn, Graphene and its derivatives for solar cells applica-
     tion, Nano Energy. 47 (2018) 51–65. doi:10.1016/j.nanoen.2018.02.047.

[57] W. Yang, G. Chen, Z. Shi, C.-C. Liu, L. Zhang, G. Xie, M. Cheng, D. Wang, R. Yang,
     D. Shi, K. Watanabe, T. Taniguchi, Y. Yao, Y. Zhang, G. Zhang, Epitaxial growth of
     single-domain graphene on hexagonal boron nitride, Nat. Mater. 12 (2013) 792–797.
     doi:10.1038/nmat3695.

[58] R. Papon, C. Pierlot, S. Sharma, S.M. Shinde, G. Kalita, M. Tanemura, Optimization
     of CVD parameters for graphene synthesis through design of experiments, Phys. Status
     Solidi. 254 (2017) 1600629.

[59] H. Liu, Y. Liu, Controlled chemical synthesis in CVD graphene, Phys. Sci. Rev. 2 (2017)
     1–28. doi:10.1515/psr-2016-0107.

[60] S.S. Shams, L.S. Zhang, R. Hu, R. Zhang, J. Zhu, Synthesis of graphene from bio-
     mass: A green chemistry approach, Mater. Lett. 161 (2015) 476–479. doi:10.1016/
     j.matlet.2015.09.022.

[61] Z.-Y. Juang, C.-Y. Wu, C.-W. Lo, W.-Y. Chen, C.-F. Huang, J.-C. Hwang, F.-R. Chen,
     K.-C. Leou, C.-H. Tsai, Synthesis of graphene on silicon carbide substrates at low tem-
     perature, Carbon N. Y. 47 (2009) 2026–2031. doi:10.1016/j.carbon.2009.03.051.

[62] Y. Pan, H.G. Zhang, D.X. Shi, J.T. Sun, S.X. Du, F. Liu, H.J. Gao, Highly ordered, millimeter-scale, continuous, single-crystalline graphene monolayer formed on Ru (0001), Adv. Mater. 21 (2009) 2739. https://www.cheric.org/research/tech/periodicals/view.php?seq=754494.

[63] M. Aliofkhazraei, N. Ali, W.I. Milne, C.S. Ozkan, S. Mitura, J.L. Gervasoni, Graphene Science Handbook: Fabrication Methods, CRC Press, Boca Raton (2016).

[64] R. Singh, V.S.K. Yadav, M.K. Purkait, Cu2O photocatalyst modified antifouling polysulfone mixed matrix membrane for ultrafiltration of protein and visible light driven photocatalytic pharmaceutical removal, Sep. Purif. Technol. 212 (2019) 191–204. doi:10.1016/j.seppur.2018.11.029.

[65] S. Kim, Y. Song, T. Takahashi, T. Oh, M.J. Heller, An aqueous single reactor arc discharge process for the synthesis of graphene nanospheres, Small. 11 (2015) 5041–5046. doi:10.1002/smll.201501022.

[66] Y. Wu, B. Wang, Y. Ma, Y. Huang, N. Li, F. Zhang, Y. Chen, Efficient and large-scale synthesis of few-layered graphene using an arc-discharge method and conductivity studies of the resulting films, Nano Res. 3 (2010) 661–669. doi:10.1007/s12274-010-0027-3.

[67] S. Kim, Y. Song, J. Wright, M.J. Heller, Graphene bi- and trilayers produced by a novel aqueous arc discharge process, Carbon N. Y. 102 (2016) 339–345. doi:10.1016/j.carbon.2016.02.049.

[68] G.W. Cheng, K. Chu, J.S. Chen, J.T.H. Tsai, Fabrication of graphene from graphite by a thermal assisted vacuum arc discharge system, Superlattices Microstruct. 104 (2017) 258–265. doi:10.1016/j.spmi.2017.02.040.

[69] X. Wu, Y. Liu, H. Yang, Z. Shi, Large-scale synthesis of high-quality graphene sheets by an improved alternating current arc-discharge method, RSC Adv. 6 (2016) 93119–93124. doi:10.1039/c6ra22273k.

[70] T. Ohta, A. Bostwick, T. Seyller, K. Horn, E. Rotenberg, Controlling the electronic structure of bilayer graphene, Sci. 313 (2006) 951–954. doi:10.1126/science.1130681.

[71] Q.H. Wang, M.C. Hersam, Room-temperature molecular-resolution characterization of self-assembled organic monolayers on epitaxial graphene, Nat. Chem. 1 (2009) 206–211. doi:10.1038/nchem.212.

[72] S.K. Min, W.Y. Kim, Y. Cho, K.S. Kim, Fast DNA sequencing with a graphene-based nanochannel device, Nat. Nanotechnol. 6 (2011) 162–165. doi:10.1038/nnano.2010.283.

[73] Y. Wang, Z. Li, J. Wang, J. Li, Y. Lin, Graphene and graphene oxide: Biofunctionalization and applications in biotechnology, Trends Biotechnol. 29 (2011) 205–212. doi:10.1016/j.tibtech.2011.01.008.

[74] V. Georgakilas, Covalent attachment of organic functional groups on pristine graphene, Funct. Graphene. (2014) 21–58. doi:10.1002/9783527672790.ch2.

[75] X. Zhang, W.R. Browne, B.L. Feringa, Preparation of dispersible graphene through organic functionalization of graphene using a zwitterion intermediate cycloaddition approach, RSC Adv. 2 (2012) 12173. doi:10.1039/c2ra22440b.

[76] X. Xu, Q. Luo, W. Lv, Y. Dong, Y. Lin, Q. Yang, A. Shen, D. Pang, J. Hu, J. Qin, Z. Li, Functionalization of graphene sheets by polyacetylene: Convenient synthesis and enhanced emission, Macromol. Chem. Phys. 212 (2011) 768–773. doi:10.1002/macp.201000608.

[77] H. He, C. Gao, General approach to individually dispersed, highly soluble, and conductive graphene nanosheets functionalized by nitrene chemistry, Chem. Mater. 22 (2010) 5054–5064. doi:10.1021/cm101634k.

[78] S. Vadukumpully, J. Gupta, Y. Zhang, G.Q. Xu, S. Valiyaveettil, Functionalization of surfactant wrapped graphene nanosheets with alkylazides for enhanced dispersibility, Nanoscale. 3 (2011) 303–308. doi:10.1039/C0NR00547A.

[79] T.A. Strom, E.P. Dillon, C.E. Hamilton, A.R. Barron, Nitrene addition to exfoliated graphene: A one-step route to highly functionalized graphene, Chem. Commun. 46 (2010) 4097. doi:10.1039/c001488e.

[80] H. Ismaili, D. Geng, A.X. Sun, T.T. Kantzas, M.S. Workentin, Light-activated covalent formation of gold nanoparticle–graphene and gold nanoparticle–glass composites, Langmuir. 27 (2011) 13261–13268. doi:10.1021/la202815g.

[81] X. Zhong, J. Jin, S. Li, Z. Niu, W. Hu, R. Li, J. Ma, Aryne cycloaddition: Highly efficient chemical modification of graphene, Chem. Commun. 46 (2010) 7340. doi:10.1039/c0cc02389b.

[82] A. Sinitskii, A. Dimiev, D.A. Corley, A.A. Fursina, D. V Kosynkin, J.M. Tour, Kinetics of diazonium functionalization of chemically converted graphene nanoribbons, ACS Nano. 4 (2010) 1949–1954. doi:10.1021/nn901899j.

[83] S. Niyogi, E. Bekyarova, M.E. Itkis, H. Zhang, K. Shepperd, J. Hicks, M. Sprinkle, C. Berger, C.N. Lau, W.A. deHeer, E.H. Conrad, R.C. Haddon, Spectroscopy of covalently functionalized graphene, Nano Lett. 10 (2010) 4061–4066. doi:10.1021/nl1021128.

[84] J.R. Lomeda, C.D. Doyle, D.V. Kosynkin, W.-F. Hwang, J.M. Tour, Diazonium functionalization of surfactant-wrapped chemically converted graphene sheets, J. Am. Chem. Soc. 130 (2008) 16201–16206. doi:10.1021/ja806499w.

[85] E. Bekyarova, M.E. Itkis, P. Ramesh, C. Berger, M. Sprinkle, W.A. de Heer, R.C. Haddon, Chemical modification of epitaxial graphene: Spontaneous grafting of aryl groups, J. Am. Chem. Soc. 131 (2009) 1336–1337. doi:10.1021/ja8057327.

[86] R. Sharma, J.H. Baik, C.J. Perera, M.S. Strano, Anomalously large reactivity of single graphene layers and edges toward electron transfer chemistries, Nano Lett. 10 (2010) 398–405. doi:10.1021/nl902741x.

[87] Z. Sun, S. Kohama, Z. Zhang, J.R. Lomeda, J.M. Tour, Soluble graphene through edge-selective functionalization, Nano Res. 3 (2010) 117–125. doi:10.1007/s12274-010-1016-2.

[88] J. Shen, Y. Hu, C. Li, C. Qin, M. Ye, Synthesis of amphiphilic graphene nanoplatelets, Small. 5 (2009) 82–85. doi:10.1002/smll.200800988.

[89] V. Chandra, J. Park, Y. Chun, J.W. Lee, I.-C. Hwang, K.S. Kim, Water-dispersible magnetite-reduced graphene oxide composites for arsenic removal, ACS Nano. 4 (2010) 3979–3986. doi:10.1021/nn1008897.

[90] Y. Chun, N. Jiten Singh, I.-C. Hwang, J. Woo Lee, S.U. Yu, K.S. Kim, Calix[n]imidazolium as a new class of positively charged homo-calix compounds, Nat. Commun. 4 (2013) 1797. doi:10.1038/ncomms2758.

[91] S.D. Chakarova-Käck, E. Schröder, B.I. Lundqvist, D.C. Langreth, Application of van der Waals density functional to an extended system: Adsorption of benzene and naphthalene on graphite, Phys. Rev. Lett. 96 (2006) 146107. doi:10.1103/PhysRevLett.96.146107.

[92] Y. Cho, S.K. Min, J. Yun, W.Y. Kim, A. Tkatchenko, K.S. Kim, Noncovalent interactions of DNA bases with naphthalene and graphene, J. Chem. Theory Comput. 9 (2013) 2090–2096. doi:10.1021/ct301097u.

[93] J. Malig, C. Romero-Nieto, N. Jux, D.M. Guldi, Graphene: Integrating water-soluble graphene into porphyrin nanohybrids, Adv. Mater. 24 (2012) 799. doi:10.1002/adma.201290023.

[94] V.K. Kodali, J. Scrimgeour, S. Kim, J.H. Hankinson, K.M. Carroll, W.A. de Heer, C. Berger, J.E. Curtis, Nonperturbative chemical modification of graphene for protein micropatterning, Langmuir. 27 (2011) 863–865. doi:10.1021/la1033178.

[95] A. Ghosh, K.V. Rao, S.J. George, C.N.R. Rao, Noncovalent functionalization, exfoliation, and solubilization of graphene in water by employing a fluorescent coronene carboxylate, Chem. A Eur. J. 16 (2010) 2700–2704. doi:10.1002/chem.200902828.

[96] Q. Su, S. Pang, V. Alijani, C. Li, X. Feng, K. Müllen, Composites of graphene with large aromatic molecules, Adv. Mater. 21 (2009) 3191–3195. doi:10.1002/adma.200803808.

[97] H.-C. Cheng, R.-J. Shiue, C.-C. Tsai, W.-H. Wang, Y.-T. Chen, High-quality graphene p–n junctions via resist-free fabrication and solution-based noncovalent functionalization, ACS Nano. 5 (2011) 2051–2059. doi:10.1021/nn103221v.

[98] M. Sharma, P. Mondal, A.D. Sontakke, A. Chakraborty, M.K. Purkait, High performance graphene-oxide doped cellulose acetate based ion exchange membrane for environmental remediation applications, Int. J. Environ. Anal. Chem. (2021) 1–22. doi:10.1080/03 067319.2021.1975276.

[99] D. Parviz, S. Das, H.S.T. Ahmed, F. Irin, S. Bhattacharia, M.J. Green, Dispersions of non-covalently functionalized graphene with minimal stabilizer, ACS Nano. 6 (2012) 8857–8867. doi:10.1021/nn302784m.

[100] C.B. K. C., S.K. Das, K. Ohkubo, S. Fukuzumi, F. D'Souza, Ultrafast charge separation in supramolecular tetrapyrrole–graphene hybrids, Chem. Commun. 48 (2012) 11859. doi:10.1039/c2cc36262g.

[101] W. Zhang, Z. Guo, D. Huang, Z. Liu, X. Guo, H. Zhong, Synergistic effect of chemo-photothermal therapy using PEGylated graphene oxide, Biomaterials. 32 (2011) 8555–8561. doi:10.1016/j.biomaterials.2011.07.071.

[102] Y. Guo, L. Deng, J. Li, S. Guo, E. Wang, S. Dong, Hemin–graphene hybrid nanosheets with intrinsic peroxidase-like activity for label-free colorimetric detection of single-nucleotide polymorphism, ACS Nano. 5 (2011) 1282–1290. doi:10.1021/nn1029586.

[103] L. Wu, L. Feng, J. Ren, X. Qu, Electrochemical detection of dopamine using porphyrin-functionalized graphene, Biosens. Bioelectron. 34 (2012) 57–62. doi:10.1016/ j.bios.2012.01.007.

[104] H. Zhang, Y. Han, Y. Guo, C. Dong, Porphyrin functionalized graphene nanosheets-based electrochemical aptasensor for label-free ATP detection, J. Mater. Chem. 22 (2012) 23900. doi:10.1039/c2jm35379b.

[105] H. Bai, Y. Xu, L. Zhao, C. Li, G. Shi, Non-covalent functionalization of graphene sheets by sulfonated polyaniline, Chem. Commun. (2009) 1667. doi:10.1039/b821805f.

[106] H. Wu, W. Zhao, H. Hu, G. Chen, One-step in situball milling synthesis of polymer-functionalized graphene nanocomposites, J. Mater. Chem. 21 (2011) 8626–8632. doi:10.1039/C1JM10819K.

[107] G.Y. Kim, M.C. Choi, D. Lee, C.S. Ha, 2D-aligned graphene sheets in transparent polyimide/graphene nanocomposite films based on noncovalent interactions between poly(amic acid) and graphene carboxylic acid, Macromol. Mater. Eng. 297 (2012) 303–311. doi:10.1002/mame.201100211.

[108] M. Fang, J. Long, W. Zhao, L. Wang, G. Chen, pH-responsive chitosan-mediated graphene dispersions, Langmuir. 26 (2010) 16771–16774. doi:10.1021/la102703b.

[109] J. Liu, S. Guo, L. Han, W. Ren, Y. Liu, E. Wang, Multiple pH-responsive graphene composites by non-covalent modification with chitosan, Talanta. 101 (2012) 151–156. doi:10.1016/j.talanta.2012.09.013.

[110] Q. Yang, X. Pan, F. Huang, K. Li, Fabrication of high-concentration and stable aqueous suspensions of graphene nanosheets by noncovalent functionalization with lignin and cellulose derivatives, J. Phys. Chem. C. 114 (2010) 3811–3816. doi:10.1021/ jp910232x.

[111] S. Matsumura, A.R. Hlil, C. Lepiller, J. Gaudet, D. Guay, Z. Shi, S. Holdcroft, A.S. Hay, Stability and utility of pyridyl disulfide functionality in RAFT and conventional radical polymerizations, J. Polym. Sci. Part A Polym. Chem. 46 (2008) 7207–7224. doi:10.1002/pola.

[112] S. Park, N. Mohanty, J.W. Suk, A. Nagaraja, J. An, R.D. Piner, W. Cai, D.R. Dreyer, V. Berry, R.S. Ruoff, Biocompatible, robust free-standing paper composed of a TWEEN/graphene composite, Adv. Mater. 22 (2010) 1736–1740. doi:10.1002/adma. 200903611.

[113] T. Kim, H. Lee, J. Kim, K.S. Suh, Synthesis of phase transferable graphene sheets using ionic liquid polymers, ACS Nano. 4 (2010) 1612–1618. doi:10.1021/nn901525e.

[114] J. Liu, Y. Li, Y. Li, J. Li, Z. Deng, Noncovalent DNA decorations of graphene oxide and reduced graphene oxide toward water-soluble metal–carbon hybrid nanostructures via self-assembly, J. Mater. Chem. 20 (2010) 900–906. doi:10.1039/B917752C.

[115] Y. Xu, Q. Wu, Y. Sun, H. Bai, G. Shi, Three-dimensional self-assembly of graphene oxide and DNA into multifunctional hydrogels, ACS Nano. 4 (2010) 7358–7362. doi:10.1021/nn1027104.

[116] J.N. Tiwari, K. Nath, S. Kumar, R.N. Tiwari, K.C. Kemp, N.H. Le, D.H. Youn, J.S. Lee, K.S. Kim, Stable platinum nanoclusters on genomic DNA–graphene oxide with a high oxygen reduction reaction activity, Nat. Commun. 4 (2013) 2221. doi:10.1038/ncomms3221.

[117] F. Lu, S. Zhang, H. Gao, H. Jia, L. Zheng, Protein-decorated reduced oxide graphene composite and its application to SERS, ACS Appl. Mater. Interfaces. 4 (2012) 3278–3284. doi:10.1021/am300634n.

[118] Y. Wang, P. Zhang, C. Fang Liu, L. Zhan, Y. Fang Li, C.Z. Huang, Green and easy synthesis of biocompatible graphene for use as an anticoagulant, RSC Adv. 2 (2012) 2322. doi:10.1039/c2ra00841f.

[119] S. Hashemzadeh, Y. Omidi, H. Rafii-Tabar, Amperometric lactate nanobiosensor based on reduced graphene oxide, carbon nanotube and gold nanoparticle nanocomposite, Microchim. Acta. 186 (2019) 680. doi:10.1007/s00604-019-3791-0.

[120] Y. Chen, H. Chen, J. Shi, Inorganic nanoparticle-based drug codelivery nanosystems to overcome the multidrug resistance of cancer cells, Mol. Pharm. 11 (2014) 2495–2510. doi:10.1021/mp400596v.

[121] N. Bertrand, J. Wu, X. Xu, N. Kamaly, O.C. Farokhzad, Cancer nanotechnology: The impact of passive and active targeting in the era of modern cancer biology, Adv. Drug Deliv. Rev. 66 (2014) 2–25. doi:10.1016/j.addr.2013.11.009.

[122] S. Mura, J. Nicolas, P. Couvreur, Stimuli-responsive nanocarriers for drug delivery, Nat. Mater. 12 (2013) 991–1003. doi:10.1038/nmat3776.

[123] H. Shen, L. Zhang, M. Liu, Z. Zhang, Biomedical applications of graphene, Theranostics. 2 (2012) 283–294. doi:10.7150/thno.3642.

[124] S.R. Shin, Y.C. Li, H.L. Jang, P. Khoshakhlagh, M. Akbari, A. Nasajpour, Y.S. Zhang, A. Tamayol, A. Khademhosseini, Graphene-based materials for tissue engineering, Adv. Drug Deliv. Rev. 105 (2016) 255–274. doi:10.1016/j.addr.2016.03.007.

[125] R. Imani, F. Mohabatpour, F. Mostafavi, Graphene-based nano-carrier modifications for gene delivery applications, Carbon N. Y. 140 (2018) 569–591. doi:10.1016/j.carbon.2018.09.019.

[126] K.P. Loh, Q. Bao, P.K. Ang, J. Yang, The chemistry of graphene, J. Mater. Chem. 20 (2010) 2277–2289. doi:10.1039/B920539J.

[127] J. Liu, L. Cui, D. Losic, Graphene and graphene oxide as new nanocarriers for drug delivery applications, Acta Biomater. 9 (2013) 9243–9257. doi:10.1016/j.actbio.2013.08.016.

[128] Y. Pan, N.G. Sahoo, L. Li, The application of graphene oxide in drug delivery, Expert Opin. Drug Deliv. 9 (2012) 1365–1376. doi:10.1517/17425247.2012.729575.

[129] L. Feng, S. Zhang, Z. Liu, Graphene based gene transfection, Nanoscale. 3 (2011) 1252–1257. doi:10.1039/C0NR00680G.

[130] K. Vinothini, N.K. Rajendran, A. Ramu, N. Elumalai, M. Rajan, Folate receptor targeted delivery of paclitaxel to breast cancer cells via folic acid conjugated graphene oxide grafted methyl acrylate nanocarrier, Biomed. Pharmacother. 110 (2019) 906–917. doi:10.1016/j.biopha.2018.12.008.

[131] A. Deb, R. Vimala, Natural and synthetic polymer for graphene oxide mediated anticancer drug delivery—a comparative study, Int. J. Biol. Macromol. 107 (2018) 2320–2333. doi:10.1016/j.ijbiomac.2017.10.119.

[132] A.D. Sontakke, A. Bhattacharjee, R. Fopase, L.M. Pandey, M.K. Purkait, One-pot, sustainable and room temperature synthesis of graphene oxide-impregnated iron-based metal-organic framework (GO/MIL-100(Fe)) nanocarriers for anticancer drug delivery systems, J. Mater. Sci. (2022). doi:10.1007/s10853-022-07773-w.

[133] H. Vovusha, D. Banerjee, M.K. Yadav, F. Perrozzi, L. Ottaviano, S. Sanyal, B. San-yal, Binding characteristics of anticancer drug doxorubicin with two-dimensional graphene and graphene oxide: Insights from density functional theory calculations and fluorescence spectroscopy, J. Phys. Chem. C. 122 (2018). doi:10.1021/acs.jpcc.8b04496.

[134] K. Priyadarshini, A.U. Keerthi, Paclitaxel against cancer: A short review, Med. Chem. (Los. Angeles). 2 (2012). doi:10.4172/2161-0444.1000130.

[135] D. Dorniani, B. Saifullah, F. Barahuie, P. Arulselvan, M.Z. Bin Hussein, S. Fakurazi, L.J. Twyman, Graphene oxide-gallic acid nanodelivery system for cancer therapy, Nanoscale Res. Lett. 11 (2016). doi:10.1186/s11671-016-1712-2.

[136] S. Tiwari, A.D. Sontakke, K. Baruah, M.K. Purkait, Development of graphene oxide-based nano-delivery system for natural chemotherapeutic agent (Caffeic Acid), Mater. Today Proc. (2022). doi:10.1016/j.matpr.2022.11.373.

[137] F. Barahuie, B. Saifullah, D. Dorniani, S. Fakurazi, G. Karthivashan, M.Z. Hussein, F.M. Elfghi, Graphene oxide as a nanocarrier for controlled release and targeted deliv-ery of an anticancer active agent, chlorogenic acid, Mater. Sci. Eng. C. 74 (2017) 177–185. doi:10.1016/j.msec.2016.11.114.

[138] E. Quagliarini, R. Di Santo, D. Pozzi, P. Tentori, F. Cardarelli, G. Caracciolo, Mech-anistic insights into the release of doxorubicin from graphene oxide in cancer cells, Nanomat. 10 (2020). doi:10.3390/nano10081482.

[139] W. Guo, Z. Chen, X. Feng, G. Shen, H. Huang, Y. Liang, B. Zhao, G. Li, Y. Hu, Graphene oxide (GO)-based nanosheets with combined chemo/photothermal/photodynamic ther-apy to overcome gastric cancer (GC) paclitaxel resistance by reducing mitochondria-derived adenosine-triphosphate (ATP), J. Nanobiotechnol 19 (2021) 146. doi:10.1186/s12951-021-00874-9.

[140] R. Gu, M. Zhang, H. Meng, D. Xu, Y. Xie, Gallic acid targets acute myeloid leukemia via Akt/mTOR-dependent mitochondrial respiration inhibition, Biomed. Pharmacother. 105 (2018) 491–497. doi:10.1016/j.biopha.2018.05.158.

[141] T. Zhang, L. Ma, P. Wu, W. Li, T. Li, R. Gu, X. Dan, Z. Li, X. Fan, Z. Xiao, Gallic acid has anticancer activity and enhances the anticancer effects of cisplatin in non-small cell lung cancer A549 cells via the JAK/STAT3 signaling pathway, Oncol. Rep. 41 (2019). doi:10.3892/or.2019.6976.

[142] A.D. Sontakke, R. Fopase, L.M. Pandey, M.K. Purkait, Development of graphene oxide nanoscrolls imparted nano-delivery system for the sustained release of gallic acid, Appl. Nanosci. (2022). doi:10.1007/s13204-022-02582-8.

[143] M. Hoseini-Ghahfarokhi, S. Mirkiani, N. Mozaffari, M.A. Abdolahi Sadatlu, A. Ghasemi, S. Abbaspour, M. Akbarian, F. Farjadain, M. Karimi, Applications of graphene and graphene oxide in smart drug/gene delivery: Is the world still flat? Int. J. Nanomed. 15 (2020) 9469–9496. doi:10.2147/IJN.S265876.

[144] A. Shah, S. Aftab, J. Nisar, M.N. Ashiq, F.J. Iftikhar, Nanocarriers for targeted drug delivery, J. Drug Deliv. Sci. Technol. 62 (2021). doi:10.1016/j.jddst.2021.102426.

[145] Y.T. Fong, C.H. Chen, J.P. Chen, Intratumoral delivery of doxorubicin on folate-conjugated graphene oxide by in-situ forming thermo-sensitive hydrogel for breast can-cer therapy, Nanomater. 7 (2017) 1–24. doi:10.3390/nano7110388.

[146] A. Pourjavadi, S. Asgari, S.H. Hosseini, Graphene oxide functionalized with oxygen-rich polymers as a pH-sensitive carrier for co-delivery of hydrophobic and hydrophilic drugs, J. Drug Deliv. Sci. Technol. 56 (2020) 101542. doi:10.1016/j.jddst.2020.101542.

[147] T. Zhou, X. Zhou, D. Xing, Controlled release of doxorubicin from graphene oxide based charge-reversal nanocarrier, Biomaterials. 35 (2014) 4185–4194. doi:10.1016/j.biomaterials.2014.01.044.

[148] C.L. Weaver, J.M. LaRosa, X. Luo, X.T. Cui, Electrically controlled drug delivery from graphene oxide nanocomposite films, ACS Nano. 8 (2014) 1834–1843. doi:10.1021/nn406223e.

[149] J. Wang, J. Fang, P. Fang, X. Li, S. Wu, W. Zhang, S. Li, Preparation of hollow core/shell Fe3O4 @graphene oxide composites as magnetic targeting drug nanocarriers, J. Biomater. Sci. Polym. Ed. 28 (2017) 337–349. doi:10.1080/09205063.2016.1268463.

[150] J. Liang, B. Chen, J. Hu, Q. Huang, D. Zhang, J. Wan, Z. Hu, B. Wang, pH and thermal dual-responsive graphene oxide nanocomplexes for targeted drug delivery and photothermal-chemo/photodynamic synergetic therapy, ACS Appl. Bio Mater. 2 (2019) 5859–5871. doi:10.1021/acsabm.9b00835.

[151] R. Imani, S. Prakash, H. Vali, J.F. Presley, S. Faghihi, Microencapsulated multifunctionalized graphene oxide equipped with chloroquine for efficient and sustained siRNA delivery, Biomed Res. Int. 2022 (2022) 1–16. doi:10.1155/2022/5866361.

[152] M.K. Laufer, P.C. Thesing, N.D. Eddington, R. Masonga, F.K. Dzinjalamala, S.L. Takala, T.E. Taylor, C. V. Plowe, Return of chloroquine antimalarial efficacy in Malawi, N. Engl. J. Med. 355 (2006) 1959–1966. doi:10.1056/NEJMoa062032.

[153] W. Chen, S. Li, Y. Shen, Y. Cai, J. Jin, Z. Yang, Polyethylenimine modified graphene oxide for effective chemo-gene-photothermal triples therapy of triple-negative breast cancer and inhibits metastasis, J. Drug Deliv. Sci. Technol. 74 (2022) 103521. doi:10.1016/j.jddst.2022.103521.

[154] N.S. Wind, I. Holen, Multidrug resistance in breast cancer: from in vitro models to clinical studies, Int. J. Breast Cancer. 2011 (2011) 1–12. doi:10.4061/2011/967419.

[155] Z. Xie, X. Zeng, DNA/RNA-based formulations for treatment of breast cancer, Expert Opin. Drug Deliv. 14 (2017) 1379–1393. doi:10.1080/17425247.2017.1317744.

[156] E. Keles, Y. Song, D. Du, W.J. Dong, Y. Lin, Recent progress in nanomaterials for gene delivery applications, Biomater. Sci. 4 (2016) 1291–1309. doi:10.1039/c6bm00441e.

[157] H. Dong, W. Dai, H. Ju, H. Lu, S. Wang, L. Xu, S.-F. Zhou, Y. Zhang, X. Zhang, Multifunctional poly(l-lactide)–polyethylene glycol-grafted graphene quantum dots for intracellular MicroRNA imaging and combined specific-gene-targeting agents delivery for improved therapeutics, ACS Appl. Mater. Interfaces. 7 (2015) 11015–11023. doi:10.1021/acsami.5b02803.

[158] Y. Zeng, Z. Yang, H. Li, Y. Hao, C. Liu, L. Zhu, J. Liu, B. Lu, R. Li, Multifunctional nanographene oxide for targeted gene-mediated thermochemotherapy of drug-resistant tumour, Sci. Rep. 7 (2017) 1–10. doi:10.1038/srep43506.

[159] A. Khademhosseini, J.P. Vacanti, R. Langer, Progress in tissue engineering, Sci. Am. 300 (2009) 64–71.

[160] A. Tamayol, M. Akbari, N. Annabi, A. Paul, A. Khademhosseini, D. Juncker, Fiber-based tissue engineering: Progress, challenges, and opportunities, Biotechnol. Adv. 31 (2013) 669–687. doi:10.1016/j.biotechadv.2012.11.007.

[161] M.P. Lutolf, J.A. Hubbell, Synthetic biomaterials as instructive extracellular microenvironments for morphogenesis in tissue engineering, Nat. Biotechnol. 23 (2005) 47–55. doi:10.1038/nbt1055.

[162] S.R. Shin, B. Aghaei-Ghareh-Bolagh, T.T. Dang, S.N. Topkaya, X. Gao, S.Y. Yang, S.M. Jung, J.H. Oh, M.R. Dokmeci, X. Tang, A. Khademhosseini, Cell-laden microengineered and mechanically tunable hybrid hydrogels of gelatin and graphene oxide, Adv. Mater. 25 (2013) 6385–6391. doi:10.1002/adma.201301082.

[163] C. Wang, J. Li, C. Amatore, Y. Chen, H. Jiang, X.-M. Wang, Gold Nanoclusters and graphene nanocomposites for drug delivery and imaging of cancer cells, Angew. Chemie Int. Ed. 50 (2011) 11644–11648. doi:10.1002/anie.201105573.

[164] C. Cha, S.R. Shin, X. Gao, N. Annabi, M.R. Dokmeci, X. Tang, A. Khademhosseini, Controlling mechanical properties of cell-laden hydrogels by covalent incorporation of graphene oxide, Small. 10 (2014) 514–523. doi:10.1002/smll.201302182.

[165] Z. Tang, H. Wu, J.R. Cort, G.W. Buchko, Y. Zhang, Y. Shao, I.A. Aksay, J. Liu, Y. Lin, Constraint of DNA on functionalized graphene improves its biostability and specificity, Small. 6 (2010) 1205–1209. doi:10.1002/smll.201000024.

[166] S. Goenka, V. Sant, S. Sant, Graphene-based nanomaterials for drug delivery and tissue engineering, J. Control. Release. 173 (2014) 75–88. doi:10.1016/j.jconrel.2013.10.017.

[167] N. Nayerossadat, P. Ali, T. Maedeh, Viral and nonviral delivery systems for gene delivery, Adv. Biomed. Res. 1 (2012) 27. doi:10.4103/2277-9175.98152.

[168] B. Chen, M. Liu, L. Zhang, J. Huang, J. Yao, Z. Zhang, Polyethylenimine-functionalized graphene oxide as an efficient gene delivery vector, J. Mater. Chem. 21 (2011) 7736–7741. doi:10.1039/c1jm10341e.

[169] S.D. Purohit, H. Singh, R. Bhaskar, I. Yadav, S. Bhushan, M.K. Gupta, A. Kumar, N.C. Mishra, Fabrication of graphene oxide and nanohydroxyapatite reinforced gelatin–alginate nanocomposite scaffold for bone tissue regeneration, Front. Mater. 7 (2020) 1–10. doi:10.3389/fmats.2020.00250.

[170] A. Sharma, S. Gupta, T.S. Sampathkumar, R.S. Verma, Modified graphene oxide nanoplates reinforced 3D printed multifunctional scaffold for bone tissue engineering, Biomater. Adv. 134 (2022) 112587. doi:10.1016/j.msec.2021.112587.

[171] S.B. Ryu, K.M. Park, K.D. Park, In situ graphene oxide-gelatin hydrogels with enhanced mechanical property for tissue adhesive and regeneration, Biochem. Biophys. Res. Commun. 592 (2022) 24–30. doi:10.1016/j.bbrc.2022.01.010.

[172] P. Dibajnia, C.M. Morshead, Role of neural precursor cells in promoting repair following stroke, Acta Pharmacol. Sin. 34 (2013) 78–90. doi:10.1038/aps.2012.107.

[173] S.Y. Park, J. Park, S.H. Sim, M.G. Sung, K.S. Kim, B.H. Hong, S. Hong, Enhanced differentiation of human neural stem cells into neurons on graphene, Adv. Mater. 23 (2011) 263–267. doi:10.1002/adma.201101503.

[174] G. Keller, H.R. Snodgrass, Human embryonic stem cells: The future is now, Nat. Med. 5 (1999) 151–152. doi:10.1038/5512.

[175] D. Yang, T. Li, M. Xu, F. Gao, J. Yang, Z. Yang, W. Le, Graphene oxide promotes the differentiation of mouse embryonic stem cells to dopamine neurons, Nanomedicine. 9 (2014) 2445–2455.

4 Drug Delivery with Graphene Oxide-Based Nanocarriers

4.1 AN OVERVIEW OF GO-BASED NANOCARRIERS

Carbon-based nanomaterials were extensively used in a variety of engineering fields owing to their large surface area and affordable production cost. Graphite, a member of the carbon allotropes, is a soft, elastic, and commonly accessible pure version of carbon. Each carbon atom in graphite is covalently bonded to three adjacent carbon atoms to produce the hexagonal layer. Graphene is designated as a single layer of carbon atoms of graphite. Graphene has been widely employed for supercapacitors [1,2], catalysis [3], hydrogen storage materials [2,4,5], battery electrodes [1], and biosensors [2] ever since its discovery because of its remarkable physicochemical characteristics, including electrical, thermal, optical, and mechanical characteristics. Precisely, the higher surface area and the optical properties of graphene nanomaterials have attracted great interest in biomedical applications such as biosensing and drugs and gene delivery [6,7]. However, the poor water solubility of graphene due to the π-π staking limits its utilization for biomedical applications. Fortunately, the oxidative and hydrophilic derivatives of hydrophobic graphene, such as graphene oxide (GO) and reduced graphene oxide(rGO), are enriched in epoxy, carboxyl, and hydroxyl functional entities, which provide them better stability and dispersibility in water [6].

Graphene, along with its derivative like graphene oxide, is currently being extensively researched, not only because of its fundamental physicochemical characteristics but also because of its agitating potential of applications in varied arenas of biomedical engineering such as drug delivery, biosensing, cancer therapeutics, and tissue engineering [8]. The modulation of defects in graphene-based nanomaterials is directly relevant to a variety of applications. In the family of graphene-derived materials, GO and rGO are considered generic nanomaterials [9–11]. The oxidation of graphene yields graphene oxide (GO), which has a variety of physicochemical characteristics. It is a 2D single atomic thick honeycomb-like structure that is indeed a hydrophilic derivative of graphene [12,13]. Other characteristics of GO, such as controllable shape and biocompatibility, make it suitable for biomedical applications [14–16]. It can be used for bioimaging and biosensing as it exhibits fluorescence in the visible and infrared regions of the EM spectrum and Raman signals in the D, G, and 2D regions [14]. As illustrated in **Figure 4.1** [17], the oxygenated functional entities are located at the trailing edge and basal planes of the GO nanosheets. In addition to the attributes listed previously, GO may be incorporated with polymers and other additives such as polyacrylic acid (PAA), polyethylene glycol (PEG), folic

 DOI: 10.1201/9781003358114-4

acid, and chitosan to improve their biocompatibility, loading capacity, targetability as well as structural properties.

Though the basic structure of rGO and GO are identical to that of graphene, they also encompass oxygen-enriched functional regions in lower and higher quantities, correspondingly [12,18]. The GO is made up of single-layer nanostructures that are loaded with oxygen-rich functional groups, offering it excellent hydrophilicity. For the preparation of GO, a conventional Hummers methodology and its variants are commonly implemented. The GO preparation method involves the use of strong acids and oxidants that incorporate oxygenated functional entities into the GO. Nonetheless, GO has been prepared using a variety of methodologies, the earliest of which was described by Brodie (1859) [19] and was pursued by Staudenmaier (1898) [20], Hummers (1958) [21], Tour (2010) [22], Sun (2013) [23] and Peng (2015) [24]. The reduced degree of oxidation, challenging reaction environments, harmful gases releases such as NO_2, N_2O_4, or ClO_2, the need for purification processes, and the high production cost are some of the drawbacks of these methods. Nonetheless, the Hummers approach and its modifications have alleviated many of the constraints to a certain degree. The specifics are presented in the succeeding section. The better water solubility of GO is attributed to the existence of hydroxyl, carboxyl, and epoxy functional groups; nonetheless, these are insufficient for biomedical applications without surface modifications. Importantly, these oxygen-containing functional units give a number of active sites for doping the elements or grafting additional functional entities to improve the surface characteristics of GO while retaining its fundamental features. [12,25]. In addition, the aqueous stability of GO is also a foremost issue for its application in drug delivery. GO has an aggregation tendency in

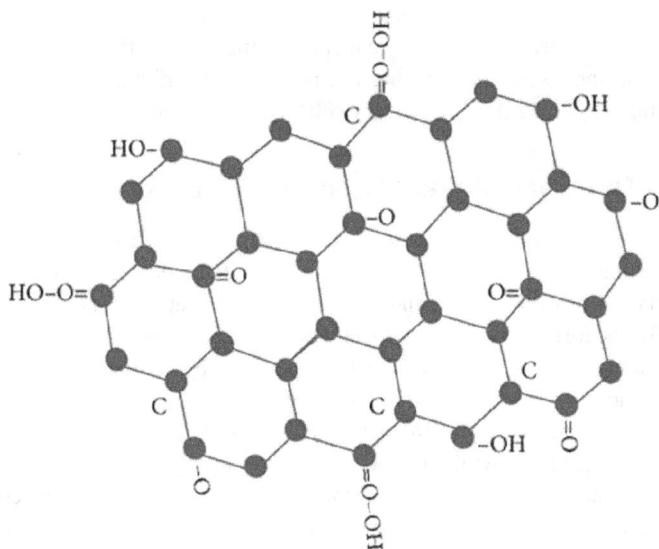

FIGURE 4.1 Chemical Structure of GO. [Replicated with permission from *Song et al. (2014)*] [17].

the physiological solutions with proteins and salt due to the nonspecific binding and electrostatic interactions, which produces a hindrance to the development of biological probes [26]. The precise functionalization of GO boosts its solubility under physiological circumstances and optimizes it for biological applications. In addition, its unrivaled properties, such as higher surface area, have made GO one of the most popular and extensively researched nanomaterials for environmental remediation and drug delivery-related applications [27–29]. Meanwhile, another graphene derivative, rGO, has been employed for diverse real-world applications, including drug delivery, and can be simply produced by reducing the oxygenated function groups of GO. The reduction mechanism can be accomplished using thermal and chemical processes, mostly for stimuli-responsive functionalization [8,30]. Previously, GO and rGO were extensively explored for energy, environmental, and drug delivery-related applications, including cancer therapeutics, neurodegenerative diseases, gene delivery, and tissue engineering [27,31–33].

The present chapter offers substantial evidence associated with the synthesis of pristine GO and rGO nanocarriers. It also debates their advantages, process features, and inadequacies besides their chronological developments. This chapter elucidates the significance, physicochemical properties, and benefits over the utilization of GO in drug delivery-related applications. Various covalent and non-covalent functionalization approaches are also explored critically in considering the inadequacies of GO in terms of aqueous stability and aggregation tendency, as well as biocompatibility for its application in the biomedical sector. Furthermore, the recent advances in the structural, functional, and morphological modifications of GO for enhancing its therapeutic efficacy in cancer and other infirmities therapy are described in detail. In addition, recommendations are made to minimize the shortcoming of GO-based nanocarriers for their synthesis functionalization and to improve the adaptability of GO in modern therapeutics. Ultimately, the outcomes of application-driven research on GO-based nanocarriers related to cancer treatment, gene therapy, neurodegenerative diseases, and tissue engineering are reviewed to offer exhaustive knowledge about its efficiency toward drug delivery-related applications.

4.2   PREPARATION OF GRAPHENE OXIDE (GO)

Since GO is indeed a quasi-molecule, it developed in a synthetic product. Graphite, the primary material, comprises many planes of hexagonal honeycomb-like structure. Exfoliation, on the other hand, can synthesize graphene as a single sheet of graphite. GO is formed when pristine graphene sheets are oxidized. As a result, GO is described as a graphene sheet or layer adorned by oxygenated functionalities. During the oxidation of graphite, the oxidizing agent such as $KMnO_4$ reacts with the carbon skeleton of graphite and further weakens the van der Waals force within the stacked sheets of graphite while increasing the interlayer spacings, subsequently [34].

The extent and the degree of oxidation firmly affect an elemental composition GO. The graphene sheets are completely exfoliated from graphite, hence depicting the absence (0 at. wt. %) of oxygen (O). Meanwhile, in the case of GO, the highest O content cannot exceed 50 at. wt.% as a result of sp^2 hybridization of the carbon atom. The atomic weight % of oxygen in the GO and hence its solubility is also dependent on the temperature conditions. GO with higher solubility in physiological conditions is generally recommended for biomedical applications [6,35]. GO was found to have an oxygen content of about 10 to 50 % atomic weight % when restricted at temperatures of around 50 to 70 °C, with higher solubility and lower reduction at 35–50 °C. Conversely, reduced graphene oxide (rGO) might be found to include up to 10% atomic weight of oxygen (O), which can be accomplished by thermal or chemical reduction processes [36]. The following section provides a comprehensive description of the processes for synthesizing GO and rGO.

4.2.1 Synthesis of Pristine GO

Typically, two processes, dry media and wet medium, are used to synthesize graphene oxide. During the dry media synthesis, graphene nanosheets are oxidized in a vacuum chamber with atomic oxygen. This method of fabrication is expensive since it necessitates the use of graphene sheets as a carbon source, an ultra-high vacuum condition, and molecular oxygen. [20,37]. On the other hand, the wet medium technique is a less expensive option since it employs natural and easily available synthetic graphite as a precursor to graphene/carbon and does not need exhaustive experimentation.

The key chemical routes for the synthesis of GO are shown in **Figure 4.2** [27]. The first method employs graphite for exfoliation to produce graphene sheets, which are subsequently followed by the oxidation process. Furthermore, the oxidation process in the subsequent technique is driven by acoustic exfoliation in an aqueous phase [38,39]. The last and third strategy is currently a well-known and commonly utilized technology for producing GO. In this scenario, graphite is oxidized using powerful oxidizing chemicals and exfoliated in an acidic media. The well-known Hummers, Brodie, and Staudenmaier approaches have also applied this methodology.

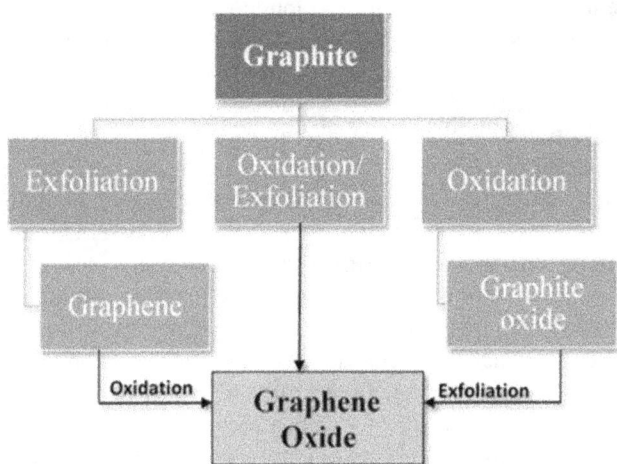

FIGURE 4.2 Schematics for the Synthesis of GO.

Although all three methods contribute to the synthesis of GO, the functional and physicochemical characteristics of each method differ, including the degree of oxidation, composition, solubility, structure, reactive sites, and water solubility.

Over the past century, a variety of methods for synthesizing GO have been investigated. The three main ways are Brodie [19], Staudenmaier [20], and Hummers [21]; each of these approaches is a replacement for the earlier method. However, Sun et al. (2013) [23] and Peng et al. (2015) [24] improved Hummers's approach by utilizing free water oxidation techniques to improve the quality and yield of GO, which is currently the main method utilized for GO synthesis. A modified version of each of these essential GO synthesis methods was developed by Tour et al. (2010). The details of these methods are as follows.

Brodie Method: The first such description of a water-soluble GO was made by Brodie in 1859. His investigation, as was customary at that period, was used to determine the weight of graphite. A number of chemical reaction experiments were undertaken to highlight the physicochemical characteristics of this unique material. Here, fumic HNO_3 was used to oxidize the graphite after mixing it with $KClO_3$. The oxidation that was taking place was monitored for any noticeable changes. The blend of GO that was produced has an elemental makeup of carbon (60%), hydrogen (2%), with oxygen (38%) [19].

Staudenmaier Method: Staudenmaier used sulfuric acid to further modify Brodie's process, which was employed in 1898 to oxidize graphite. Sulfuric acid and a number of serial dilutions of KClO3 were added to the solution well before the reaction to make the solution more acidic. However, much as in Brodie's reaction, explosive ClO_2 gas was produced throughout the reaction and contributed to the explosions since it decomposed quickly in the air. Staudenmaier's modifications, on the other hand, were effective in producing a highly oxidized variant of graphite [20].

Hummers Method: Hummers and Offeman (1958) had established an alternate method for the oxidation of graphite to produce GO by taking into account the sluggish and risky reaction conditions of Staudenmaier's method. A water-soluble brownish-gray paste of GO was produced by combining sodium nitrate ($NaNO_3$), potassium permanganate ($KMnO_4$), and concentrated H_2SO_4 in different stoichiometric ratios and mixing with graphite. A yellowish-brown mixture was produced when the reaction was subsequently suspended with water, and contaminants like manganese were removed using hydrogen peroxide (H_2O_2). Eventually, the combination underwent further filtration and water washing. Although the degree of oxidation in GO attained by Hummers techniques is comparable to Staudenmaier, there is a significant decrease in reaction time under secured reaction circumstances. The time-consuming separating procedure was the main flaw in the Hummers approach [21]. The further improvements to Hummers's technique are mostly concentrated on over-reaction time, quality, yield, and quantity of GO with an improved degree of oxidation. As a modified Hummers method, several variants and optimization techniques are established over GO synthesis.

Tour Method: By substituting sodium nitrate with phosphoric acid and introducing excess $KMnO4$, Marcano et al. (2010) established a modified version of the Hummers technique to increase the oxidation and reduce the
production of harmful gases like NO_2, N_2O_4, or ClO_2. It was asserted that
phosphoric acid offers graphite more integral basal planes. The GO that
was produced exhibits improved hydrophilicity, oxidation level, and reaction efficiency [22]. **Figure 4.3** depicts a quick comparison of conventional
procedures with Hummers and its modified versions.

Due to the inertness of the inorganic carbon found in graphite, expanding graphite and
dispersing it in a solvent upon oxidation both necessitate strong protic or warm acids [36].

The Hummers method is augmented by the free water oxidation techniques,
which benefit from the robust interaction among expanded graphite and oxidizing
reagents. The free water oxidation-based modified Hummers technique was recently
developed by Sun et al. (2013) and Peng et al. (2015). These approaches overcome
the limitations of the conventional Hummers method, including producing poisonous
gases and using toxic chemicals.

Sun Method: Sun and Fugetsu (2013) recently unveiled the first-ever environmentally friendly strategy and more straightforward technology for synthesizing GO. Sulfuric acid was utilized as an acid media, while potassium
permanganate served as both an intercalator and an oxidizer. It was suggested that the volumetric proliferation of graphitic layers was caused by
the complexation of potassium permanganate, which increased the degree
of oxidation into the layers. They performed the oxidation reaction using
graphite: H_2SO_4 weight ratio of 1:20 and eliminated all other chemicals
from the GO reaction mechanism [23].

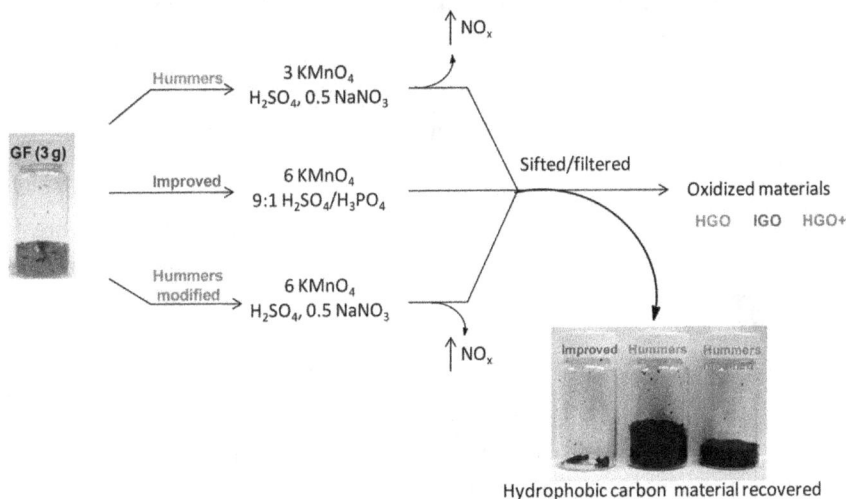

FIGURE 4.3 A Quick Comparison between Hummers's Technique and Its Modified Versions.
[Replicated with permission from *Marcano et al. (2010)*] [22].

Peng Method: Peng et al. (2015) have succeeded in synthesizing a substantially water-soluble GO with a higher degree of oxidation. They presented a sustainable and scalable manner GO synthesis technique that relied on sulfuric acid and potassium ferrate (K_2FeO4) as an oxidant. The proposed approach was successful in preventing the reaction's generation of hazardous gases and heavy metals. Here, sulfuric acid was used to make a suspension of graphite and potassium ferrate, which was then agitated at room temperature for roughly an hour. Additionally, the combination underwent centrifugation and water washing to produce a pure form of GO as the end product [24]. The specifics of the parameters and the features of the techniques that have been proposed for the synthesis of GO are outlined in **Table 4.1** [19–24,40].

4.2.2 SYNTHESIS OF REDUCED GO (rGO)

Graphene, being a robust nanomaterial, presents several prospects for its real-world applications like drug delivery, gene therapy, biosensors, and bioimaging due to its structural and optical characteristics. Unfortunately, large-scale graphene production is a costly as well as time-consuming approach. Numerous initiatives have been taken to eradicate the oxygen functional sites within GO in order to produce a substance with characteristics analogous to graphene [41]. GO can be reduced via chemical, thermal, and electrochemical treatments. Nevertheless, the rGO produced by each of the aforementioned methods exhibits distinct surface features, structure, and additional optical and electrical attributes [39,41,42]. The important variables to be considered for GO reduction are the following:

- The elemental composition of obtained rGO (C/O atomic ratio).
- Precision toward the elimination of oxygen group and reduction of oxygenated functional entities.
- Mitigation of surface defects of GO.
- Employing environmentally friendly reducing agents.
- Maintaining and enhancing the desirable chemical and physical attributes of the parental GO.

Apart from oxygen functionalities, GO comprises a persistent sp^2 carbon structure that could be used for C-C bonding and is augmented by the chemical reduction of GO.

At elevated temperatures, the thermal reduction of GO is reliant upon the breakdown of oxygen-containing groups. Following the thermal reduction of GO, CO and CO_2 gases developed, resulting in nanosheet exfoliation. Other strategies for thermal reduction of GO include increased temperature annealing in an inert environment, microwave heating, and high energy light-assisted flash reduction of GO [43]. Perhaps the chemical reduction of GO is currently the simplest and most widely used method for producing reduced graphene oxide (rGO). Chemicals like amino acids, hydrazine, pyrrole, hydroxylamine, hydroquinone, hydrohalic acid, and metal hydrides have been extensively used as reducing agents.

TABLE 4.1
Specifics of Process Conditions and Attributes of Various Methods for GO Synthesis [19–24,40].

Method	Reagents	Reaction temperature and time	Characteristics	GO thickness (nm)	Reference
Brodie	$KClO_3$, HNO_3	60 °C, 3-4 h	The very first methodology for GO synthesis. Evolution of toxic gas ClO_2	-	[19]
Staudenmaier	$KClO_3$, HNO_3, H_2SO_4	Room Temperature, 96 h	Successfully enhanced the graphite oxidation. Evolution of toxic gas ClO_2	-	[20]
Hummers	H_2SO_4, $NaNO_3$, $KMnO_4$	35°C, 20 h	Safe reaction conditions. Reduced reaction time	-	[21]
Tour	H_3PO_4, $NaNO_3$, $KMnO_4$	35-40 °C, 12h	Restraining the discharge of toxic gases like NO_2, N_2O_4, or ClO_2. A higher dose of $KMnO_4$	1.1	[22]
Sun	H_2SO_4, $KMnO_4$	Room Temperature, 2 h	Free water oxidation method. Safe and efficient in scalable applications	1.2	[23]
Peng	H_2SO_4, K_2FeO_4	Room Temperature, 1 h	Free water oxidation. Heavy metals and hazardous gases were prevented	0.9	[24]
Panwar	H_2SO_4, H_3PO_4, HNO_3, $KMnO_4$	50°C, 3 h	High yield	-	[40]

Shin et al. (2009) employed different amounts of sodium borohydride ($NaBH_4$) to chemically reduce GO. The rGO produced upon reduction was further examined using XRD; the 2Θ was found at 23.98°, confirming a substantial reduction of GO [44]. Stankovich et al. (2007) employed hydrazine hydrate as a reducing agent to reduce a homogeneous dispersion of exfoliated GO. The resulting rGO exhibited a BET surface area of 466 m²/g, and elemental composition revealed a considerable increase in the C/O ratio of rGO (10.2) upon GO reduction (2.7) [39]. Similarly, various reducing agents and thermal treatments were applied for the reduction of GO and have been successfully used for drug delivery-related applications [45–47].

Diverse characterization techniques may be employed to explore the structural and morphological properties of GO, rGO, and GO-based nanocarriers. These characterization methods include transmission electron microscopy (TEM), X-ray photoelectron spectroscopy (XPS), Fourier transform infrared spectroscopy (FTIR), atomic force microscopy (AFM), energy dispersive X-ray analysis (EDX), X-ray diffraction, and Raman spectroscopy. The single-layer geometry of GO and GO-based nanocarriers may be observed through TEM, and AFM analysis can be used to determine the thickness of the GO sheets. The elemental composition may be confirmed by EDX; however, FTIR was utilized to demonstrate the existence of carboxyl, hydroxyl, and epoxy functional entities present within GO. The extent and stage of GO hybridization are investigated using XPS and Raman spectroscopic studies. After graphite has been oxidized, the defect concentration over GO nanosheets can also be determined by Raman spectroscopy. However, the XPS survey offers details about the degree of oxidation, bonding, functional groups, and elemental makeup. The X-ray diffraction analysis may be employed to ascertain the interlayer spacing, crystal structure, and crystal size of GO along with GO-based nanocarriers.

4.3 FUNCTIONALIZATION AND MODIFICATION OF GO

In real-world applications, GO has displayed significant advantages due to its oxygen-rich functional sites, large interfacial area, hydrophilic nature, and surface alteration potential. However, the aqueous stability and inclination for aggregation of GO nanosheets have prompted serious questions about their uses in the biomedical field [12,48]. Moreover, morphological and surface modification of GO to increase its physiochemical properties is an important aspect of applications-driven studies, which is another vast and fast-increasing field of study. The tendency of GO to aggregate can be reduced with adequate functionalization. GO can be functionalized by introducing additional moieties or sites that might deliver distinctive and enhanced features to the parent GO despite losing its core characteristics [27,49,50]. Even though the various oxygen functional groups in GO have varied properties, functionalizing GO causes a modest decrease in their oxygenated sites, which causes its reduction and forms rGO.

The GO was functionalized via various inorganic and organic molecules to improve its solubility and biocompatibility under physiological conditions for biomedical and drug-delivery applications. Currently, there are two techniques for functionalizing graphene oxide: covalent and non-covalent conjugation. The subsequent sections describe the specifics of each form of functionalization.

4.3.1 COVALENT FUNCTIONALIZATION OF GO

The GO has an abundance of oxygenated sites of carboxy, hydroxy, and epoxy functional groups. In GO, covalent bonding is used to link existing functional groups to newly introduced functional groups. Covalent cross-linking is primarily used to enhance the surface properties, bio-compatibility, loading effectiveness, and release behavior of GO in drug delivery systems (DDS) [6]. A number of typical reactions, including acetylation, isocyanation, diazotization, and others, may be carried out using the functional groups located in GO. Covalent function-alization of GO may be achieved in various ways, including by functionalizing hydroxyl, carboxyl groups, and aromatic rings. The covalent functionalization approach entails binding polymers with excellent solubility and biocompatibility via esterification, click chemistry, amidation, nitrene chemistry, and radical addi-tion [51]. Polyethylene glycol (PEG) is the most common and established polymer that has been utilized for the functionalization of GO. Alongside, poly (vinyl alco-hol) (PVA), polyacrylic acid (PAA), chitosan, and dextran are some of the other polymers that have been extensively explored for GO functionalization in line with drug delivery[6].

4.3.1.1 Carboxyl Group Functionalization

Due to its availability and excellent reactivity, the carboxyl functional group has been frequently utilized to functionalize GO, which is found in enormous proportions near the edges in GO nanosheets. The most common kind of carboxyl functionalization comprises reaction activation, proceeded by the dehydration of hydroxyl and amino groups to produce amide or ester couplings. Several reagents, including hexafluo-rophosphate, thionyl chloride (SOCl$_2$), N,N-dicyclohexylcarbodiimide (DCC), and 1-ethyl-3 (3dimethylaminopropyl)-carbodiimide (EDC), are used to carry out the activation. Recently, Liu et al. (2019) have developed highly biocompatible and stim-uli-responsive nanoparticle-assisted anticancer DDS. The nanocarrier was obtained via covalent cross-linking of carboxyl functional groups of GO with chitosan oli-gosaccharide (CO), which was further adorned with γ-polyglutamic acid (γ-PGA). The GO–CO–γ-PGA composites were obtained by an amidation coupling reaction, and the activation of carboxylic groups of γ-PGA and GO was done with the help of NHS and EDC. The impregnation of CO and γ-PGA on GO was further confirmed by XPS and FTIR analysis. A well-known anticancer agent Doxorubicin (DOX) was also loaded over the synthesized nanosystems. The designed nanocarrier had shown superior solubility in physiological conditions with sustainable and controlled delivery of DOX. *In-vitro* analysis of the synthesized nanocomposite revealed easier transfer of nanocarriers within the HeLa cells with good compatibility to the normal cells and higher anticancer activity for the tumor cells. The stated formulation was found to be suitable for their future application in anticancer biomedicines [52].

In the other study, Sousa et al. (2018) developed a carboxyl-activated and func-tionalized nanocarrier based on the folic acid (FA) and GO of potential and targeted drug delivery of Camptothecin (CPT) for anticancer activity. Initially, FA was conju-gated with the PEG, and later it was coupled with the surface of GO. The respective conjugation and coupling of FA-PEG and GO were confirmed via FTIR, magic-angle spinning carbon-13 nuclear magnetic resonance (CP/MAS 13C NMR) spectroscopy, and electrospray ionization (ESI) mass spectrometry. In FTIR spectra, the intensity of the carboxyl functional groups declined significantly during the functionaliza-tion process, which confirms the successful impregnation of FA-PEG conjugate on the GO surface. The toxicity of GO-FA and GOFA + CPT was evaluated in two extensively researched preclinical cell models: J774 and HepG2. It was observed that the toxicity of the nanocarrier without a drug is cell type-dependent, with a higher survival rate for J774 and toxicity for HepG2 tumor cells. Also, the existence of FA in the nanocarrier loaded with CPT was found to be critical for inducing apoptosis in both cancer cell types [53].

Similarly, various other biocompatible polymers, such as PAA and PVA, have been used for the carboxylic functionalization of GO [54]. However, the major concern regarding their application in the drug is the lack of targetability, adaptability, and sustainable and controlled release behavior, which must be addressed.

4.3.1.2 Hydroxy Group Functionalization

A substantial proportion of hydroxyl functional groups, like carboxyl groups, were located on the surface of GO nanosheets. The presence of the hydroxyl group not just gives GO substantial hydrophilicity as well as better surface characteristics, but it also serves as a spacer for the covalent bonding of other ligands at the perimeter of GO nanosheets. Through selectively functionalizing hydroxyl groups toward orthogonal reactions under mild circumstances, Vachhi et al. (2018) examined the reactivity of graphene oxide (GO). A Williamson process with an amino-terminated linker was used to functionalize the hydroxyl functional sites of GO. The acquired data revealed the formation of ether bonds. The study described previously was also extended to ketones in order to investigate their derivatization through the Wittig reaction. Unfortunately, the ineffective reactions suggested that the surface of GO lacked a substantial number of ketone functional sites. [55]. Namvari et al. (2017) demonstrated the cutting-edge innovative Reversible addition-fragmentation chain-transfer RAFT-CTA adapted rGO for the esterification process. The proposed nanomaterial was utilized to polymerize methacrylamide (N-acryloyl-L-phenylalanine methyl ester) monomer based on amino acids. The thermogravimetric investigation validated nanoparticles' thermal stability over GO. In addition, the aqueous stability was examined using zeta potential analysis; the findings were much more acceptable. It was discovered that the polydispersity index (PDI) diminishes as the number of monomers rises, suggesting a well-controlled polymerization [56]. Such improvement in the hydrophilicity and the aqueous stability of GO via hydroxyl group functionalization may provide significant advantages for their application in the biomedical sector, including drug delivery.

4.3.1.3 Aromatic Ring Functionalization

The functionalization of the carbon skeleton is brought on by the C=C in graphene oxide's aromatic rings. One example of aromatic ring functionalization is the fundamental reaction that produces diazonium salt or its derivatives inside the aromatic rings of GO through diazotization. In a study by Jin et al. (2011), 4-propargyloxy diazobenzene tetrafluoroborate was mixed with 2% sodium cholate as a surfactant for eight hours at 45 °C to functionalize graphene. Later, click chemistry was used to elucidate the addition process in the carbon skeleton for functionalization. The suggested technique is most advantageous, adaptable, and practical and may be utilized to develop GO composites for cancer therapeutics [57]. Unfortunately, there is limited information in the literature on the functionalization of aromatic rings inside GO; as a result, further investigation will be necessary.

4.3.2 Non-covalent Functionalization of GO

Non-covalent functionalization is the better cross-linking approach in terms of electrostatic force and hydrogen bonding between GO and GO functional compounds for preserving the core structure and distinctive characteristics of GO while improving stability and dispersibility in an aqueous solution. The key components of non-covalent functionalization include hydrogen bonds, electrostatic interactions, and π-π bonds. The notable characteristics of these types of functionalization approach are the gentle working conditions, which preserve the parent structure and characteristics of GO. Various research outputs have claimed significant improvements in the drug loading capacity, controlled and sustainable release behavior with better biocompatibility and anticancer activity of the nanocarriers synthesized via non-covalent bonding of functional entities to the GO. Some of them are discussed subsequently, along with the details of the functionalization mechanism.

4.3.2.1 Hydrogen Bond Functionalization

The most adaptable approach for the functionalization of GO and rGO in the non-covalent functionalization approach is hydrogen bond functionalization. The importance of GO functionalization via hydrogen bonding has been demonstrated by a number of research findings. Xie et al. (2016) synthesized chitosan (CS)/dextran (Dex) functionalized GO via a non-covalent layer-by-layer self-assembly method. The cationic and anionic polyelectrolytes, namely, CS and Dex, were deposited directly over the surface of GO, and the process was conducted through both hydrogen bonding and electrostatic interactions. Both of these polyelectrolytes are biocompatible, providing suitable adaptability for drug delivery. In this regard, the GO/CS/Dex nanocomposites were further used for the loading of the anticancer drug DOX. It was observed that the polyelectrolyte deposition had upgraded the dispersibility of both the DOX-loaded and pristine GO in physiological surroundings, along with the reduction in the nonspecific protein adsorption of GO. The DOX-loaded nanocomposites showed prominent pH-responsive drug release behavior and exhibited significant anticancer activity toward the MCF-7 cancer cells [58].

Similarly, Hu et al. (2016) demonstrated a novel one-pot synthesis of Dex-coated rGO nanocomposites for the targeted photo-chemotherapy, where rGO was synthesized using Dex as a reducing agent. During the reduction process, the Dex was directly coupled with the rGO nanoparticles via hydrogen bonding to form a self-assembled rGO/Dex nanocomposite. In this study, the Dex conjugation improved the DOX loading capacity (10.85%) and the aqueous dispersibility and biocompatibility of the rGO/Dex nanocomposite. The DOX-loaded rGO/Dex nanocomposite displayed efficient anticancer activity for B16F10 cells and achieved the therapeutic level in a short time with a lower concentration of DOX. In addition, the oligopeptide molecules (RGD) were introduced over the rGO/Dex nanocomposite to improve the intracellular uptake. The DOX-loaded rGO/DOX/Dex and rGO/DOX/RDex nanocomposites exhibit greater cytotoxicity under NIR irradiation than the control groups, indicating their efficacy in photo-chemotherapy [59]. Overall, the functionalization of GO with CS/Dex via hydrogen bonding resulted in improved dispersibility and stability in aqueous conditions, as well as sustained and regulated drug release, which is enormously helpful for biomedical applications. Nevertheless, the drug loading capacity of the GO functionalized nanocarriers was not satisfactory for the DOX, which can be improved via the impregnation of nanomaterials such as metal-organic frameworks (MOFs) of porous structure and higher surface area.

4.3.2.2 Electrostatic Interaction

An additional approach for the functionalization of GO is the electrostatic inter-actions among the negatively charged surface of GO and other nanomaterials or functional entities with a positive surface charge, such as chitosan, liposomes, and metal nanoparticles. Prasad et al. (2019) recently developed novel graphene oxide-fortified liposomal (GOF-Lipo) nanohybrids for the red emissive nano delivery system. The nanohybrid was further functionalized with the tumor-targeting ligand, folic acid (FA). The functionalization was established via electrostatic interaction among the negatively charged GOF and positively charged dipalmitoylphosphati-dylcholine (DPPC) lipids. The obtained GOF-Lipo and GOF-Lipo-FA conjugates were loaded with a chemotherapeutic agent, DOX-HCL, and studied further for the *in-vitro* cytotoxicity over the breast cancer cell lines, MDA-MB-231 and 4T1 for combined chemo-photothermal therapy (PTT). The nanohybrids have shown superior aqueous dispersibility, quick photothermal response with 90% cell viability and hemocompatibility. The combined Chemo-PPT was more effective than the sole chemo or PTT therapy [60].

Kavinkumar et al. (2017) proposed a green chemical approach for the synthesis of silver nanoparticles (AgNP) and the composites of GO and rGO with AgNP using vitamin C as a reducing agent. The functionalization was established via electrostatic interaction between negatively charged GO, rGO surface, and positively charged AgNP. Further, the anticancer activity of AgNP, GO, rGO, GO-AgNP, and rGO-AgNP nanocomposites were demonstrated for the human lung cancer cell line. The rGO-AgNP nanocomposites have displayed superior anticancer for A549 cells among the other nanocomposites, with an IC_{50} value of 30 µg/mL. The higher anti-cancer activity of the rGO-AgNP was accomplished due to its de-agglomeration tendency. In addition, the electrostatically functionalized rGO-AgNP nanocomposite was found to be more biocompatible while reducing the toxicity and corrosiveness of AgNP [61].

It was found that in cancer therapeutics studies, the electrostatic interaction phenomenon was extensively used for material functionalization. However, the drug loading capacity of the functionalized materials was not very significant, which can be improved via the introduction of micro-mesoporous materials. As the loading capacity and sustainable release are important parameters for reducing the dosing frequency of chemotherapeutic agents/drugs, further efforts must be made to address these issues.

4.3.2.3 π-π Bond Functionalization

As the structure of GO comprises sp^2 hybridized carbon atoms, additionally, the GO sheets offer strong π-π bond interactions, which render them favorable for protein adsorption, photodynamic treatments, and interfacial adhesion for the reinforcement of polymer matrix. Recently, Zhao et al. (2018) developed various polymer chain configurations to explore the interactions across polymers and rGO through π-π bonds. Several polymers of diverse chain configurations were used for the investigation, including 2-vinyl naphthalene with naphthalene rings and 4-cyanostyrene with substituted phenyl rings. The polymer-rGO nanocomposite has been developed by utilizing the solution blending technique with chloroform as a solvent. To assess the strength of π-π bond interactions, Raman spectroscopy and TGA analyses were conducted to examine the developed nanocomposites [62]. The π-π stacking was observed as a common phenomenon for drug loading. In most of the studies, the hydrophobic interaction and π-π bond functionalization are considered a mechanism behind the attachment of drug molecules to the hydrophilic surface of GO [63,64]. There is no direct evidence over the functionalization of GO by certain additives via π-π bond functionalization for the drug delivery-related application.

4.4 GO-BASED NANOCARRIERS AS DRUG DELIVERY SYSTEMS

The procedure of administering a pharmaceutical ingredient within an organism to obtain a therapeutic effect is called drug delivery. Synthesis of the active pharmaceutical ingredient, mode of administration, target site selection, metabolism, and toxicity are all aspects of drug delivery that fall under this category. Some current initiatives in the arena of drug delivery focus on enhancing the efficiency of the drug in a resistant system or developing tailored delivery systems that are only active in their intended location.

Graphene oxide (GO) has several characteristics that make it appealing for therapeutic and biomedical pertinence. The most attractive is its water solubility. It also enables hassle-free attachment of drugs through functional group linkages. The enormous surface area of GO aggrandizes the drug loading efficiency. GO at the nanoscale level has been used to deliver anticancer medicines and aptamers for gene delivery directly in living cells [65]. This section discusses the different approaches in which GO-based nanocarriers are employed to release therapeutic moieties at specific places within an organism to alleviate calamitous ailments like cancer, genetic disorders, and neurodegenerative diseases.

4.4.1 Cancer Treatment

The practice in which chemicals are used to destroy cancerous cells is known as chemotherapy. Chemotherapy is one of the most prevalent cancer treatment options, among others, such as radiation therapy, hormone therapy, surgery, etc. The mainstream drugs used in this procedure are insoluble or less soluble in water. Thus, the capacity to properly administer nonsoluble cancer medications has emerged as a critical focus of research [6].

In 2008, Liu et al. used GO as a nanocarrier to convey insoluble chemo-drugs for the first time [66]. SN38, Camptothecin (CPT) analog, was loaded onto GOPEG via physical adsorption to create GOPEG-SN38. In this situation, water-soluble GOPEG-SN38 demonstrated identical toxicity to SN38 in DMSO and considerably greater effectiveness than iriotecan, with a loading drug percent estimated at 10%

(CPT-11). The first-time doxorubicin (DOX) binds to an NGO PEG was reported by Sun et al. in the NGO PEG/DOX DDS [67]. The previously mentioned studies are considered pioneers in the GO-polymer drug delivery system. Various other drugs were investigated for chemotherapy that was delivered via GO nanocarriers. Pham et al. (2019) employed alendronate (AL), an FDA-approved second-generation bis-phosphonate for treating tumor-associated hypercalcemia and various bone-related disorders, coupled with PEGylated graphene oxide nanocarriers to increase DOX accumulation. The DOX@PEG-GO-Al was reported to release more than 60% of the load at pH 4.5. In comparison, about 14–18% of DOX was released in a pH 7.4 environment, demonstrating the pH selectivity of the nanocarrier. According to these findings, PEG-GO-ALs seem to be helpful in treating bone cancer by increasing antitumor effects and reducing off-target toxicity [68].

Kakran et al. (2011) functionalized biocompatible and hydrophilic moieties such as Maltodextrin (MD), Pluronic F38 (F38), and Tween 80 (T80), to GO in 2011 for loading and delivery of ellagic acid (EA), a sparingly water-soluble antioxidant and anticancer medication. This system had a 114% load capacity for the GOMD, a 100% loading capacity for GO-F38, and a 122% loading capacity for the GO-T80. In human breast cancer cells (MCF-7) and human colon adenocarcinoma cells, the EA release rate was pH-dependent and reported to have a more potent cytotoxic effect than free EA dissolved in DMSO (HT29) [69].

Although *in-vitro* and *in-vivo* studies have been carried out successfully for several chemo-agent loaded onto GO-based nanocarriers, clinical trial studies have not been concluded yet due to the government's stringent regulations worldwide.

4.4.2 GENE THERAPY

Gene therapy refers to any method that involves genetically altering a patient's cells to combat the ailment. Genes oligonucleotides or gene fragments that have essentially been introduced into patient cells are the drugs in this situation. Vectors that can be used to deliver genetic material within a host cell may be viral or nonviral. Overall, there has been some success with very few adverse effects. For instance, compared to the former cancer treatment via gene delivery, retrovirus integration into the human genome with the danger of mutagenesis and subsequent malignancies, risk of virus or tumor immunogenicity, and treatment resistance followed by resumption of the disease are some of the factors that have all been considerably lowered [6]. With great biocompatibility, the ability to identify cancer cells by surface alterations, and controlled release techniques, GO-based nanocarriers seem to be a compelling option as a nonviral vector for delivering genes into cancer cells.

Feng et al. (2011) developed GO-PEI complexes with two distinct PEI molecular weights, GOPEI-1.2k and GOPEG-10k, for the purpose of gene transfection. The GO-PEI nanocomplexes were shown to attach to plasmid DNA (pDNA) and were then utilized to transfect HeLa cells intracellularly with the enhanced green fluorescence protein (EGFP) gene. The high level of EGFP expression seen with GOPEI-1.2k/10k and the lower toxicity of the GO carriers demonstrate the systems' suitability for use in this sort of application [70]. Additionally, several studies employed the GO-PEI method to determine transfection effectiveness and the optimal transport of pDNA to the nucleus [71]. Feng et al. (2013) created a dual-polymer GO. They created a dual-polymer-GO (GO-PEG-PEI) by combining PEG and PEI. GO-PEG-PEI demonstrated better gene transfection efficacy without serum interference and decreased cytotoxicity [72]. For the first time, aided transfection was investigated using low-power NIR laser irradiation, where the photothermal effect may have increased the permeability of the cell membrane, resulting in increased transfection efficiency. The precise contribution describes utilizing the same nanocarrier to distribute siRNA under regulated conditions.

Chen et al. (2021) linked anti-EpCAM, a tumor-specific monoclonal antibody, to GO-CS via a π-π interaction after chitosan (CS) was conjugated to GO surface via amide bonds (GO—CS). To properly distribute siRNA, a new carrier GO—CS/ anti-EpCAM (GCE) was synthesized. The delivery mechanism of GCE was studied in detail using survivin-siRNA. Survivin-siRNA was well protected *in-vitro* by the GCE, which demonstrated improved loading performance, stability in various solutions, and good protection *in-vitro*. Apoptosis is enhanced by silencing survivin, which prevents cancers from developing and metastasizing. The study reported that the GCE encapsulated survivin-siRNA and slowed the growth of MCF-7 breast cancer cells [73].

The promising results from various other studies in gene therapy via GO nanocarriers have raised the hopes of those awaiting treatment. Though this is still a farfetched idea, the approvals from regulatory bodies will take substantial time since the technology and its effect on humans are relatively unfamiliar.

4.4.3 Therapy for Other Infirmities

The recent advances in biomedical and pharmaceutical research have led to expanding various systems to treat life-threatening diseases. The role of these systems was either therapeutic or diagnostic, or both in the form of theranostics. Among various nanomaterials, GO has been extensively implemented for biomedical applications due to its countless excellent properties, like facile preparation methods, higher drug loading capacity, and decent biocompatibility. Previous research findings have demonstrated that the use of GO also offers numerous benefits in treating severe brain disorders of neurodegenerative diseases like Parkinson's and Alzheimer's disease, along with tissue engineering and regenerative medication. The neurodegenerative diseases (NDs) are characterized by continuous damage of brain neurons, resulting in vocal, cognitive, and motor dysfunction. Such neuron dysfunction can be recovered via sustainable delivery of the natural drug puerarin (Pue) via nanocarriers to the brain cells. GO, with a 2D structure and higher surface area with its functionalized form, can be used as a biocompatible drug nanocarrier for NDs as well as a substrate for cellular interactions and can carry biomolecules, including DNAs for tissue engineering (TE).

Recently, Xiong et al. (2021) developed a GO-based targeted DDSs for Parkinson's disease (PD). The GO nanosheets were loaded with the Pue, which has shown superior drug loading efficiency of 69.01% with modified surface functional groups and better biocompatibility. The Pue was successfully carried across the blood-brain barriers (BBBs) into the brain with the help of lactoferrin (Lf) targeting ligand. The obtained Lf-GO-Pue nanosystems presented reasonable efficiency for brain targeting in both the *in-vitro* and *in-vivo* analyses. In addition, this nanoplatform did not show any toxicity or adverse effects on the major organs, indicating its potential for treating Parkinson's disease [74]. Wang et al. (2021) demonstrated a dauricine (Dau) loaded GO nanoformulation for investigating the collective antioxidative and anti-inflammatory stress effects of Dau with avoiding the aggregation and misfolding of amyloid-β (Aβ) protein by GO. Aβ1–42 was used to induce in both the *in-vitro* and *in-vivo* models, and the nanoformulation was delivered nasally to mice. The results showed that for *in-vitro*, GO-loaded with Dau significantly decreased oxidative stress by raising superoxide dismutase levels and lowering malondialdehyde and reactive oxygen species (ROS) levels. In addition, nanoformulation has lightened cognitive memory deficits and activated the brain glial cells in mice. The study had proven the effectiveness of GO loaded with Dau for protecting against Aβ1–42-induced oxidative damage for Alzheimer's disease [75].

The tissue engineering (TE) field regenerates or reproduces the damaged organs or tissues by engineering scaffolds, a combination of cells and biologically active molecules. A perfect scaffold may transport active biomolecules, provide appropriate physiological signals, stimulate the mechanical features of native tissue, and serve as a platform for live cells to connect, proliferate, and differentiate. The use of GO as a biocompatible material for tissue regeneration and drug delivery has recently piqued the interest of investigators. GO has the capacity to adsorb numerous proteins and stick to cells due to its huge surface area and π-conjugated structure, making it an effective and viable candidate for use in ligament tissue regeneration. The specific application of GO in tissue engineering is presented in **Figure 4.4** [76].

Recently, Purohit et al. (2020) synthesized graphene oxide-nanohydroxyapatite (GO-nHAp) nanocomposites as reinforcing agents for developing gelatin-alginate (GA)-based 3D polymeric scaffold. The scaffold was made by freeze-drying, which demonstrated the collaborative influence of each component in tissue regeneration and established significant physicochemical properties. The substantial swelling of the scaffold in the presence of water suggests that it is much hydrophilic, implying that it is suitable for tissue regeneration. It was found that the incorporation of GO-nHAp nanocomposites has improved the compressive strength of the scaffold to 14.72 MPa while reducing the biodegradation rate. The biocompatible and less biodegradable property of the scaffold provides significant advantages for bone tissue engineering [77].

Similarly, numerous studies have demonstrated the effective utilization of GO-based nanocarriers for skin regeneration [78], cardiac tissue regeneration [79], and muscle regeneration [76,80]. Overall, GO presented superior performance and ability for drug delivery in cancer therapeutics, gene delivery, and regenerative medication, which could signify a versatile solution for diseased patients. Despite the encouraging results of biocompatibility studies of GO, further investigations are required on the side effects and toxicity aspects of GO.

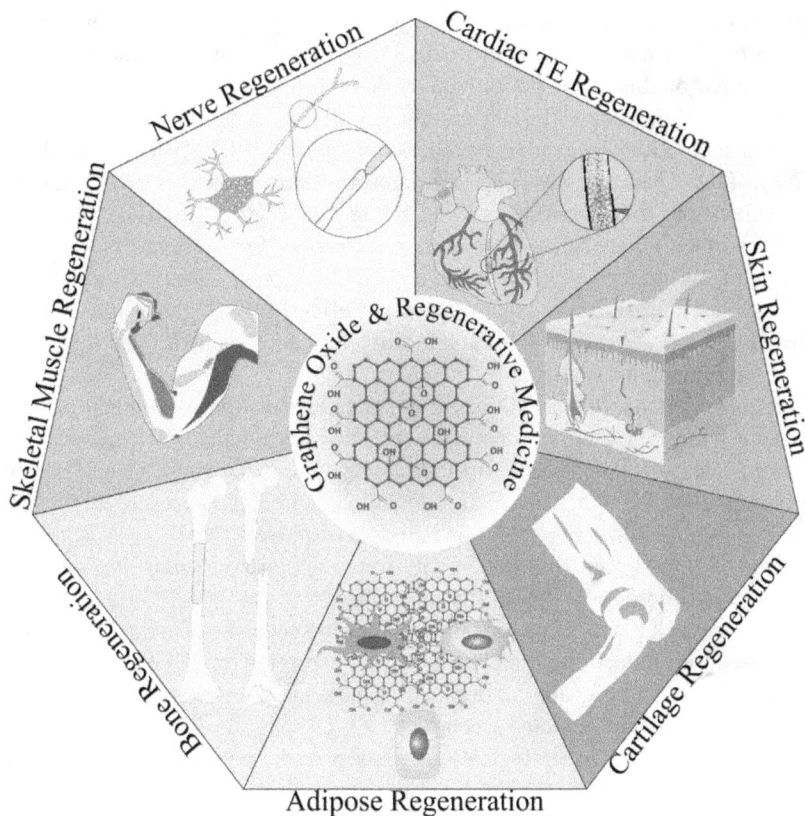

FIGURE 4.4 Application of GO in Tissue Engineering. [Reprinted with permission from *Maleki et al. (2021)*] [76].

4.5 SUMMARY AND FUTURE PROSPECTIVE

The unique characteristics of graphene-based nanomaterials have encouraged the world community for their application in various scientific and technological sectors, including the biomedical field. Specifically, GO, with its oxygen-enriched functional entities, better surface area, and functionalization abilities, is a standout candidate for biological application where the interaction/combination of molecules with the surface of nanocarriers is obligatory. At the initial stages, GO-based nanocarriers suffered from low solubility and aqueous stability issues, limiting their use as drug delivery vehicles for biomedical applications. However, covalent and non-covalent functionalization approaches can resolve these issues, fortifying GO as an effective nanocarrier for the DDS. The present chapter elaborated on the details related to the synthesis, functionalization, and application of graphene oxide, graphene oxide-based nanocarriers in drug delivery for cancer treatment, neurodegenerative treatment, and tissue engineering. GO, rGO, and functionalization of GO through covalent bonding and non-covalent bonding interactions were also discussed in this chapter. It was discovered that the superior quality of GO is defined by a higher level of oxidation with abundant oxygenated functional groups. Based on this, it can be stated that the modified Hummers technique, which includes the Tour, Sun, and Peng methods, is the most appropriate approach for the synthesis of GO in the current predicament. The challenges for the application of GO in DDSs have mostly been alleviated by the appropriate functionalization via covalent and non-covalent bonding while conserving the fundamental characteristics of GO. Especially for cancer treatment, GO seemed to be the perfect nanocarrier for numerous poorly soluble chemotherapeutic drugs while improving their loading characteristics, release behavior, effectiveness, and bioavailability. In addition, GO has shown suitable targetability for cancer cells guided through cellular receptors and aptamers.

The future perspective of GO-based nanocarriers involves additional perfection in surface features via novel functional molecules best suited for improving their controlled release behavior and biocompatibility. The major challenges to overcome for the synthesis of GO include a better oxidation degree, higher yield, sluggish purification steps, and cost. Therefore, it is obligatory to investigate these aspects further by means of suitable substitutes. The GO-based nanocarriers must be investigated frequently and thoroughly due to the uniqueness and complexity of each nanocarrier. The investigation of these nanocarriers is also necessary for the same delivery system because all the critical mechanisms of absorption, metabolism, distribution, and excretion in the body are not defined. Also, detailed investigations are required on the side effects and toxicity aspects of GO. Despite the fact that GO has been extensively studied for its biological uses, based on its physicochemical characteristics, more studies into its employment in the fields of nanotechnology, catalysis, and hydrogen storage might be undertaken.

REFERENCES

[1] Y. Zhu, S. Murali, W. Cai, X. Li, J.W. Suk, J.R. Potts, R.S. Ruoff, Graphene and graphene oxide: Synthesis, properties, and applications, Adv. Mater. 22 (2010) 3906–3924. doi:10.1002/adma.201001068.

[2] W. Ren, H.M. Cheng, The global growth of graphene, Nat. Nanotechnol. 9 (2014) 726–730. doi:10.1038/nnano.2014.229.

[3] S. Kumbhar, M. De, Carbon quantum dots modified Bi2WO6 nanosheets for photo-oxidation of glycerol to value-added product, Mater. Today Proc. (2022). doi:10.1016/j.matpr.2022.11.230.

[4] P. Dhar, S.S. Gaur, A. Kumar, V. Katiyar, Cellulose nanocrystal templated graphene nano-scrolls for high performance supercapacitors and hydrogen storage: An experimental and molecular simulation study, Sci. Rep. 8 (2018) 1–15. doi:10.1038/s41598-018-22123-0.

[5] S.B. Singh, M. De, Scope of doped mesoporous (<10 nm) surfactant-modified alumina templated carbons for hydrogen storage applications, Int. J. Energy Res. 43 (2019) 4264–4280. doi:10.1002/er.4552.

[6] R. Muñoz, D.P. Singh, R. Kumar, A. Matsuda, Graphene oxide for drug delivery and cancer therapy, Nanostruct. Poly. Composit. Biomed. Appl. (2019). doi:10.1016/b978-0-12-816771-7.00023-5.

[7] L. Zhang, J. Xia, Q. Zhao, L. Liu, Z. Zhang, Functional graphene oxide as a nanocarrier for controlled loading and targeted delivery of mixed anticancer drugs, Small. 6 (2010) 537–544. doi:10.1002/smll.200901680.

[8] L. Liu, Q. Ma, J. Cao, Y. Gao, S. Han, Y. Liang, T. Zhang, Y. Song, Y. Sun, Recent progress of graphene oxide-based multifunctional nanomaterials for cancer treatment, Cancer Nanotechnol. 12 (2021) 1–31. doi:10.1186/s12645-021-00087-7.

[9] H.M. Hegab, L. Zou, Graphene oxide-assisted membranes: Fabrication and potential applications in desalination and water purification, J. Memb. Sci. 484 (2015) 95–106. doi:10.1016/j.memsci.2015.03.011.

[10] S.I. Siddiqui, S.A. Chaudhry, A review on graphene oxide and its composites preparation and their use for the removal of As3+and As5+ from water under the effect of various parameters: Application of isotherm, kinetic and thermodynamics, Process Saf. Environ. Prot. 119 (2018) 138–163. doi:10.1016/j.psep.2018.07.020.

[11] P. Jha, A. Sontakke, Biodiesel production from waste cooking oil selecting a solid catalyst derived from activated coconut coir, Int. J. Energy Prod. Manag. 3 (2018) 122–131. doi:10.2495/EQ-V3-N2-122-131.

[12] A.D. Sontakke, M.K. Purkait, Fabrication of ultrasound-mediated tunable graphene oxide nanoscrolls, Ultrason. Sonochem. 63 (2020) 104976. doi:10.1016/j.ultsonch.2020. 104976.

[13] A.D. Sontakke, M.K. Purkait, A brief review on graphene oxide nanoscrolls: Structure, synthesis, characterization and scope of applications, Chem. Eng. J. 420 (2021) 129914. doi:10.1016/j.cej.2021.129914.

[14] F. Alemi, R. Zarezadeh, A.R. Sadigh, H. Hamishehkar, M. Rahimi, M. Majidinia, Z. Asemi, A. Ebrahimi-Kalan, B. Yousefi, N. Rashtchizadeh, Graphene oxide and reduced graphene oxide: Efficient cargo platforms for cancer theranostics, J. Drug Deliv. Sci. Technol. 60 (2020) 101974. doi:10.1016/j.jddst.2020.101974.

[15] A.D. Sontakke, R. Fopase, L.M. Pandey, M.K. Purkait, Development of graphene oxide nanoscrolls imparted nano-delivery system for the sustained release of gallic acid, Appl. Nanosci. (2022). doi:10.1007/s13204-022-02582-8.

[16] A.D. Sontakke, A. Bhattacharjee, R. Fopase, L.M. Pandey, M.K. Purkait, One-pot, sustainable and room temperature synthesis of graphene oxide-impregnated iron-based metal-organic framework (GO/MIL-100(Fe)) nanocarriers for anticancer drug delivery systems, J. Mater. Sci. (2022). doi:10.1007/s10853-022-07773-w.

[17] J. Song, X. Wang, C.-T. Chang, Preparation and characterization of graphene oxide, J. Nanomater. 2014 (2014) 1–6. doi:10.1155/2014/276143.

[18] A.D. Sontakke, P. Mondal, M.K. Purkait, Graphene oxide-based advanced nanomaterials for environmental remediation applications, in: S.J. Ikhmayies (Ed.), Advanced Nanomaterials Advanced Materials Research Technology, Springer International Publishing, Cham (2022): pp. 155–190. doi:10.1007/978-3-031-11996-5_6.

[19] B.C. Brodie XIII, On the atomic weight of graphite, Philos. Trans. R. Soc. London. 149 (1859) 249–259. doi:10.1098/rstl.1859.0013.

[20] L. Staudenmaier, Verfahren zur darstellung der graphitsäure, Berichte Der Dtsch. Chem. Gesellschaft. 31 (1898) 1481–1487. doi:10.1002/cber.18980310237.

[21] W.S. Hummers, R.E. Offeman, Preparation of graphitic oxide, J. Am. Chem. Soc. 80 (1958) 1339. doi:10.1021/ja01539a017.

[22] D.C. Marcano, D.V. Kosynkin, J.M. Berlin, A. Sinitskii, Z. Sun, A. Slesarev, L.B. Alemany, W. Lu, J.M. Tour, Improved synthesis of graphene oxide, ACS Nano. 4 (2010) 4806–4814. doi:10.1021/nn1006368.

[23] L. Sun, B. Fugetsu, Mass production of graphene oxide from expanded graphite, Mater. Lett. 109 (2013) 207–210. doi:10.1016/j.matlet.2013.07.072.

[24] L. Peng, Z. Xu, Z. Liu, Y. Wei, H. Sun, Z. Li, X. Zhao, C. Gao, An iron-based green approach to 1-h production of single-layer graphene oxide, Nat. Commun. 6 (2015) 5716. doi:10.1038/ncomms6716.

[25] X. Pan, J. Ji, N. Zhang, M. Xing, Research progress of graphene-based nanomaterials for the environmental remediation, Chinese Chem. Lett. 31 (2020) 1462–1473. doi:10.1016/j.cclet.2019.10.002.

[26] Y. Pan, N.G. Sahoo, L. Li, The application of graphene oxide in drug delivery, Expert Opin. Drug Deliv. 9 (2012) 1365–1376. doi:10.1517/17425247.2012.729575.

[27] A.D. Sontakke, S. Tiwari, M.K. Purkait, A comprehensive review on graphene oxide-based nanocarriers: Synthesis, functionalization and biomedical applications, FlatChem. 38 (2023) 100484. doi:10.1016/j.flatc.2023.100484.

[28] P. Jha, A. Sontakke, Biodiesel production from waste cooking oil selecting a solid catalyst derived from activated coconut coir, Int. J. Energy Prod. Manag. 3 (2018). doi:10.2495/EQ-V3-N2-122-131.

[29] A.D. Sontakke, P.P. Das, P. Mondal, M.K. Purkait, Thin-film composite nanofiltration hollow fiber membranes toward textile industry effluent treatment and environmental remediation applications: Review, Emergent Mater. (2021). doi:10.1007/s42247-021-00261-y.

[30] X. Liu, X. Wu, Y. Xing, Y. Zhang, X. Zhang, Q. Pu, M. Wu, J.X. Zhao, Reduced graphene oxide/mesoporous silica nanocarriers for pH-triggered drug release and photothermal therapy, ACS Appl. Bio Mater. 3 (2020) 2577–2587. doi:10.1021/acsabm.9b01108.

[31] A.D. Sontakke, P. Mondal, M.K. Purkait, Green synthesis of metallic nanoparticles for biofuel production, in: M. Srivastava, M.A. Malik, P.K. Mishra (Eds.), Green Nano Solution for Bioenergy Production Enhancement, Springer Nature, Singapore (2022): pp. 51–77. doi:10.1007/978-981-16-9356-4_3.

[32] A.D. Sontakke, A. Tiwari, M.K. Purkait, Fabrication of borate cross-linked graphene oxide framework (GOF)-laminated UF membrane for heavy metal removal, in: D. Deka, S.K. Majumder, M.K. Purkait (Eds.), Sustainable Environment, Springer Nature, Singapore (2023): pp. 135–149. doi:10.1007/978-981-19-8464-8_8.

[33] A.D. Sontakke, S. Tiwari, A. Bhattacharjee, P. Mondal, M.K. Purkait, Recent advances in biochar production and its applications toward textile industry effluent treatment, in: Designer Biochar Assisted Bioremediation of Industrial Effluents, CRC Press, Boca Raton (2022): pp. 1–21. doi:10.1201/9781003203438-1.

[34] B. Paulchamy, G. Arthi, B.D. Lingesh, A simple approach to stepwise synthesis of graphene oxide nanomaterial, J. Nanomed. Nanotechnol. 6 (2015) 1–4. doi:10.4172/2157-7439.1000253.

[35] D. Dorniani, B. Saifullah, F. Barahuie, P. Arulselvan, M.Z. Bin Hussein, S. Fakurazi, L.J. Twyman, Graphene oxide-gallic acid nanodelivery system for cancer therapy, Nanoscale Res. Lett. 11 (2016). doi:10.1186/s11671-016-1712-2.

[36] F. Pendolino, N. Armata, Graphene Oxide in Environmental Remediation Process, Springer, Cham (2017). doi:10.1007/978-3-319-60429-9.

[37] E. Starodub, N.C. Bartelt, K.F. McCarty, Oxidation of graphene on metals, J. Phys. Chem. C. 114 (2010) 5134–5140. doi:10.1021/jp912139e.

[38] C. Bosch-Navarro, F. Busolo, E. Coronado, Y. Duan, C. Martí-Gastaldo, H. Prima-Garcia, Influence of the covalent grafting of organic radicals to graphene on its magnetoresistance, J. Mater. Chem. C. (2013). doi:10.1039/c3tc30799a.

[39] S. Stankovich, D.A. Dikin, R.D. Piner, K.A. Kohlhaas, A. Kleinhammes, Y. Jia, Y. Wu, Synthesis of graphene-based nanosheets via chemical reduction of exfoliated graphite oxide, Carbon. 45 (2007) 1558–1565. doi:10.1016/j.carbon.2007.02.034.

[40] V. Panwar, A. Kumar, R. Singh, P. Gupta, S.S. Ray, S.L. Jain, Nickel-decorated graphene oxide/polyaniline hybrid: A robust and highly efficient heterogeneous catalyst for hydrogenation of terminal alkynes, Ind. Eng. Chem. Res. 54 (2015) 11493–11499. doi:10.1021/acs.iecr.5b02888.

[41] A.T. Smith, A. Marie, S. Zeng, B. Liu, L. Sun, Nano materials science synthesis, properties, and applications of graphene oxide/reduced graphene oxide and their nanocomposites, Nano Mater. Sci. 1 (2019) 31–47. doi:10.1016/j.nanoms.2019.02.004.

[42] K.K.H. De Silva, H. Huang, R.K. Joshi, M. Yoshimura, Chemical reduction of graphene oxide using green reductants, Carbon N. Y. 119 (2017) 190–199. doi:10.1016/j.carbon.2017.04.025.

[43] R.K. Singh, R. Kumar, D.P. Singh, Graphene oxide: Strategies for synthesis, reduction and frontier applications, RSC Adv. (2016) 64993–65011. doi:10.1039/c6ra07626b.

[44] B.H. Shin, K.K. Kim, A. Benayad, S. Yoon, K. Park, I. Jung, M.H. Jin, H. Jeong, J.M. Kim, J. Choi, Y.H. Lee, Efficient reduction of graphite oxide by sodium borohydride and its effect on electrical conductance, Adv. Funct. Mater. (2009) 1987–1992. doi:10.1002/adfm.200900167.

[45] M.J. Molaei, Two-dimensional (2D) materials beyond graphene in cancer drug delivery, photothermal and photodynamic therapy, recent advances and challenges ahead: A review, J. Drug Deliv. Sci. Technol. 61 (2021) 101830. doi:10.1016/j.jddst.2020.101830.

[46] S. Priyadarsini, S. Mohanty, S. Mukherjee, S. Basu, M. Mishra, Graphene and graphene oxide as nanomaterials for medicine and biology application, J. Nanostructure Chem. 8 (2018) 123–137. doi:10.1007/s40097-018-0265-6.

[47] S. Gurunathan, J. Woong Han, E. Kim, D.N. Kwon, J.K. Park, J.H. Kim, Enhanced green fluorescent protein-mediated synthesis of biocompatible graphene, J. Nanobiotechnol. 12 (2014) 1–16. doi:10.1186/s12951-014-0041-9.

[48] W. Yu, L. Sisi, Y. Haiyan, L. Jie, Progress in the functional modification of graphene/graphene oxide: A review, RSC Adv. (2020) 15328–15345. doi:10.1039/d0ra01068e.

[49] E.N. Zare, A. Mudhoo, M.A. Khan, M. Otero, Z.M.A. Bundhoo, C. Navarathna, M. Patel, A. Srivastava, C.U. Pittman, T. Mlsna, D. Mohan, P. Makvandi, M. Sillanpää, Water Decontamination Using Bio-Based, Chemically Functionalized, Doped, and Ionic Liquid-Enhanced Adsorbents: Review, Springer International Publishing, Cham (2021). doi:10.1007/s10311-021-01207-w.

[50] P. Jha, A. Sontakke, Application of crop-residue biomass as a catalyst for bio-diesel production from waste cooking oil, SSRN Electron. J. (2020). doi:10.2139/ssrn.3705099.

[51] R.K. Layek, A.K. Nandi, A review on synthesis and properties of polymer functionalized graphene, Polymer (Guildf). 54 (2013) 5087–5103. doi:10.1016/j.polymer.2013.06.027.

[52] B. Liu, C. Che, J. Liu, M. Si, Z. Gong, Y. Li, J. Zhang, G. Yang, Fabrication and antitumor mechanism of a nanoparticle drug delivery system: Graphene oxide/chitosan oligosaccharide/γ-polyglutamic acid composites for anticancer drug delivery, ChemistrySelect. 4 (2019) 12491–12502. doi:10.1002/slct.201903145.

[53] M. De Sousa, L.A. Visani De Luna, L.C. Fonseca, S. Giorgio, O.L. Alves, Folic-acid-functionalized graphene oxide nanocarrier: Synthetic approaches, characterization, drug delivery study, and antitumor screening, ACS Appl. Nano Mater. 1 (2018) 922–932. doi:10.1021/acsanm.7b00324.

[54] H. Sharma, S. Mondal, Functionalized graphene oxide for chemotherapeutic drug delivery and cancer treatment: A promising material in nanomedicine, Int. J. Mol. Sci. 21 (2020) 6280. doi:10.3390/ijms21176280.

[55] I.A. Vacchi, J. Raya, A. Bianco, C. Ménard-Moyon, Controlled derivatization of hydroxyl groups of graphene oxide in mild conditions, 2D Mater. 5 (2018) 035037.

[56] M. Namvari, C.S. Biswas, Q. Wang, W. Liang, F.J. Stadler, Crosslinking hydroxylated reduced graphene oxide with RAFT-CTA: A nano-initiator for preparation of well-defined amino acid-based polymer nanohybrids, J. Colloid Interface Sci. 504 (2017) 731–740. doi:10.1016/j.jcis.2017.06.007.

[57] Z. Jin, T.P. Mcnicholas, C. Shih, Q.H. Wang, G.L.C. Paulus, A.J. Hilmer, S. Shimizu, M.S. Strano, Click chemistry on solution-dispersed graphene and monolayer CVD graphene, Chem. Mater. (2011) 3362–3370.

[58] M. Xie, H. Lei, Y. Zhang, Y. Xu, S. Shen, Y. Ge, H. Li, J. Xie, Non-covalent modification of graphene oxide nanocomposites with chitosan/dextran and its application in drug delivery, RSC Adv. 6 (2016) 9328–9337. doi:10.1039/c5ra23823d.

[59] Y. Hu, L. He, J. Ding, D. Sun, L. Chen, X. Chen, One-pot synthesis of dextran decorated reduced graphene oxide nanoparticles for targeted photo-chemotherapy, Carbohydr. Polym. 144 (2016) 223–229. doi:10.1016/j.carbpol.2016.02.062.

[60] R. Prasad, A.S. Yadav, M. Gorain, D.S. Chauhan, G.C. Kundu, R. Srivastava, K. Selvaraj, Graphene oxide supported liposomes as red emissive theranostics for phototriggered tissue visualization and tumor regression, ACS Appl. Bio Mater. 2 (2019) 3312–3320. doi:10.1021/acsabm.9b00335.

[61] T. Kavinkumar, K. Varunkumar, V. Ravikumar, S. Manivannan, Anticancer activity of graphene oxide-reduced graphene oxide-silver nanoparticle composites, J. Colloid Interface Sci. 505 (2017) 1125–1133. doi:10.1016/j.jcis.2017.07.002.

[62] D. Zhao, Construction of a different polymer chain structure to study π - π interaction between polymer and reduced graphene oxide, Polymers. (2018). doi:10.3390/polym10070716.

[63] Y. Li, H. Dong, Y. Li, D. Shi, Graphene-based nanovehicles for photodynamic medical therapy, Int. J. Nanomedicine. 10 (2015) 2451–2459. doi:10.2147/IJN.S68600.

[64] S. Tiwari, A.D. Sontakke, K. Baruah, M.K. Purkait, Development of graphene oxide-based nano-delivery system for natural chemotherapeutic agent (Caffeic Acid), Mater. Today Proc. (2022). doi:10.1016/j.matpr.2022.11.373.

[65] E. Campbell, M.T. Hasan, C. Pho, K. Callaghan, G.R. Akkaraju, A. V. Naumov, Graphene oxide as a multifunctional platform for intracellular delivery, imaging, and cancer sensing, Sci. Rep. 9 (2019) 1–9. doi:10.1038/s41598-018-36617-4.

[66] Z. Liu, J.T. Robinson, X. Sun, H. Dai, PEGylated nanographene oxide for delivery of water-insoluble cancer drugs, J. Am. Chem. Soc. 130 (2008) 10876–10877. doi:10.1021/ja803688x.

[67] X. Sun, Z. Liu, K. Welsher, J.T. Robinson, A. Goodwin, S. Zaric, H. Dai, Nano-graphene oxide for cellular imaging and drug delivery, Nano Res. 1 (2008) 203–212. doi:10.1007/s12274-008-8021-8.

[68] T.T. Pham, H.T. Nguyen, C.D. Phung, S. Pathak, S. Regmi, D.H. Ha, J.O. Kim, C.S. Yong, S.K. Kim, J.E. Choi, S. Yook, J.B. Park, J.H. Jeong, Targeted delivery of doxorubicin for the treatment of bone metastasis from breast cancer using alendronate-functionalized graphene oxide nanosheets, J. Ind. Eng. Chem. 76 (2019) 310–317. doi:10.1016/j.jiec.2019.03.055.

[69] M. Kakran, N. G. Sahoo, H. Bao, Y. Pan, L. Li, Functionalized graphene oxide as nanocarrier for loading and delivery of ellagic acid, Curr. Med. Chem. 18 (2011) 4503–4512. doi:10.2174/092986711797287548.

[70] L. Feng, S. Zhang, Z. Liu, Graphene based gene transfection, Nanoscale. 3 (2011) 1252–1257. doi:10.1039/c0nr00680g.

[71] B. Chen, M. Liu, L. Zhang, J. Huang, J. Yao, Z. Zhang, Polyethylenimine-functionalized graphene oxide as an efficient gene delivery vector, J. Mater. Chem. 21 (2011) 7736–7741. doi:10.1039/c1jm10341e.

[72] L. Feng, X. Yang, X. Shi, X. Tan, R. Peng, J. Wang, Z. Liu, Polyethylene glycol and polyethylenimine dual-functionalized nano-graphene oxide for photothermally enhanced gene delivery, Small. 9 (2013) 1989–1997. doi:10.1002/smll.201202538.

[73] S. Chen, S. Zhang, Y. Wang, X. Yang, H. Yang, C. Cui, Anti-EpCAM functionalized graphene oxide vector for tumor targeted siRNA delivery and cancer therapy, Asian J. Pharm. Sci. 16 (2021) 598–611. doi:10.1016/j.ajps.2021.04.002.

[74] S. Xiong, J. Luo, Q. Wang, Z. Li, J. Li, Q. Liu, L. Gao, S. Fang, Y. Li, H. Pan, H. Wang, Y. Zhang, Q. Wang, X. Chen, T. Chen, Targeted graphene oxide for drug delivery as a therapeutic nanoplatform against Parkinson's disease, Biomater. Sci. 9 (2021) 1705–1715. doi:10.1039/d0bm01765e.

[75] K. Wang, L. Wang, L. Chen, C. Peng, B. Luo, J. Mo, W. Chen, Intranasal administration of dauricine loaded on graphene oxide: Multi-target therapy for Alzheimer's disease, Drug Deliv. 28 (2021) 580–593. doi:10.1080/10717544.2021.1895909.

[76] M. Maleki, R. Zarezadeh, M. Nouri, A.R. Sadigh, F. Pouremamali, Z. Asemi, H.S. Kafil, F. Alemi, B. Yousefi, Graphene oxide: A promising material for regenerative medicine and tissue engineering, Biomol. Concepts. 11 (2021) 182–200. doi:10.1515/bmc-2020-0017.

[77] S.D. Purohit, H. Singh, R. Bhaskar, I. Yadav, S. Bhushan, M.K. Gupta, A. Kumar, N.C. Mishra, Fabrication of graphene oxide and nanohydroxyapatite reinforced gelatin–alginate nanocomposite scaffold for bone tissue regeneration, Front. Mater. 7 (2020) 1–10. doi:10.3389/fmats.2020.00250.

[78] S. Shahmoradi, H. Golzar, M. Hashemi, V. Mansouri, M. Omidi, F. Yazdian, A. Yadegari, L. Tayebi, Optimizing the nanostructure of graphene oxide/silver/arginine for effective wound healing, Nanotechnol. 29 (2018). doi:10.1088/1361-6528/aadedc.

[79] S. Saravanan, N. Sareen, E. Abu-El-Rub, H. Ashour, G.L. Sequiera, H.I. Ammar, V. Gopinath, A.A. Shamaa, S.S.E. Sayed, M. Moudgil, J. Vadivelu, S. Dhingra, Graphene oxide-gold nanosheets containing chitosan scaffold improves ventricular contractility and function after implantation into infarcted heart, Sci. Rep. 8 (2018) 1–13. doi:10.1038/s41598-018-33144-0.

[80] S.H. Ku, C.B. Park, Myoblast differentiation on graphene oxide, Biomater. 34 (2013) 2017–2023. doi:10.1016/j.biomaterials.2012.11.052.

5 Carbon Nanotubes for Drug Delivery System

5.1 INTRODUCTION TO CARBON NANOTUBES: STRUCTURE AND PROPERTIES

The last 20 years have seen a boom in the biomedical and nanomedicine sectors due to advances in nanoscience technology. There has been substantial growth in the significance of nanotechnology for biomedicines, drug and gene delivery, biosensors, and tissue engineering-related applications. Various nanomaterials, including carbon-based nanomaterials (CBNs) with their distinct physicochemical characteristics, morphological advancements, and functionalization ability, have unlocked novel avenues in the biomedical field [1]. In addition, applications of CBNs in the realms of energy, the environment, electronics, optics, and health care all show considerable potential. Carbon could bond in various ways to form structures with utterly unique characteristics. The chemical element carbon contains six electrons that are located in the $1s^2$, $2s^2$, and $2p^2$ atomic orbitals and are capable of forming sp, sp^2, or sp^3 hybrids. The biomedical sector has been stimulated by the discovery of sp^2 carbon-bonded materials with relatively constant nanoscale sizes, such as graphene, graphene oxide (GO), graphene quantum dots (GQDs) fullerenes, and carbon nanotubes (CNTs). Graphene is the source of most of the physical characteristics of CBNs. The consistent atomic-scale hexagonal honeycomb (sp^2-bonded) arrangement of the carbon atoms in graphene serves as the fundamental framework for its sp^2 carbon-bonded allotropes, including fullerenes and carbon nanotubes. Theoretically, a carbon nanotube is unique since it is made of a rolled-up graphene sheet, which can be of single or multiple wells [2]. Nanotubes having a single well are known as single-wall carbon nanotubes (SWCNTs) and were originally documented in 1993 [3], whereas those with multiple wells are recognized as multiwall carbon nanotubes (MWCNTs) and were discovered in 1991 by Iijima [4].

CNTs are one-dimensional graphitic morphologies formed by rolling graphite/graphene sheets, which may form diverse carbon allotropes along with graphite and fullerenes. Nanotubes resemble buckytubes with a cylindrical shape and feature unique properties that make CNTs valuable for numerous real-world applications. CNTs exhibit superior mechanical, electrical, thermal, and optical properties. Nanotubes are integrated with extraordinary stiffness and resilience, as well as reversible folding and collapsing. CNTs are one of the most rigid substances known and yet have the potential of elastic deformation after exerting compressive stresses. This is due to the strong C-C bond stiffness of the hexagonal network, which results in an axial Young's modulus (E) of ~1 TPa with tensile strength (σ) of 150 GPa [5]. In addition to simple elements, these carbon assemblages may generate a variety of configurations and forms [3–7]. Beneath high pressure, nanotubes can merge, exchanging numerous

DOI: 10.1201/9781003358114-5

sp^2 links for sp^3 bonds, allowing high-pressure nanotube linking to produce strong, infinite-length wires [5,6].

Since the dawn of the 21st century, CNTs have been extensively utilized in pharmaceutical and biomedical applications as drug delivery. They stand out beyond bulk counterparts with the similar constitution (in microscale) due to their ultra-small size, high reactivity, needle-like morphology, significant strength, adaptable interaction with cargo, higher drug loading efficiency, exceptional electrical and optical properties, good stability, biocompatibility, and potential to deliver therapeutic molecules at specific or targeted sites and enormous surface area to mass ratio [6,7]. Furthermore, CNTs have been discovered to be an effective drug delivery vehicle since they directly enter cells and maintain the drug molecules intact without metabolizing them during delivery. CNTs, including SWCNTs and MWCNTs, can conjugate or absorb numerous therapeutic molecules, including drugs, antibodies, nucleic acids, proteins, and enzymes. Although these characteristics are linked to highly desirable attributes, CNTs exhibit toxicity and biodegradability-related issues, which further limit their adaptability for biomedical applications. Nevertheless, despite certain drawbacks, CNTs remain to perform admirably in the field of medicine, particularly in the areas of drug delivery systems (DDSs), gene therapy, bioimaging, and biosensors [5,7].

The major challenges related to the application of CNTs in biomedical fields include lack of solubility, dispersibility, biodistribution, bioactivity, biodegradability, and toxicity. These inadequacies are mainly attributed to the hydrophobic structure, van der Waals interactions, and the length of the CNTs, along with the nonuniformity in their surface characteristics. However, the functionalization of CNTs with hydrophilic and more biocompatible functional elements such as biopolymers and targeting ligands can overcome these challenges. Also, it is much obligatory to tune the dimensions of the CNTs utilizing suitable synthesis approaches and process parameters to counter their agglomeration tendency while improving the aqueous stability.

Considering the significant surface characteristics and potential of CNTs in the biomedical field, this chapter describes the recent advancement in the synthesis and functionalization of CNTs for oncological and other therapeutic applications. This chapter also highlights the classifications and purification process for CNTs. Various covalent and non-covalent functionalization strategies employed to improve the solubility, biocompatibility, and targeting ability of CNTs are illustrated with recent developments. Recommendations are provided to overcome the criticalities related to the synthesis and functionalization of CNTs. The present chapter also highlights the applications of various CNTs in cancer therapeutics, biosensing, tissue engineering, and other infirmities. The toxicological aspects of CNTs are discussed in the last section.

5.2   CLASSIFICATION

The CNTs are mainly classified as SWCNT and MWCNT based on the existence of the number of graphene sheets within the nanotubes and the type of chirality. The SWCNT encompasses the alignment of a single layer of graphene nanosheets. It can be synthesized via a catalyst-assisted method such as chemical vapor deposition

(CVD) and twisted easily. However, it does not exhibit the purest form. SWCNT exhibits a simple structure and exists in a fluffy black powder or granular and sometimes shiny metallic form [8]. SWCNTs may be trundled up in various forms of a seamless tube and exist in a range of configurations. This configuration may allow SWCNTs to function more unambiguously as a semiconducting, semimetallic, or metallic structure, depending on their chirality and diameter [9]. In one of the US patents for the production of SWCNTs, new methods for synthesizing an array or densely packed bundle of SWCNTs were reported that meet reaction parameters that are economically feasible and have ideally smaller diameters than 0.2μ [10]. The lengths of SWCNTs generally fall within the micrometers range, with diameters ranging from 0.4 to 2 to 3 nm. SWCNTs may often be bundled together and can be arranged hexagonally to produce a crystal-like structure. As shown in **Figure 5.1** [2,11], the SWCNTs are further classified into three distinct forms based on their way of wrapping into the cylindrical configuration, namely, armchair, chiral, and zigzag. The chiral vectors and their direct impact on the electrical characteristics of nanotubes are described by a set of indexes (n, m) that are employed to define the configuration of an SWCNT. The numbers n and m define the number of unit vectors across two orientations in the graphene honeycomb crystal structure. According to pervasive impressions, nanotubes are known as zigzag nanotubes if m = 0, armchair nanotubes with n = m, and chiral in other states [2].

MWCNTs are made of multilayered graphene nanosheets that were wrapped over one another; their diameter ranges from 2 to 50 nm depending on the number

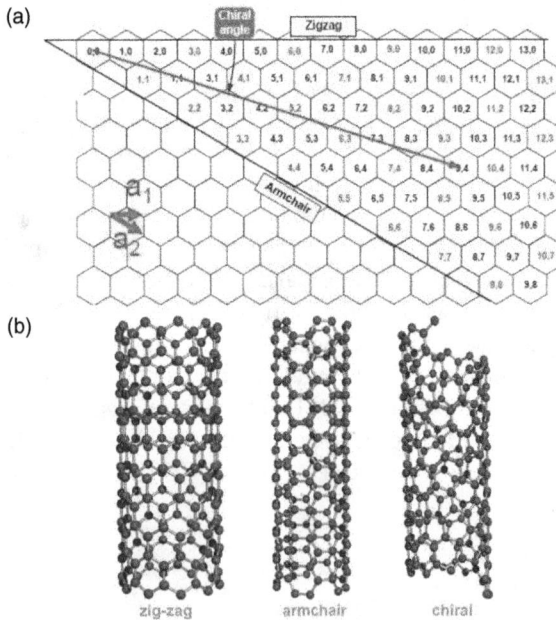

FIGURE 5.1 (a) The Chiral Vector C and Chiral Angle θ Defining a Nanotube on a Graphene Sheet [2], (b) Classification of SWCNTs Based on the Chirality. [Reprinted with permission from *N. Grobert (2007)*] [11].

of tubes rolled together. In contrast to SWCNTs, the production of MWCNTs does not require any catalyst and exhibits a complex structure as well as a pure form. Also, the MWCNTs are difficult to twist and often appear in a granular or black fluffy powder form [3]. The interlayer spacing in these tubes is roughly 0.34 nm [2,5]. There are two significant structural models for MWCNTs, namely, Russian Doll and Parchment models. The Russian Doll model occurs whenever a carbon nanotube comprises additional nanotubes beneath it, and the outer nanotube has a larger diameter than the thinner one. In contrast, the Parchment model refers to wrapping a single graphene sheet over itself several times to resemble a scroll of paper. The characteristics of MWCNTs and SWCNTs are comparable. MWCNTs' multilayer structure allows the outside walls to insulate not only the inner carbon nanotubes against chemical interactions with external contaminants but also demonstrates high tensile strength characteristics, which are missing in SWCNTs [2,12]. In addition to this, there is another sort of CNTs that is structurally comparable to SWCNTs. These nanotubes are made up of two concentric sheets that encapsulate an inner cylindrical tube inside an outer tube and are known as Dual or Double-walled carbon nanotubes (CNTs) [13].

5.3   SYNTHESIS OF CARBON NANOTUBES

The CNTs, including SWCNTs and MWCNTs, can be synthesized using chemical vapor deposition, laser ablation, arc discharge, and flame-assisted synthesis methods. As stated before, in contrast to MWCNTs, the SWCNTs required certain metallic catalysts as a substrate for their synthesis. Certainly, each of the methods mentioned earlier demands specified precursors and process conditions. In line with this, the details related to the fabrication methods of CNTs are described as follows.

5.3.1   CHEMICAL VAPOR DEPOSITION

Chemical vapor deposition (CVD) is one of the prevalent processes used to synthesize CNTs. Employing CVD techniques, nanotubes may be synthesized from a variety of elements, allowing them to contribute more productively to numerous applications, including biomedical and electronics. The aforementioned method may also be further broken down into four categories: catalytic (CCVD) [14], oxygen-mediated CVD [15], microwave plasma (MPECVD) [16], and plasma-assisted (PE-CVD) [17]. The CVD approach entails the catalyzed breakdown of volatile or other gaseous compounds utilizing metallic nanoparticles, which appropriately serve as the nucleation site meant for the induction of CNT development. Compared to the other methods for CNT synthesis, CVD is a promising approach for producing on a broad scale that is also cost-effective [18]. The formation of CNTs may take place at a relatively low temperature, and their size can also be controlled by adjusting the catalyst's particle size. Carbon monoxide (CO), acetylene, methane (CH_4), etc., are often utilized sources of carbon in this process. Small catalyst particle sizes are difficult to synthesize; however, with small catalyst particle sizes, a variety of catalyst sizes can be obtained, leading to the production of nanotubes with a variety of diameters [5]. This method includes the chemical decomposition of hydrocarbons on a substrate and enables CNTs to grow on various materials. Similar to the arc discharge approach, the first step in this technique for synthesizing CNTs is to excite carbon atoms that are in conjunction with metallic catalyst particles.

Generally, tubes are bored through silicon and subsequently loaded with iron nanoparticles at the bottom. The substrates are later heated to break down a hydrocarbon. As soon as the carbon is in interaction with the metal atoms that have been inserted into the holes, it starts to form nanotubes that take on the structure of the tunnel. These characteristics allow CNTs to develop exceptionally long and perfectly aligned forms in the tunnel's angle. A substrate is prepared and processed in the CVD method at a temperature of around 700 °C by coating the particles of metal catalysts. Iron, nickel, cobalt, or a mixture of these metals are typical metal catalyst particles used in CVD processing [2,19]. The purpose of utilizing metal nanoparticles in conjunction with catalyst support like Magnesium oxide (MgO) or Alumina (Al_2O_3) is to increase the active surface area for increasing by-products of the catalytic reaction of the metal particles and pure carbon. A carbon-containing gas, like ethylene, acetylene, methane, and process gas, including ammonia, nitrogen, or hydrogen, was utilized as the reactor's fuel during the initial stage of nanotube growth. The fluidized bed reactors (FBRs) are most frequently employed in the process of CVD [20,21]. The carbon-containing gas is fragmented across the catalyst particle's surface, and as a result, the carbon is now exposed around the edges of the nanoparticle, wherein nanotubes could proliferate. However, the discussions over the mechanism of this method are still under investigation. According to studies, the most widely recognized theories are the base growth and the tip growth models [22]. The catalyst particles may remain at the bottom or within the nanotubes throughout their development and expansion, relying on the attachment and adhesion of these particles with the substrate [2]. The schematics of the CVD method for the fabrication of CNTs are presented in **Figure 5.2a** [23].

This method leads to the formation of CNTs of requisite size and characteristics if the pertinent factors are considered. Basically, the CVD process involves two steps: 1. catalyst nucleation and deposition through chemical etching or thermal annealing [24,25]; 2. nanotube growth onto the substrate at temperatures between 500 to 1000 °C [26]. Overall size and the length of the nanotubes depend mostly on the reaction time; however, nanotubes of a maximum of 60 mm in length can be established through CVD [27].

5.3.2 LASER ABLATION

The laser ablation method demonstrates the synthesis of CNTs through targeting carbonaceous feedstock gas using a continuous laser pulse or extremely powerful laser beam. The schematic of the laser ablation technique is illustrated in **Figure 5.2b** [5]. It is made up of graphitic rods and a catalytic mixture of Co and Ni (50:50), which is heated to around 1200 °C with argon gas flowing through it. Graphite is used as a source of carbon; however, this method is quite costly [28,29]. The employment of a continuous laser has caused the graphite target to vaporize at 1200 °C in an oven. To maintain the pressure at roughly 500 Torr, inert gases such as argon and helium gas are employed within the reactor chamber. This technique is quite similar to the arc discharge approach. Due to the high cost of this process, it is typically utilized to produce SWCNTs and is able to synthesize SWCNTs with higher yields [30].

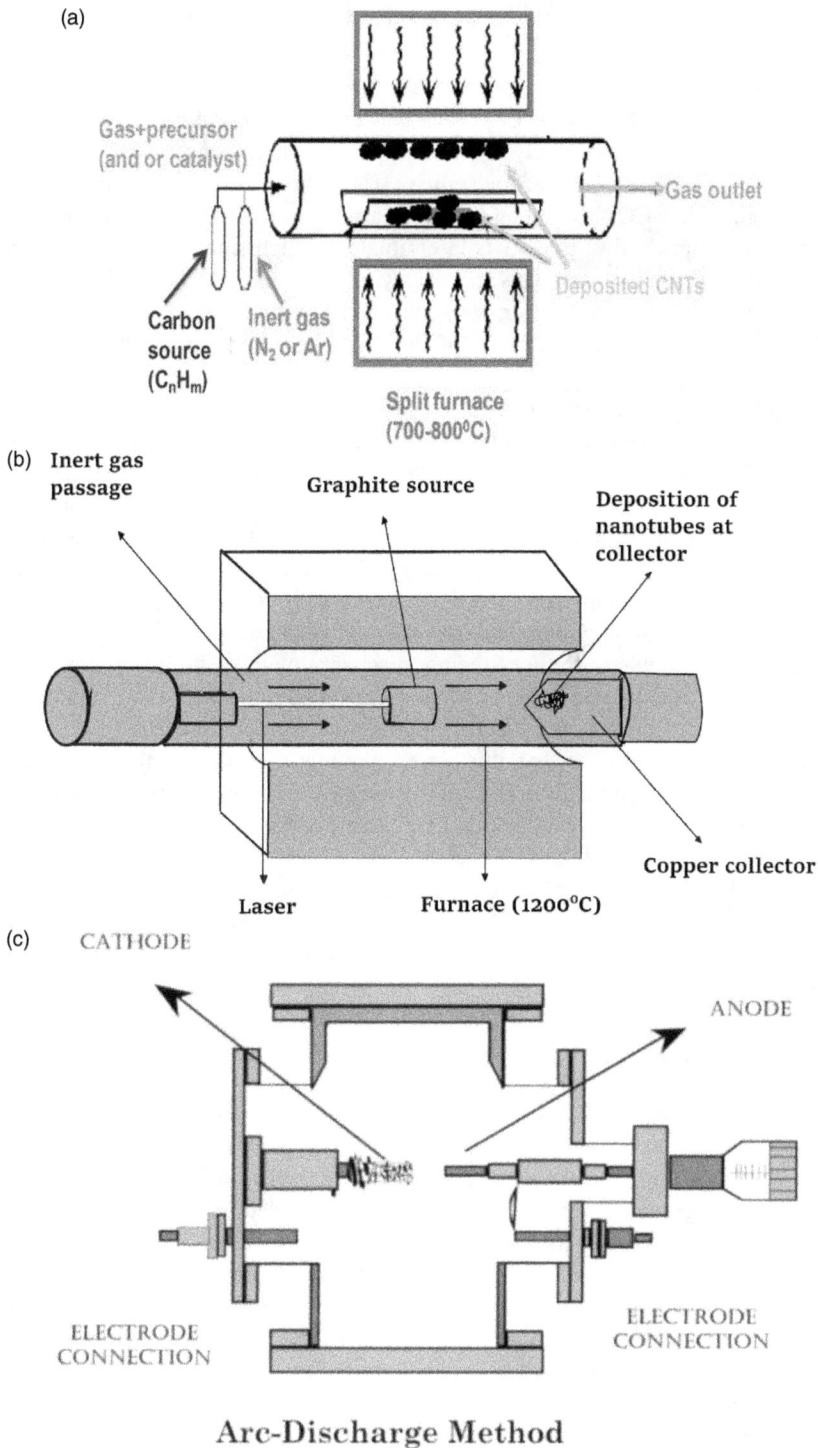

(a)

Gas+precursor
(and or catalyst)

Gas outlet

Carbon source (C_nH_m)   Inert gas (N_2 or Ar)

Deposited CNTs

Split furnace
(700–800°C)

(b) Inert gas passage

Graphite source

Deposition of nanotubes at collector

Copper collector

Laser   Furnace (1200°C)

(c) CATHODE

ANODE

ELECTRODE CONNECTION

ELECTRODE CONNECTION

Arc-Discharge Method

FIGURE 5.2 Schematic Representation for the Synthesis of Carbon Nanotubes (CNTs) by (a) Chemical Vapor Deposition [23], (b) Laser Ablation, and (c) Arc Discharge Methods. [Reprinted with permission from *Jha et al. (2020)*] [5].

Various laser ablation-assisted techniques were employed for the synthesis CNTs, such as the free electron laser (FEL) technique and laser powder method. The FEL method employs a pulse width of ~400 and a preheated argon gas jet to disperse carbon soot from the front of the carbon source [31]. At the same time, the laser powder approach employs a CO_2 laser in an argon stream. In this method, a combination of carbon source and catalyst powder is laser-ablated, which significantly reduces the losses in thermal conductivity. This approach yields around 5 gm/hr of CNTs using a Ni: Co (1:1) catalyst [32]. Moreover, with an increase in the laser power, the diameter of CNTs decreases; therefore, the size of CNTs can be tailored through altering the power provided by laser beams [2].

The properties CNTs synthesized via laser ablations techniques are strongly affected by the chemical and structural characteristics of the target material along with the characteristics of the laser beam such as power, wavelength, cw versus frequency, and energy fluence. In addition, the spacing between the substrate and target, flow velocity and pressure of the inert gases, the chemical composition of the chamber, and the ambient temperature also influence the yield and characteristics of CNTs. This process has the ability to produce SWCNTs with a high degree of purity and quality. Although the fundamentals and mechanisms of the laser ablation method are comparable to those of the arc discharge method, in this approach, the required energy is delivered by a laser that strikes a pure graphite pellet containing catalyst elements [2]. Since the metallic atoms display their tendency to evaporate out from the tip of the tube when it is closed, the major benefits of this technology include reasonably high yields and fairly lower metallic contaminants. The fundamental drawback of this method is that the nanotubes produced are not always consistently straight but occasionally branched.

Nevertheless, the laser ablation approach is not economically viable since it involves high-grade graphite rods, demands strong laser power (in certain situations, two laser beams are involved), and produces fewer nanotubes per day than the arc discharge approach.

5.3.3 Arc Discharge

Compared to previous approaches, the arc discharge process employs elevated temperatures (over 1700°C) for the synthesis of CNTs, resulting in CNTs with lower structural flaws. One of the most popular techniques involves arc discharge for high-purity graphite electrodes, typically water-cooled and spaced 1 to 2 mm apart in a helium chamber at sub-atmospheric pressure [11]. The chamber includes a cathode and anode composed of graphite, vaporized carbon molecules, and a tiny proportion of metallic catalysts. The helium gas in the chamber can be replaced with methane or hydrogen gas. The iron, cobalt, or nickel metallic particle are employed as catalysts for synthesizing SWCNTs. The schematics of the arc discharge process are illustrated in **Figure 5.2c** [5].

The chamber is compressed, heated to about 4000 K, and direct current is transmitted across the arch during the arcing process. The anode was consumed throughout this process of arcing, and nearly half of the carbon accumulated over the cathode electrode. The accumulated layer is known as a cylindrical hard deposit, which continues to grow at the rate of ~1 mm/min. The residual carbon, which forms a hard-gray coating on edge, crystallizes to form "cathode soot" near the cathode and "chamber soot" adjacent to the chamber walls. The SWCNTs or MWCNTs and stacked polyhedral graphene nanosheets may be produced from the inner core, chamber soot, and cathode soot that are both soft and dark. The morphology and the texture of the cathode deposit can be investigated via scanning electron microscopic (SEM) analysis. Generally, two distinct textures are yielded by the cathode deposit. The gray exterior shell is made up of curved and rigid graphene nano layers, while the interior, softer, and dark core deposits are made up of bundle-like structures that comprise irregularly distributed nanotubes [2].

There are two basic methods for the production and deposition of CNTs using arc discharge: one uses various catalyst precursors, and the other does not. In overall, the formation of MWCNTs may be carried out in the absence of catalyst precursors; however, the formulation of SWCNTs uses various catalyst precursors. The complex anode electrodes have mostly been employed for the expansion in arc discharge, which can be formulated by the varied composite of metals such as iron, cobalt, nickel, silver, palladium platinum, and graphite [12]. According to previous reports, Ni-Y-graphite combinations may produce high yields (around 90%) of SWCNTs with an average size of 1.4 nm [33], and this combination is presently utilized all over the world to produce SWCNTs with a great yield. The ability and possibility for producing a significant number of nanotubes is the major benefit of the arc discharge method. In contrast, this method's major drawback is that it gives very limited control over the nanotubes' alignment, or chirality, which is crucial for their classification, characteristics, and function. Furthermore, it is imperative to purify the resulting products due to the metallic catalyst required for the reaction. The developed SWCNTs thought this method exhibits a 1.2 to 1.4 nm diameter. The efficiency of CNTs produced using the arc discharge method depended on factors such as 1. selectivity of the inert gas, 2. inert gas pressure, and 3. catalyst [34,35].

Similarly, MWCNTs of higher crystallinity and yield can be synthesized through this arc discharge method. This approach may yield MWCNTs from pure graphite arcs with an estimated inner diameter of 1–3 nm and an outside diameter of 10 nm [36]. Since the catalyst is not employed in this process, there are no prerequisites for a severe acidic purification process. Consequently, this method highlights the fabrication of MWCNTs with fewer defects. It has been demonstrated that the introduction of hydrogen gas into the formation zone allows for the best possible production of MWCNTs with few intrinsically entangled CNTs and high crystallinity [37]. MWCNTs can be synthesized using a variety of methods, including 1. liquid nitrogen nanotube synthesis, 2. magnetic field synthesis, 3. arc discharge by plasma rotation, etc. [35].

5.3.4 FLAME SYNTHESIS METHOD

In a regulated flame atmosphere, SWCNTs can be synthesized from hydrocarbons and thin metallic aerosol catalysts [38]. In comparison to other processes, flames are significantly less costly for producing nanotubes in bulk. Three essential elements are required for the production of CNTs: a carbon precursor, metal catalyst particles, and a heating element. This process also nucleates and ultimately condenses the catalytic precursors, which are typically introduced via the flame process, into solid metal spherical nanoparticles. Both the catalytic characteristics and the modification of the flame parameters may influence the structure of the final product [39]. As a result, several flame configurations, such as inverse diffusion, partly mixed, and premixed flames, would have been used to produce nanotubes and nanofibers [40,41]. In the post-flame region of the premixed argon/oxygen/acetylene flame, performed at around 50 Torr, SWCNTs may have been identified by using the vapor of pentacarbonyl and iron as a source of a metal catalyst. In the space of around 30 ms, nanotubes have been seen to coalesce and assemble into clusters between 40 and 70 nm just above the burner [42].

5.4   PURIFICATION METHODS

Along with the large-scale synthesis, the purification of CNTs is a significant issue. The CNTs contain a number of contaminants whose concentrations vary depending on the CNT production procedure. Depending on the approach utilized, quality and quantity may vary. Carbonaceous compounds are the most prevalent impurities in CNTs, although metals are the other sorts of impurities that are typically observed [13,43].

Numerous contaminants can be found in the CNT soot as it is formed. Amorphous carbon, metal catalyst, smaller fullerenes, and graphite (wrapped up) sheets are the primary contaminants in the soot. The majority of the CNTs' desirable qualities will be hindered by these contaminants. It is essential to produce CNTs that are as pure as feasible for basic research as well. The CNT specimens must also be as homogenous as reasonable to comprehend the measurements effectively. The oxidation and acid-refluxing methods were used in typical industrial processes for the purification of CNT, which affects the structural integrity of nanotubes. The CNTs' insoluble nature limits the use of liquid chromatography and makes purification challenges rather severe. According to the kind of purification process, the purification stage of CNTs eliminates amorphous carbon from CNTs, promotes or reduces mesopore or micropore volume, breaks down the functional groups obstructing the pores' entry, or induces new functional groups. For instance, CNT purification processes, including heat or NH_3 treatment, may be modified to improve mesopore volume and surface area in the event of bacterial adsorption. These methods essentially fall into two categories: size- and structure-selective separations. The first will isolate the CNTs from contaminants, while the next will result in a relatively uniform distribution of size or diameter of CNTs. Most of these processes are coupled with other techniques to enhance purification and eliminate many contaminants at once [13].

It has been demonstrated that the CNTs produced by CVD are typically between 5 and 10% pure. Consequently, considerable purification is necessary before their usage in biological applications [44]. The nanoparticulate systems contain several residual metals, including Co, Ni, Mo, and Fe, in addition to specific organic contaminants and other impurities, including magnesium oxide, alumina, and silica. These impurities and other carbonaceous contaminants present within the CNTs can be removed through various purification techniques, which are discussed subsequently.

5.4.1 AIR OXIDATION

This method is the most effective for getting rid of amorphous carbon and metal catalysts like Co, Fe, and Ni. Typically, the ideal air oxidation conditions have been discovered as 40 minutes at 673 K [44]. Carbonaceous contaminants on the metal surface may be effortlessly eliminated by utilizing oxidative processing. Since the nanotubes are also oxidized during this process along with the impurities, it has several disadvantages [45]. Fortunately, CNT breakdown is not as severe as impurity damage. These contaminants are more exposed or have higher defects. The fact that such impurities are frequently bonded to the metal catalyst, which also serves as an oxidizing catalyst, is another factor promoting impurity oxidation.

Overall, the variety of variables, including metal content, oxidation period, environment, oxidizing agent, and temperature, have a significant impact on the effectiveness and yield of the process [13].

5.4.2 ACID TREATMENT

The acid treatment is one of the simplest ways to reduce the concentration of impurities from the nanotubes. The higher concentrations of metal particles and amorphous carbon (soot) can be successfully reduced by refluxing the sample in strong acids such as HCl, H_2SO_4, and HNO_3, although HCl has been proven to be the best refluxing agent [44]. The metal should initially undergo the oxidation or sonication process to expose its surface. The metallic catalyst is subsequently solvated and subjected to acid treatment. In this process, the CNTs remain in suspended form. Only the acid affects the metallic catalyst, particularly when applying an HNO_3 treatment; however, the CNTs and additional carbon atoms remain unaffected. The HNO_3 reflux and the moderate acid treatments through 4 M HCl solution are essentially the same, except that the metal must be completely subjected to the acid to solvate it. According to the state-of-art literature, the influence of important factors, including type and concentration of acid, temperature, time, and pressure, are not defined thoroughly. As per their dependency, it must be explored with adequate experimental design to demonstrate the possible interactions and effects [13,46].

5.4.3 ULTRASONICATION

The foundation of this method is the segregation of particles brought on by ultrasonic vibrations. In this method, diverse nanoparticle aggregations will be compelled to vibrate and spread more widely. The choice of surfactants, solvents, or reagents utilized is a crucial factor in separating the particles. The stability of the scattered tubes in the system is affected by the solvent. If the CNTs are coupled to the metal particles, they will be more stable in weak solvents [47].

However, monodispersed nanoparticles are highly persistent in certain solvents, like alcohols. The purity of the CNTs relies on the irradiation time once an acid is applied. Only the metal particles get dissolved when the tubes are in the solution for a short period; however, if the tubes are in the acid for a prolonged period of time, the tubes will also undergo chemical degradation [13].

5.4.4 Micro-Filtration

The principle behind microfiltration is particle or size separation. In this method, filters are used to capture CNTs and a limited number of carbon nanoparticles. The filter allows the additional particles, such as catalytic metal nanoparticles, carbon nanoparticles, and fullerenes, to pass across. Soaking the freshly made CNTs in a CS_2 solution is one method of using microfiltration to separate fullerenes from CNTs. Afterward, a filter traps the CS_2 insoluble and allows the solubilized fullerenes from the CS_2 to trickle across [48–50].

Cross-flow filtration is a unique type of filtration technique used for the separation of CNTs. This technique uses a hollow fiber as the membrane. The solution can pass through the membrane. The filtrate is continuously recycled through the fiber by pumping the filtrate through the fiber's bore under some head pressure. The majority of the fast-flowing solution that does not leak out on the sides of the fiber is then supplied directly to the reservoir. The membrane surface is swept by a rapid hydrodynamic flow along the fiber bore (cross flow), avoiding the formation of a filter cake [51,52].

5.4.5 Surfactant-Based Annealing

Although the CNTs produced by the acid reflux approach are generally pure, numerous contaminants may be trapped when the tubes converge and may not be effectively removed by a straightforward filtration procedure. Therefore, the surfactant-based annealing method is used. In general, organic solvents like methanol or ethanol are utilized within this technique when sodium dodecyl benzene sulphate (SDBS) is employed. The ultra-filtration process is followed by annealing at a very high temperature (1273 K) for four hours since the nanotubes require more time to settle. In addition, annealing is an efficient method for improving CNT structure [44,53].

5.5 FUNCTIONALIZATION OF CARBON NANOTUBES

Perhaps one of the challenges associated with nanotubes for their application in the biomedical field is their tendency to aggregate due to weaker intermolecular interactions, which makes it difficult to disperse them into the suitable polymeric medium and in various organic solvents. Such inadequacy of CNTs to dissolve in aqueous media for biomedical and biological applications has been a significant technical barrier [54]. To prevent the development of bundles owing to their aggregation tendency, CNTs are frequently functionalized to further enhance their diffusion in solvents and other mediums. Functionalization refers to the addition of distinct functional groups to the side chains or ends of CNTs [55]. This may be accomplished by making the CNTs more hydrophilic with improved solubility, utterly altering their biocompatibility profile by anchoring various functional groups, biomolecules, and other biocompatible nanomaterials to them via covalent or non-covalent functionalization approaches.

Along with improving aqueous solubility, the functionalization of CNTs demonstrates their potential to minimize toxicity, improve biological compatibility, and even offer the opportunity to load drug molecules, genes, or biomolecules for effective drug delivery systems (DDSs) [5]. Till now, numerous scientific studies have presented surface functionalization strategies for CNTs with different molecules. As stated, two approaches have been frequently used for the functionalization of CNTs, namely, covalent and non-covalent functionalization, which conjugates the functionalization molecules through the chemical bonding and physical adsorption phenomenon. The details related to these approaches are provided subsequently.

5.5.1 Covalent Functionalization

In the covalent functionalization method, the desirable functional groups can be firmly and irrevocably bound to the sidewalls or ends of the CNTs. Multiple functional entities, including the secondary dichloro-carbon groups, the fluorine carboxylic group, and p-aminobenzoic acid, have been attached to the outer surface or to the extremities of the nanotubes. The main advantages of chemical functionalization are its ability to covalently bond with polymeric materials and its ability to diffuse easily in a wide range of solvents. However, the development of defects in CNTs is among the significant disadvantages of this sort of functionalization [5,56].

There are two distinct methods for the covalent functionalization of CNTs, such as the direct functionalization of side walls and indirect functionalization of the exterior of CNTs with oxygenated functional groups such as hydroxyl and carboxylic functional groups [57]. Regarding the two different types of CNTs, SWCNTs and MWCNTs, SWCNTs were discovered to be significantly convenient to functionalize since MWCNTs possess an outermost part with comparatively higher radii, and the interior layers of graphene sheets are protected by the superficial layers, which inevitably prevent those from being paired with the exterior surface via the functional groups. The CNTs are not particularly reactive and typically require extreme conditions for the reaction to occur. As a result, it has only been shown that the surface chemistry of the CNTs may produce relatively modest chemical reactions. Furthermore, it might be challenging to categorize functionalized SWCNTs, pinpoint the precise position of functionalized entities, and comprehend their anchoring mechanism [58]. Although the covalent functionalization techniques are not entirely distinctive, the final compounds vary greatly depending on the properties of the conjugated group or moieties.

The CNTs can be covalently functionalized through oxidation reactions, cycloaddition reactions, polymerization, and reaction with sulfoxides or acyl peroxides, which are described as follows.

5.5.1.1 Oxidation

It is the most common method for the covalent functionalization of CNTs, which is frequently carried out by employing different oxidizing agents such as nitric acid (HNO_3) and developing hydrophilic functional entities like carboxylic or hydroxyl groups within CNTs. These groups were typically spotted at the terminal along with the sidewall or surface of the CNTs [59]. After oxidation, the SWCNTs adopt the sp^3 carbon atom configuration, which allows their subsequent functionalization with diverse biomolecules like proteins or amino acids [60].

The solubility of CNT has certainly been augmented through oxidation; however, this also causes an issue with CNT aggregation since it has been found that oxidized

CNTs aggregate mostly in the vicinity of salts, which may be caused by the process of charge screening. As a result, the CNTs are unstable in living organisms due to the presence of various salts in the biological fluid. The oxidized CNTs are employed to address this agglomeration issue together with introducing a hydrophilic polymer to its surface, such as polyethylene glycol (PEG), which renders nanotubes much soluble and viable both in the *in-vivo* and *in-vitro* environment [61]. It has been demonstrated that the oxidation of CNTs is a potential method of functionalization suitable for small-scale manufacturing as well as the development of functionalized CNTs on a large scale. Although oxidation using an acidic solution might shorten the nanotubes by compromising specific properties, it is frequently required for specific biomedical applications like oral drug delivery [62].

5.5.1.2   Reaction with Acyl Peroxides or Sulfoxides

As with oxidized CNTs, this reaction may also be utilized to functionalize CNTs on the surface. It has the capacity to covalently bind the variety of functional groups at the edges or sidewalls of the CNTs, without causing defects or disrupting the structure of CNTs [59]. As a result of the development of radicals with a carbon core, acyl peroxide potentially contains terminal units for additional functionalization. For instance, an amide could have resulted whenever the acyl chloride interacts with the organic group comprising a carboxylic acid. Sulfoxides are also utilized for this purpose in addition to acyl peroxides [5]. In addition to improving solvent dispersibility, these reacting functional groups linked to CNTs provide reactive sites for the incorporation of monomers into polymeric structures. The major characteristics of this free radical approach are its simplicity and sensible selection of radical-forming compounds [1,63].

5.5.1.3   Cycloaddition Reaction

The cycloaddition reaction differs from the reaction discussed previously, as it occurs near the sidewalls of CNTs rather than next to its defects or ends. This method is also commonly employed for the covalent functionalization of CNTs. This reaction can be split into three categories: 1. photoinduced cyclo addition, which is a photochemical reaction involving azides [64]; 2. Bingel reaction, which takes place when a strong base is involved in the reaction and produces carbenes and which is also known as the [2 + 1] cycloaddition process [65]; and 3. 1,3-dipolar cycloaddition reaction, which has extensively been employed to functionalize CNTs in the current scenarios [66].

5.5.1.4   Functionalization of CNTs with Polymers

Typically, the polymer molecules are employed to improve the dispersion of CNTs and to develop CNT-based compounds in order to investigate their novel properties. The main methods for modifying CNTs using polymer are covalent and non-covalent attachments [57]. However, the covalent attachment of polymeric molecules through their grafting on the CNTs is the most popular and adaptable method. The in-situ monomer polymerization, in which the monomer interacts with the elements already present on the CNTs surface, has been used to attach the polymers to the CNT's surface in the presence of initiators [67]. In 2008, Ford and Qin developed a technique for synthesizing polymer/CNTs composites that allow polymers to be covalently attached to CNTs [68]. The end-product composites can be easily dissolved in an aqueous medium and develop stable colloidal dispersions without separating for longer time frames. CNTs that have been polymer functionalized can also be disseminated into the parent polymer. CNTs have been functionalized, solubilized, and purified using this approach efficiently and economically; however, the stability of these dispersions is highly reliant on specific colloidal systems. Barrera et al. (2014) have suggested a three-step process in which functionalized CNTs are first employed to make polymer composites before being defunctionalized and then reverting to their natural chemistry. In the first step, functionalized CNTs are dispersed in a solvent to obtain dispersion. In the second step, the obtained dispersion is incorporated further into a polymer host matrix to produce a functionalized CNTs-polymer composite. In the third step, the functionalized CNTs-polymer composite is modified with radiation, in which the alteration involves defunctionalizing the functionalized CNTs using radiation chosen from the group composed of cosmic radiation, heavy ions, protons, neutrons, and alpha particles [69].

The covalent functionalization of CNTs with polymers is primarily based on two strategies: "grafting to" or "grafting from" approaches. The "grafting to" approach can be established through coupling, nucleophilic addition, cycloaddition, and amidation reactions. At the same time, the "grafting from" approach was achieved by atom transfer radical polymerization (ATRP), reversible addition–fragmentation chain transfer (RAFT), and free radical polymerization reactions [70]. Zhang et al. (2017) demonstrated the grafting to strategy for the functionalization of CNTs through a nucleophilic addition reaction. They have presented the thiol-ene addition process among low-density polyethylene (LDPE) with a vinyl terminal cap and MWCNTs functionalized with trimethoxysilane at the moderate reaction environment. With a high grafting degree of 18 weight percent, this approach produced an effective reaction. It was reported that the end-grafted LDPE offered excellent compatibility while promoting the homogeneous dispersion for the CNT-polymer matrix [71]. The ATRP of polystyrene (PS) and poly(methylmethacrylate) (PMMA) from MWCNTs was demonstrated by Baskaran et al. (2005). PMMA had a covalent anchorage of 70% by weight, whereas PS had a covalent anchorage of 18–34% by weight after increasing the initiator amount. Therefore, it would seem that altering the initiator content may be used to modify the polymer's molecular weight [72].

Additionally, by derivatizing CNTs with a functional group that is an essential component of the polymerization process, it is possible to develop composite materials in which CNTs work chemically as a catalyst for polymer development. Although it does not solve the issue of CNT dispersion, this technique ensures a great connection between the matrix and CNTs since CNTs promote polymerization and the expansion of polymer chains, making them more compatible with the host polymer [1].

5.5.2 Non-covalent Functionalization

On the surface of virgin CNTs, several tiny and big polymeric anticancer drugs can be adsorbed through various non-covalent interactions. The hydrophobic and π-π stacking interactions among these molecules and the surface of the CNTs are the driving forces behind this adsorption. However, the hydrophobic forces are considered as the primary mechanism for the loading of such therapeutics into or onto the surface of CNTs seeing as many anticancer drugs are hydrophobic by nature or include hydrophobic moieties. Additionally, through electrostatic interaction, the existence of surface charge on the nanotube surface as a result of chemical processing can facilitate the adhesion of the ionized molecules [73]. Depending on the π-π stacking in between the CNT surface and aromatic bases/amino acids in the structural backbone of these functional biomolecules, aromatic compounds or molecules containing aromatic groups can be commenced to disassemble and solubilize CNTs. Non-covalent functionalization of CNTs is especially appealing since it allows for the attachment of molecule handles without altering the tubes' electronic network.

For the structured synthesis of SWCNTs, oxide interfaces modulated with pyrene via π-π stacking interactions were used [74]. Pyrene organic compounds with distinctive molecular characteristics may be employed to identify the carbon graphitic structure. An amine-covered surface can be produced via bonding among bifunctional molecules (containing amino and silane groups) and the hydroxyl groups on an oxide substrate. The next phase included coupling, which entailed enabling molecules with pyrene groups to interact with amines. Employing π-π stacking with the region occupied with pyrenyl groups, the structured fabrication of a single layer of SWCNT may be accomplished. Also, the pyrene-carboxylic acid compound was used as a chemical cross-linker to connect alkyl-modified iron oxide nanoparticles to CNT [75]. The physicochemical characteristics of the inorganic nanoparticles gave rise to a substance that was more soluble in organic media.

Non-covalent functionalization approaches are significant as they do not strongly damage or affect the configuration of CNTs [76]. This is an alternate method of adjusting the interfacial properties of CNTs. Nanotubes can maintain their aromatic structure and, consequently, their inherent electronic characteristics because of the non-covalent dispersion in the solution. Typical examples of this kind of functionalization often entail the employment of a surfactant, particularly with non-covalent interactions of protein, SWCNTs, and CNT wrapping by taking advantage of the hydrophobic or alternatively π-π stacking by most of the CNTs surface [77]. Numerous compounds, including pyrene, polyaniline, poly acrylic acid, siRNA, proteins, DNA, and other biomolecules, have effectively been immobilized across the surface of CNTs via a physical method that incorporates π-π stacking interactions [78]. Additionally, multiple anionic or cationic and non-ionic surfactants have been employed in the dispersion of CNTs. In the case of drug delivery molecular carriers, polymers are frequently utilized. Despite having a similar dispersion efficiency to surfactants, they are an excellent alternative for solubilizing CNT [79].

As per the study done by Moon et al. (2010), the serum nucleases have been able to disintegrate DNA molecules that have been immobilized on SWCNTs, which shows that CNTs functionalized simply by physical adsorption may not be entirely stable *in-vivo* [80]. The development of one hydrophilic and one hydrophobic link in between the sidewalls of the CNTs owing to π-π interaction will significantly increase the aqueous dispersion of CNTs [81]. Moreover, by taking advantage of the hydrophobic interaction phenomena, surfactant polymers are frequently employed to functionalize CNTs. The development of stable CNT dispersion often involves the application of certain surfactants [82]. Surfactants were primarily used as dispersants in the purification regimens for raw carbon material. Consequently, surfactants have been utilized to enhance the adaptability of synthetic structures and stabilize CNT dispersions for spectroscopic techniques [83]. Although the surfactants are efficient in solubilizing, they are known to be permeable to plasma membranes. These complexes may only be used in limited circumstances for biomedical applications since they are also detrimental to the biological system. Surfactants have limitations with increased critical micellar concentrations (CMCs), decreased stability, and cellular protein interactions. As a result, the optimal surfactant must be nontoxic and compatible with the biological environment, represent stable compounds with CNT, and remain resilient in both the *in-vivo* and *in-vitro* environments [5,84].

Phospholipids, a crucial component of plasma membranes, have generally been biologically compatible and might thus be used effectively in biomedical applications. They are employed as a functionalizing group due to their continued amphiphilia. Non-covalent functionalization can link a hydrophobic portion of the phospholipid to the surface of CNTs, while the polar phosphate group can alternatively be aligned to branched or linear PEG polymers. This method has led to the development of CNT compounds that may be utilized for a variety of biomedical applications, such as bioimaging, biosensing, and targeted DDS, as the CNT based on PEG complexes are much more robust and biocompatible in the biological system [5,85].

5.6   APPLICATION OF CARBON NANOTUBE IN DRUG DELIVERY SYSTEM

Due to their large surface areas, small dimensions, and high aspect ratios, CNTs can conjugate a range of therapeutic compounds. It is generally known that CNTs' needle-like structure and simplicity of adjustable functionalization assist their uptake into target cells. CNTs have consequently been recognized as potential nanocarriers for the transport and administration of drugs, biomolecules, and genes. As a result, a significant proportion of the studies on CNT-based nanocarriers have concentrated on the anticancer DDS. This is because the inherent behavior of the safety of endocytic carriers, such as liposomes, has immensely encouraged the incorporation of CNTs in cancer more than other diseases. The recent advancements in the application of CNTs and CNT-based nanocarriers for oncological and other disease therapeutics are highlighted subsequently.

5.6.1   ONCOLOGICAL APPLICATIONS

The oncological application of CNT is primarily divided into their utilization in cancer diagnosis and treatment. CNTs, with their unique optoelectronic characteristics, have been widely used for cancer detection. Also, other physicochemical properties of CNTs provided novel avenues in the targeted DDS for cancer therapeutics.

5.6.1.1 Carbon nanotubes for cancer diagnosis

Due to their distinctive physical characteristics, CNTs have been frequently employed in bioimaging. To enable NIR (wavelength 700 nm–1400 nm) fluorescence emission, SWCNTs persist in a small band gap of ~1 eV [5]. Additionally, SWCNTs have the capacity to exhibit high Raman scattering resonance, demonstrating their use as Raman probes for bioimaging and biosensing applications [54]. Similarly, CNTs are effective contrasting agents for photoacoustic (PA) imaging since they effectively absorb in the NIR range [86]. In fact, adding metal NPs to defective CNTs makes MRI easier by providing imaging contrast [76].

Fluorescence imaging is an essential biological imaging technique; however, its operational usage has been hampered by the poor penetration level of visible light within tissues [77]. To circumvent this constraint, researchers designed CNT-based fluorescent probes with emission/excitation wavelengths in the NIR range, where biological tissues are visible [87]. The SWCNTs are more suitable for the NIR bioimaging and biosensing application in comparison to the MWCNTs, owing to their superior E11 optical transitions, better optical absorption, and reduced photobleaching. Ghosh et al. (2014) developed an M13-stabilized SWCNTs probe that could accurately identify SPARC-expressing tumor clusters *in-vivo*. To avoid optical scattering and achieve a better cellular immersion impact throughout NIRF imaging, second-window NIR light (NIR-II) was employed in their study as the fluorescence source. The diagnostics findings showed that these NIR2-emitting SWCNTs probes provided exceptional signal-to-noise competitiveness and displayed remarkable precision against the in situ ovarian tumor and the transplanted tumor nodules existent on the interfaces of other peritoneal organs [88].

Further efforts have been made to assemble biodegradable SWCNTs with a high quantum yield. Welsher et al. (2009), for example, adopted a moderate approach of step ultrasonic treatment of SWCNTs with PEG and sodium cholate that could barely inflict significant degradation to the CNTs during the operations. The utilization of CNTs as contrast amplifiers allowed HR microscopy imaging of tumor arteries beneath thick skin since NIR might infiltrate interior tissues despite a minimal auto-fluorescence background. Additionally, while injecting SWCNTs as a NIR-II contrast agent, they conducted fluorescence video imaging of the mouse to further examine the mouse anatomy. The dynamic contrast imaging data examined using primary components assessment showed a significant enhancement in the anatomic precision of the organs. Additionally, they witnessed the migration of SWCNTs across the liver, lungs, spleen, and kidneys in real time. Hence, their investigation proved the significance of CNT-based NIR-II fluorescence imaging [89].

Similar to fluorescence imaging, Raman imaging was also extensively employed for cancer diagnosis. Raman scattering involves the transmission of photons' emission wavelength caused by light excitation. The radial breathing model (RBM) and tangent G-module (TGM), which can be observed with a Raman microscope [90], are two examples of the multiple high Raman peaks that CNTs display as a result of the acute electronic density of states near the van Hove singularities. To investigate the time-dependent variation in NIR fluorescence imaging of colon-26 cancer cells, Sekiyama et al. (2019) developed an epoxide-type oxygen-doped SWCNTs with the alteration of PEG (o-SWCNTs-PEG). The localization of o-SWCNTs-PEG in colon-26 cells was investigated using Raman microscopy. The experiment's findings demonstrated that, in contrast to the first day, the Raman signals generated by the developed nanostructure in colon-26 cells were significantly boosted on the fifth day [91].

Furthermore, the diagnosis of cancer *in-vitro* and *in-vivo* conditions have been successfully achieved through CNTs as an imaging probe for photoacoustic and nuclear magnetic resonance imaging (MRI) techniques. Additionally, CNTs can be used as nano-biosensors in the extremely specific early diagnosis of several cancer types, such as pancreatic cancer, colon cancer, and cervical cancer, when combined with other diagnosis markers [92,93].

5.6.1.2   Carbon nanotubes for cancer therapy

Although chemotherapy is typically used in conjunction with other therapies like radiation and surgery to shrink the quantity and volume of tumors, it may still have detrimental side effects. Since cancer drugs typically have a limited therapeutic window, they are nonspecific to cancerous cells and need higher dosages as cancer cells can develop drug resistance and limit their efficacy [93]. Consequently, there is a substantial need for innovative approaches to delivering anticancer agents selectively to tumors while reducing the side effects and increasing treatment efficacy. This part focuses on the most recent methods for using CNT-based materials as cutting-edge carriers in anticancer therapeutics.

CNTs, with their unique characteristics, have been thoroughly researched for the targeted delivery of drugs in cancer therapy. The intrinsic optical properties of CNTs make them effective activators in phototherapy, in addition to being drug carriers for a variety of anticancer cancer drugs. The versatility of CNTs allows for a wide range of therapeutic uses in the treatment of different malignancies. Many anticancer therapy approaches are currently focused on eradicating tumor cells and the environment in which they thrive. Actively targeting tumor cells can efficiently eradicate their parenchyma, but directly attacking the tumor microenvironment can prevent tumor cells from growing and metastasizing by disrupting their environment, which also kills tumor cells indirectly [92]. Recently, Zhou et al. (2022) synthesized multifunctional and PEGylated MWCNTs for the targeted delivery of the anticancer agent, Doxorubicin (DOX). Adipic acid (AA) was used as a cross-linking agent to bind the targeted ligand of folic acid (FA) to hyperbranched poly-L-lysine (HBPLL). Further, DOX was successfully integrated on the MWCNT-PEG-AA-HBPLL-FA nanocarrier, and the *in-vitro* release of drugs was examined using a UV-Vis spectrophotometer. The *in-vitro* cytotoxicity and anticancer capabilities of DOX-loaded nanocarrier were investigated in the human embryonic kidney (HEK293) and liver cancer (HepG2) cells. The presented nanocarrier demonstrated effective drug loading efficiency, pH-responsive and targeted drug release; this assessment is significant as it can get around some of the drawbacks of traditional cancer chemotherapy, like the simplicity through which obtained nanoparticles attach to cancerous cells receptors, which then quickly enter receptor-mediated endocytosis and deliver the drug to the affected regions. At acidic pH levels, intracellular endosome surroundings showed a significant proportion of drug release rate. The nanoparticles were demonstrated to be substantially cytotoxic to HepG2 cells while very mildly cytotoxic to HEK293 cells [94]. Yu et al. (2016) developed a novel SWCNTs-based DDS for the sustained delivery of Paclitaxel (PTX). To increase the biocompatibility of SWCNTs, chitosan was non-covalently coupled to the walls of SWCNTs. Additionally, biodegradable hyaluronan was incorporated into the outermost layer of chitosan to accomplish the cell-targeting characteristic. The findings demonstrated that PTX release was pH-dependent and improved at lower pH levels (pH 5.5). Intracellular reactive oxygen species (ROS) were significantly reduced in the modified SWCNTs, which might have increased the activation of mitogen-activated protein kinases and substantially encouraged cellular damage. According to the findings of western blotting, A549 cells had a high level of expression of apoptosis-related proteins. Cell viability tests and a lactate dehydrogenase (LDH) release experiment showed that PTX-loaded SWCNTs might damage cell membrane structure, which reduced the viability of the A549 cells [95].

Furthermore, the potential of CNTs for combined cancer therapy was revealed by Wang et al. (2017) [96]. To treat cancer with targeted combination chemophotothermal therapy, they have designed a bifunctional nanoplatform. The nanoplatform was developed using a simple methodology that involved coating the sliced MWCNTs with poly (N-vinyl pyrrole (PVPy). FA-PEG-SH was then coupled to MWCNT@ PVPy via thiol-ene click reaction to enhance the targeted delivery potential, aqueous stability, and biocompatibility, as well as to prolong the time for blood circulation. The PVPy shell dramatically improved the photothermal impact of MWCNTs and offered a substrate that could be customized for drugs and targeting compounds. The resultant MWCNT@ PVPy-S-PEG-FA was capable of pH-sensitive release for the DOX and had a high drug-loading ratio [96].

Recently, González-Domínguez et al. (2022) developed a functionalized SWCNTs nano cellulose platform for colon cancer cells. Folic acid, fluorescein, and capecitabine, a drug routinely used to treat colon cancer, were effectively functionalized into SWCNTs. By using their stimulatory interactions with type-II nanocrystalline cellulose (II-NCC), those functionalized SWCNTs were dissolved in water, and the resultant colloidal solution was evaluated *in-vitro* on both healthy and malignant human colon cells (Caco-2). In comparison to the reference (capecitabine), the functionalized SWCNT/II-NCC hybrids exhibit greater potency against the Caco-2 cancer cell line. Although capecitabine was not necessary, that effect seems to be inherently linked to the SWCNT/II-NCC complex, especially when fluorescein is involved [97]. In addition to the conventional chemotherapeutic application of CNTs via targeted delivery of the anticancer agent, photothermal and magnetic hyperthermia techniques have also attracted the tremendous attention of the research community. In line with this, Radzi et al. (2022) demonstrated breast cancer therapeutic regimens that include the effects of MWCNTs and hyperthermia. In their study, H_2SO_4/HNO_3 (98%/68%) with a 3:1 (v/v) ratio was employed to synthesize acid-functionalized MWCNTs (ox-MWCNTs). Ox-MWCNTs were further administered to mice with EMT6 tumors together with local hyperthermia at 43 °C. Monitoring the tumor development and assessing the impact of the immune system response, the findings of this study showed that mice treated with local hyperthermia and ox-MWCNTs had completely eliminated tumors, and their median survival had increased significantly. Especially compared to the untreated tumor, a combination treatment-treated tumor suffered cell disintegration and had a much lower number of proliferating cells, according to histological and immunohistochemistry analyses of tumor tissues. This finding is corroborated by a rise in Hsp70 expression in hyperthermia-treated tumors. In mice undergoing the combination therapy, flow cytometry assessment of the flowing lymph nodes revealed an upsurge in dendritic cell penetration and growth [98].

Although numerous research outcomes have advocated the use of CNTs for anticancer DDS, their toxicity, biodistribution, bioactivity, and colloidal and storage stability are some of the major concerns that must be addressed for their implementation in a real-world scenario. These challenges can be overcome through the functionalization of CNTs, including SWCNTs and MWCNTs with numerous biocompatible nanocomposites counting dendrimers, liposomes, and biomolecules. Additionally, further efforts must be made to improve the drug loading efficiency, release behavior, and biocompatibility of CNTs through structural and functional modifications.

5.6.2 THERAPEUTICS FOR OTHER DISEASES

The distinct surface characteristics of CNTs with numerous physicochemical characteristics enable their application in several therapeutics for other diseases, such as neurodegenerative diseases and tissue engineering. A diverse group of sporadic or genetic diseases known as neurodegenerative disorders is all characterized by a gradual nervous system failure that results in the degradation of certain central nervous system (CNS) neurons. Parkinson's disease (PD) and Alzheimer's disease (AD) are the most prevalent neurodegenerative diseases [99]. The blood-brain barrier (BBB), which makes it challenging to transfer drugs to the brain, is one reason why there are currently few effective therapies for PD. Guo et al. (2017) have investigated the viability and therapeutic potential of functional SWCNT-PEGs-Lf, which can efficiently transport and release dopamine (DA) to the brain of PD mice. SWCNTs have strong drug-loading and pH-responsive drug-release capabilities and can permeate the cell membrane with remarkable efficiency. Polyethylene glycol (PEG)-coated SWCNTs have the potential to expand the concentration gradient of SWCNTs reaching the brain by extending the circulation time. In their study, aside from an evident lactoferrin-nanoparticle (Lf-NP) buildup in the striatum, which has been identified as the pharmaceutical target location of PD, a dual functionalization of PEG and Lf onto SWCNTs was used, resulting in a particular SWCNT-PEGs-Lf to transport DA. According to the outcomes of *in-vitro* experiments, the activity of PC12 cells greatly rises when 20 mol L^{-1} DA and 100 mol L^{-1} 6-hydroxydopamine (6-OHDA) are deposited onto SWCNT-PEG, and the concentrations of lactate dehydrogenase (LDH) along with ROS significantly decrease [100]. Although the carbon nanotubes, including the SWCNTs and MWCNTs, have been extensively employed for diagnosing PD through electrochemical sensors [97], the literature related to their application in PD treatment is scant.

Alzheimer's disease (AD) is a neurological condition that advances with time. This deadly condition is accompanied by a range of neuropsychiatric symptoms, including behavioral abnormaliti es, cognitive deficits, disruption to everyday activities, and so forth. Medications like donepezil, galantamine, berberine (BRB), and rivastigmine that enhance the concentrations of acetylcholine in the brain tissue are used in the commonly accepted therapy methods for AD patients. It has been shown that transporting neuro-pharmaceutical drugs to the interior microenvironment of brain microglial cells is more successful when done with MWCNTs. MWCNTs have various benefits over SWCNTs, including easier large-scale manufacturing, cheaper production cost, and enhanced chemical stability and drug adsorption potential. To effectively alleviate Alzheimer's disease [101], Lohan et al. (2017) described the comprehensive production of berberine (BRB)-loaded MWCNTs with phospholipid and polysorbate coating (**Figure 5.3**). A central composite design (FCCD) was used for comprehensive optimization using the design of experiments (DoE), and the optimum formulation was selected using the statistical desirability function. The optimized formulation had a size of the particles of 186 nm with 68.6% drug loading and a drug release rate of 96% in 16 hours. Confocal tests confirmed the BRB-loaded MWCNT formulations' propensity to be taken up by SH-SY5Y cell lines. When compared to a pure drug, *in-vivo* pharmacokinetic experiments on rats revealed a considerable improvement in the pace and amount of drug uptake in the plasma and brain tissues. The improved performance effectiveness of the synthesized MWCNT compounds was confirmed by behavioral testing using the Morris maze test. Interestingly, the memory subsystem of the phospholipid-coated and polysorbate-coated MWCNTs significantly improved from the 18th to the 20th day compared to other groups [102].

Another significant neurologic condition brought on by an obstruction in blood supply to the brain is typically referred to as a "stroke." One-sided paralysis, paralysis of the face, arms, or legs, vision issues, a decline in balance and coordination, movement obstructions, and in severe cases, even death, are possible symptoms of the condition. They are often abrupt, occurring from seconds to hours. For the very first time, Lee et al. (2011) demonstrated the neuroprotective potential of CNTs in stroke models. In their investigation, rats were administered with aggregated SWCNTs by transverse ventricular injection. A middle cerebral arterial occlusion (MCAO) treatment to inflict ischemic brain trauma was carried out a week later. The coronal brain segments and cerebral cortex lysate analyses of the rats administered with aggregated SWCNTs revealed minimal impairments and speedy recovery of functions of the nervous system than those of the other groups.

Additionally, compared to the PBS-treated mice, the animals treated with aggregated SWCNT displayed N-cadherin at a greater level (around 1.8-fold). It was discovered that perhaps the N-cadherin cellular adhesion activity is crucial to the entire phenomenon [103]. Further investigation by Moon et al. (2012) showed the potential of hydrophobic CNTs loaded with subventricular zone neural progenitor cells to restore destroyed neural tissue after the stroke. In comparison to control groups, the rat neural progenitor cells functionalized with CNTs showed augmented behavior and a decrease in the volume and size of stroke cysts. The majority of the implanted neural progenitor cells expanded over the ischemia-wounded area and reduced microglia after being modified with CNTs. Their work opened the window for more research on innovative SWCNT-based therapies against ischemic neurological

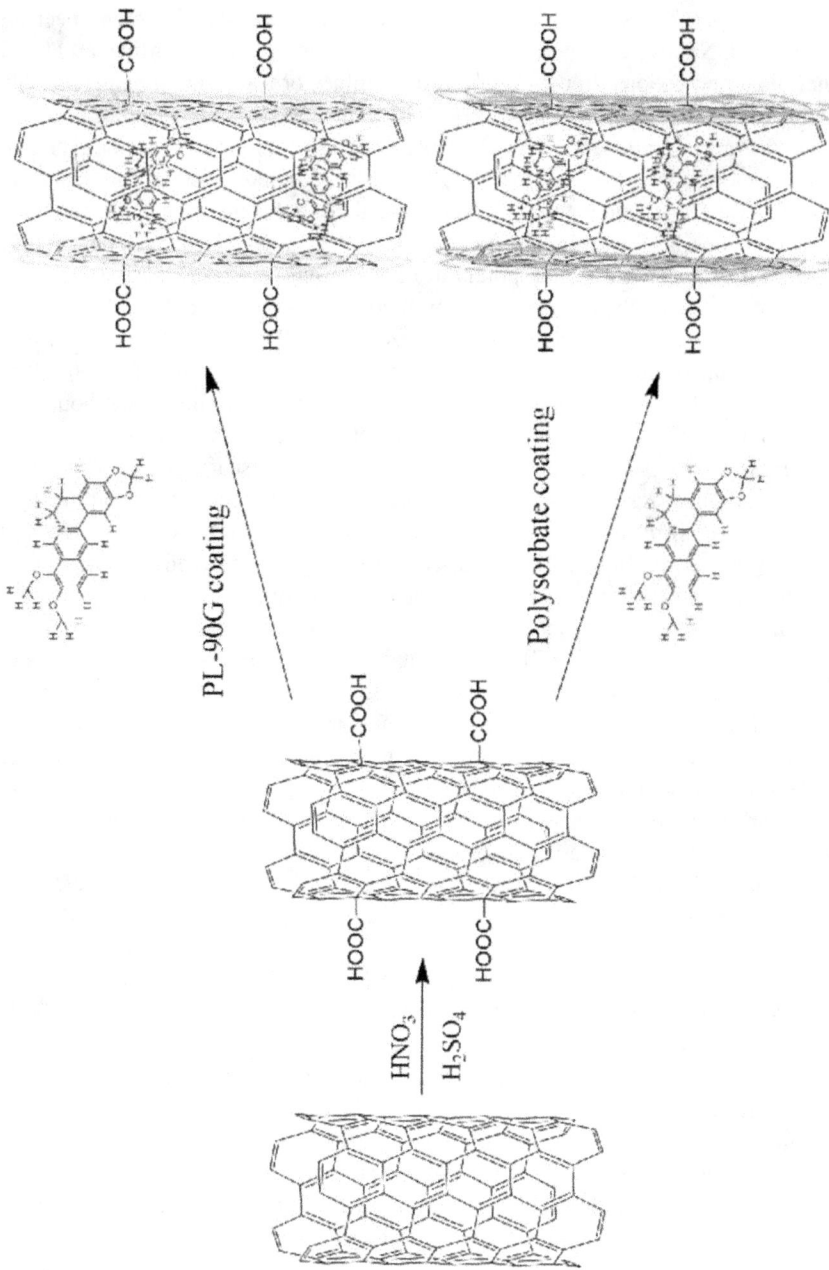

FIGURE 5.3 Synthesis of Phospholipid and Polysorbate-Coated MWCNTs. [Reprinted with permission from *Lohan et al. (2017)*][102].

damage. Nevertheless, again, their study emphasized f-CNTs as potential therapeutic alternatives for stroke [104].

Similar to neurodegenerative diseases, CNTs, with their superior mechanical and chemical properties, have displayed significant potential for tissue engineering applications. CNTs were successfully employed for the neuronal, cardiac, and bone regeneration medications. In the event of minor injury or fracturing, bone is capable of self-healing and remodeling. However, if the bone defects are larger than a threshold size (5 mm) in pathogenic injuries, acute bone attrition, or core tumor excision, bone is no more capable of healing itself [105,106]. Numerous therapies, including xenografts, allografts, and autografts, were described in this instance. Unfortunately, these approaches have significant drawbacks, notably restricted supply and donor site morbidity for autografts, the potential of resistance and transmission of infection for allografts, and the possibility of immunogenicity and poor clinical prognosis for xenografts [106]. Consequently, the utilization of 3D constructs called tissue-engineered synthetic bone scaffolds, which offer the support needed for cell adhesion, growth, and transformation, is a unique and extremely promising method.

Tanaka et al. (2017) designed a 3D block structure out of CNTs and examined its effectiveness in comparison to PET-reinforced gelatin as a scaffold for bone regeneration. Mechanical screening indicated no noticeable differences between the artificial structure and rat femoral bone, with compressive strengths of 62.1 MPa and 61.86 MPa, correspondingly. In comparison to collagen-reinforced PET scaffolds, CNT scaffolds witnessed earlier cell adherence. The addition of recombinant human BMP-2 increased the ALP activity in the CNTs block, demonstrating favorable osteogenesis characteristics [107]. *In-vitro* and *in-vivo* comparisons between CNTs and hydroxyapatite (HA) were also made by Tanaka et al. (2017). According to the findings, CNTs have improved protein release and absorption characteristics. *In-vivo* experiments revealed that the addition of recombinant human BMP-2 increased bone formation, osseointegration, and cell growth in CNT porous frameworks. Several studies have extensively discussed the use of CNTs in conjunction with bioceramics, including hydroxyapatite and bioactive glasses, for bone healing [108]. Khalid et al. (2015) explored MWCNT/HA scaffolding containing diverse CNT loadings (1wt%, 3wt%, and 5wt%). The cytotoxicity of the scaffolds was found to be dose-dependent, and findings involving human osteoblast sarcoma cell lines revealed that the CNT content increased was accompanied by a reduction in cell viability [109]. Jing et al. (2017) adopted a freeze-drying approach to manufacture MWCNT/Col/HA scaffolds by combining MWCNTs with collagen/hydroxyapatite. According to the findings, MWCNT/Col/HA scaffolds were ten times stiffer than Col/HA scaffolds. *In-vitro* studies using bone marrow mesenchymal stem cells (BMSCs) revealed that scaffolds incorporating MWCNTs elevated the proliferative activity, mRNA, and protein transcription of bone sialoprotein (BSP) and osteocalcin (OCN) **(Figure 5.4)** [110].

Similarly, the intercalated discs (IDs) linking the cardiomyocytes are not sufficiently remodeled by existing cardiac tissue engineering techniques. CNTs could help to get around this restriction. A CNT/collagen patch was designed by Sun et al. (2015) to improve intercalated disc formation in cardiac myocytes. A variety of cellular signaling pathways, notably focal adhesion kinase (FAK), integrin-linked kinase (ILK), and Src, are activated in the myocardial by the mechano-transducer

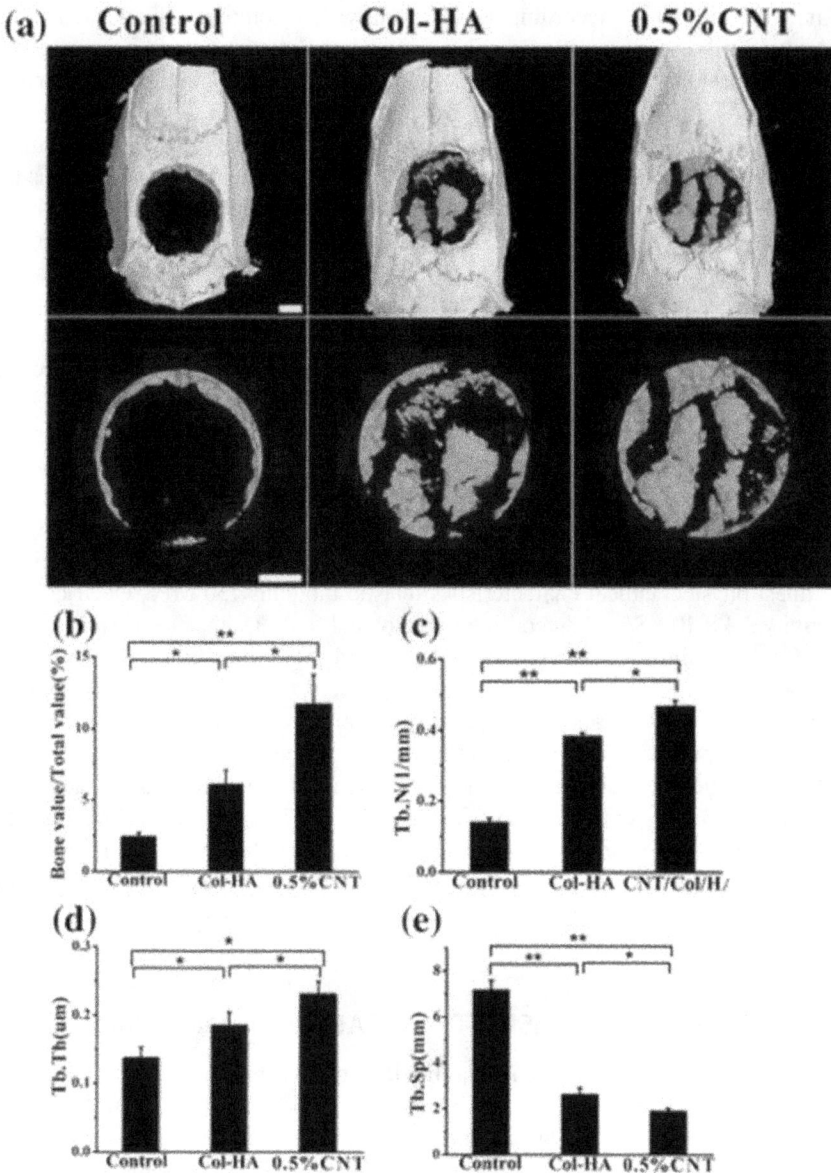

FIGURE 5.4 *In-vivo* Osteogenesis of Col-HA and 0.5%CNT for Rat Calvarial Bone Metastases Obtained After 12 Weeks of Healing: (a) 3D μ-CT Pictures of Bone Growth, (b–e) Quantitative Analysis of Bone Volume/Total Volume (BV/TV) Ratio, Mean Trabecular Number (Tb. N), Mean Trabecular Plate Thickness (Tb. Th), and Mean Trabecular Bone Spacing (Tb. Sp), Respectively. [Reprinted with permission from *Jing et al. (2017)*] [110].

β1-integrin [106,111]. According to the results, the composite platform not just improves cardiomyocyte adherence and growth but also stimulates the production of ID-related proteins while promoting ID generation and functioning. By triggering the FAK/ERK/GATA4 pathway through the β1-integrin, composite scaffolds incorporating CNTs substantially accelerated gap junction development [111]. The primary drawback of employing biopolymeric compounds to heal heart abnormalities is that the insulating walls make it challenging for electrical impulses to transmit through cardiac myocytes, which can result in arrhythmias after implanting the polymers. The previous problem was resolved by Shin et al. (2013) by developing patches for cardiac tissue engineering employing gelatin methacrylate (GelMA) and CNTs. GelMA was initially pre-coated over CNT bunches, then photo-cross-linking was employed to fabricate 50 μm thick CNT-GelMA blended hydrogels. Porous substrates were fabricated and cultivated using newborn rat cardiomyocytes. According to the findings, CNT-GelMA considerably enhanced cell attachment, order, and cell-cell linkage by possessing a threefold greater impulsive heartbeat rate and an 85% reduced excitation limit [112]. Recently, Mombini et al. (2019) synthesized electrospun cardiac conductive scaffolds by employing PVA, chitosan (CS), and distinct amounts of CNTs (1, 3, and 5 wt%). According to the findings, nanofiber with 1 wt.%CNT exhibited the finest physiochemical characteristics (elastic modulus 130 MPa, electrical conductivity 3.4×10^{-6} S/cm). According to biological findings, the electrical activity of a scaffold containing 1 wt.% of CNT has boosted the cardiac biomarker expression of genes [113].

Although CNTs are gaining popularity as reinforcing fillers for biocompatible polymer composites and are frequently utilized in the formation of neural, heart, and bone tissue, there are still a number of significant restrictions; hence additional exploration remains obligatory to fully advance the integration of CNTs into tissue engineering applications and ensure their long-term therapeutic efficacy. In the field of regenerative tissue engineering, developing nontoxic, safe, and environmentally friendly CNTs and associated polymeric nanocomposites still poses significant challenges.

5.7   TOXICOLOGICAL ASPECTS OF CARBON NANOTUBES

CNTs have demonstrated their applicability in numerous biomedical applications due to their distinct physicochemical characteristics. Also, the exposure to CNTs and CNT-based nanocomposites has increased across the population due to the enhancements in their applications in diverse sectors. Although CNTs have numerous applications, "their toxicity" is the key concern that restricts their adoption. The challenge of harmonizing the potential therapeutic impressions of CNTs with the adverse consequences brought on by their toxicity is one that researchers encounter frequently. As a result, the selection of an experimental paradigm, either *in-vitro* or *in-vivo*, must be critical in assessing the toxicity of this nanomaterial [99,114]. The toxicity of CNTs is dependent on numerous factors such as size, surface charge, route of administration, dose concentration, and exposure time. In fact, the incubating conditions, including the exposure dosage, culture period, and type of cell, in addition to the previously mentioned factors, have a direct impact on the toxicity of CNTs [5,99]. The evaluation of the cytotoxicity of CNTs is critical for their *in-vivo* biological applications. *In-vitro* tests primarily examined cell uptake, cell viability, and ROS. The size, shape, dose, and surface properties of carbon nanomaterials are all strongly correlated with their cytotoxicity. In line with this, Zhang et al. (2012) examined the effects of MWCNTs, nanodiamonds (ND), and graphene oxide (GO) on HeLa cellular uptake and toxicity. The sequence of the three different types of carbon nanomaterials' cellular uptake ratios was ND > MWCNTs > GO. The cytotoxicity of these substances, however, did not correlate well with the cellular uptake ratios. Despite MWCNTs having a greater cellular uptake than GO, no discernible variations in their cytotoxicity were detected. Compared to MWCNTs and GO, ND demonstrated superior biocompatibility. Studies have shown that the mass basis and doses have a significant impact on the cytotoxicity of CNTs, and SWCNTs are considered to be more toxic than MWCNTs [115]. Yuan et al. (2011) investigated the cell viability of HepG2 fibroblasts exposed to SWCNTs and graphene. The outcomes demonstrated that SWCNTs had a greater level of cytotoxicity, were perhaps able to cause oxidative stress, and ultimately induced apoptosis by turning on P53-mediated degradation [116].

After cytotoxicity investigation, toxicology investigation *in-vivo* is critical in validating the biocompatibility of CNTs. To thoroughly comprehend the dynamic behaviors and biocompatibility of nanomaterials *in-vivo*, biomedical studies frequently use animal models, including mice, zebrafish, and rats. To increase the biocompatibility of CNTs, some researchers have functionalized CNTs through biocompatible polymers and other biosafety compounds [99]. Liu et al. (2007) employed positron emission tomography to investigate the *in-vivo* bioavailability of SWCNTs conjugated with more compatible and hydrophilic PEG. Long blood circulation periods and minimal absorption in the reticuloendothelial system were observed in the PEG-functionalized SWCNTs. Mice did not exhibit adverse effects, including weight loss or weariness, and no evident toxicity-related circumstances were discovered [117]. Even though it was previously established that SWCNTs seemed to have a high level of cytotoxicity, Xue et al. (2016) discovered that aggregated SWCNTs effectively reduced the behavioral and neurochemical consequences of methamphetamine in mice. It is important to note that, at the dosage levels used during the study, the striatum and midbrain showed no evidence of neuronal toxicity or a substantial change in the activities of mice, like eating, drinking, and movement [118].

Although there have been numerous attempts to increase the biocompatibility of CNTs, the propensity for oxidative stress, production of free radicals, buildup of peroxidative products, DNA fragmentation, and inflammation remain barriers to the widespread prospect of CNTs in the treatment of neurological diseases. The main concern regarding using CNTs as an intrinsic drug for neurological disorder therapies is their safety, particularly brain breakdown and expulsion. To increase the brain's breakdown and expulsion of CNTs, the functionalization of CNTs deserves a significant amount of attention.

5.8 SUMMARY

In this chapter, we have addressed the potential applications of CNTs as nano-carriers for therapeutic drugs in oncological, neurological, and tissue engineering applications. The unique characteristics and great potential of CNTs in cancer diagnosis and treatment, as well as tissue and cardiovascular tissue engineering, were emphasized based on all the studies described previously. Oncological and neurological ailments are a collection of tumor development and CNS disorders that impact the functioning of the human body, specifically the lungs and brain, respectively. The compelling functionalities of CNTs make them good candidates for their adoption in the treatment of cancer and neurodegenerative diseases. To enhance the surface and physicochemical properties of CNTs, several functionalization strategies have been explored in the present chapter to outline the structure and properties of CNTs, as well as recent advancements in CNT synthesis using CVD, arc discharge, laser ablation, and flame synthesis methods. It has been noted that the variety of CNTs' sizes, structures, and functionalized forms leads to a multitude of alterations in their physical, biological, chemical, and optoelectronic properties. It was observed that CNTs, including SWCNTs and MWCNTs, with their variable size and physicochemical properties, have provided significant advantages for drug delivery. However, for their large-scale production and commercial usage, these formulations' toxicity still has to be improved. The biocompatibility of CNT-based nanocomposites can be improved by using numerous biomolecules that need to be investigated for their application.

REFERENCES

[1] W. Zhang, Z. Zhang, Y. Zhang, The application of carbon nanotubes in target drug delivery systems for cancer therapies, Nanoscale Res. Lett. (2011) 1–22.

[2] A. Eatemadi, H. Daraee, H. Karimkhanloo, M. Kouhi, N. Zarghami, A. Akbarzadeh, M. Abasi, Y. Hanifehpour, S.W. Joo, Carbon nanotubes: Properties, synthesis, purification, and medical applications, Nanoscale Res. Lett. 9 (2014) 393. doi:10.1186/1556-276X-9-393.

[3] S. Iijima, T. Ichihashi, Single-shell carbon nanotubes of 1-nm diameter, Nature. 363 (1993) 603–605. doi:10.1038/363603a0.

[4] S. Iijima, Helical microtubules of graphitic carbon, Nature. 354 (1991) 56–58. doi:10.1038/354056a0.

[5] R. Jha, A. Singh, P.K. Sharma, N.K. Fuloria, Smart carbon nanotubes for drug delivery system: A comprehensive study, J. Drug Deliv. Sci. Technol. 58 (2020) 101811. doi:10.1016/j.jddst.2020.101811.

[6] M. Lamberti, P. Pedata, N. Sannolo, S. Porto, A. De Rosa, M. Caraglia, Carbon nanotubes: Properties, biomedical applications, advantages and risks in patients and occupationally-exposed workers, Int. J. Immunopathol. Pharmacol. 28 (2015) 4–13. doi:10.1177/0394632015572559.

[7] H. Zare, S. Ahmadi, A. Ghasemi, M. Ghanbari, N. Rabiee, M. Bagherzadeh, M. Karimi, T.J. Webster, M.R. Hamblin, E. Mostafavi, Carbon Nanotubes: Smart drug/gene delivery carriers, Int. J. Nanomedicine. 16 (2021) 1681–1706. doi:10.2147/IJN.S299448.

[8] S. Beg, M. Rizwan, A.M. Sheikh, M.S. Hasnain, K. Anwer, K. Kohli, Advancement in carbon nanotubes: Basics, biomedical applications and toxicity, J. Pharm. Pharmacol. 63 (2011) 141–163. doi:10.1111/j.2042-7158.2010.01167.x.

[9] M.S. Dresselhaus, G. Dresselhaus, J.C. Charlier, E. Hernández, Electronic, thermal and mechanical properties of carbon nanotubes, Philos. Trans. R. Soc. London. Ser. A Math. Phys. Eng. Sci. 362 (2004) 2065–2098. doi:10.1098/rsta.2004.1430.

[10] X. Zhang, J. Ma, H. Tennent, R. Hoch, Method for Preparing Single Walled Carbon Nanotubes (2012). https://patents.justia.com/patent/8287836.

[11] N. Grobert, Carbon nanotubes—becoming clean, Mater. Today. 10 (2007) 28–35. doi:10.1016/S1369-7021(06)71789-8.

[12] R.L. Vander Wal, G.M. Berger, T.M. Ticich, Carbon nanotube synthesis in a flame using laser ablation for in situ catalyst generation, Appl. Phys. A Mater. Sci. Process. 77 (2003) 885–889. doi:10.1007/s00339-003-2196-3.

[13] A. Aqel, K.M.M.A. El-Nour, R.A.A. Ammar, A. Al-Warthan, Carbon nanotubes, science and technology part (I) structure, synthesis and characterisation, Arab. J. Chem. 5 (2012) 1–23. doi:10.1016/j.arabjc.2010.08.022.

[14] J.W. Seo, A. Magrez, M. Milas, K. Lee, V. Lukovac, L. Forró, Catalytically grown carbon nanotubes: From synthesis to toxicity, J. Phys. D Appl. Phys. 40 (2007) R109. doi:10.1088/0022-3727/40/6/R01.

[15] G. Rahman, Z. Najaf, A. Mehmood, S. Bilal, A. Shah, S. Mian, G. Ali, An overview of the recent progress in the synthesis and applications of carbon nanotubes, Carbon. 5 (2019) 3. doi:10.3390/c5010003.

[16] T.W. Ebbesen, P.M. Ajayan, Large-scale synthesis of carbon nanotubes, Nature. 358 (1992) 220–222. doi:10.1038/358220a0.

[17] Y. Li, D. Mann, M. Rolandi, W. Kim, A. Ural, S. Hung, A. Javey, J. Cao, D. Wang, E. Yenilmez, Q. Wang, J.F. Gibbons, Y. Nishi, H. Dai, Preferential growth of semiconducting single-walled carbon nanotubes by a plasma enhanced CVD method, Nano Lett. 4 (2004) 317–321. doi:10.1021/nl035097c.

[18] H. Dai, Carbon nanotubes: Opportunities and challenges, Surf. Sci. 500 (2002) 218–241. doi:10.1016/S0039-6028(01)01558-8.

[19] B.J. Landi, R.P. Raffaelle, S.L. Castro, S.G. Bailey, Single-wall carbon nanotube-polymer solar cells, Prog. Photovoltaics Res. Appl. 13 (2005) 165–172. doi:10.1002/pip.604.

[20] P.C. Eklund, B.K. Pradhan, U.J. Kim, Q. Xiong, J.E. Fischer, A.D. Friedman, B.C. Holloway, K. Jordan, M.W. Smith, Large-scale production of single-walled carbon nanotubes using ultrafast pulses from a free electron laser, Nano Lett. 2 (2002) 561–566. doi:10.1021/nl025515y.

[21] S.A. Steiner III, T.F. Baumann, B.C. Bayer, R. Blume, M.A. Worsley, W.J. Moberly-Chan, E.L. Shaw, R. Schlögl, A.J. Hart, S. Hofmann, B.L. Wardle, Nanoscale zirconia as a nonmetallic catalyst for graphitization of carbon and growth of single- and multiwall carbon nanotubes, J. Am. Chem. Soc. 131 (2009) 12144–12154. doi:10.1021/ja902913r.

[22] H. Tempel, R. Joshi, J.J. Schneider, Ink jet printing of ferritin as method for selective catalyst patterning and growth of multiwalled carbon nanotubes, Mater. Chem. Phys. 121 (2010) 178–183. doi:10.1016/j.matchemphys.2010.01.029.

[23] W. Khan, R. Sharma, P. Saini, Carbon Nanotube-Based Polymer Composites: Synthesis, Properties and Applications, M.R. Berber, I.H. Hafez (Eds.), InTech, Rijeka (2016): Ch. 1. doi:10.5772/62497.

[24] J. Namdeo, M.D. Shah, N. Karthik, S. Pramod, N.M. Bhatia, Methods of carbon nanotube and nanohorn synthesis: A review, Pharm. Inf. 5 (2007).

[25] R.L. Vander Wal, G.M. Berger, L.J. Hall, Single-walled carbon nanotube synthesis via a multi-stage flame configuration, J. Phys. Chem. B. 106 (2002) 3564–3567. doi:10.1021/jp012844q.

[26] M. Ishigami, J. Cumings, A. Zettl, S. Chen, A simple method for the continuous production of carbon nanotubes, Chem. Phys. Lett. 319 (2000) 457–459. doi:10.1016/S0009-2614(00)00151-2.

[27] C. Journet, P. Bernier, Production of carbon nanotubes, Appl. Phys. A Mater. Sci. Process. 67 (1998) 1–9. doi:10.1007/s003390050731.

[28] B.K. Kaushik, M.K. Majumder, B.K. Kaushik, M.K. Majumder, Carbon nanotube: Properties and applications, Carbon Nanotub. Based VLSI Interconnects Anal. Des. (2015) 17–37.

[29] S.B. Sinnott, R. Andrews, Carbon nanotubes: Synthesis, properties, and applications, Crit. Rev. Solid State Mater. Sci. 26 (2001) 145–249. doi:10.1080/20014091104189.

[30] A. Thess, R. Lee, P. Nikolaev, H. Dai, P. Petit, J. Robert, C. Xu, Y.H. Lee, S.G. Kim, A.G. Rinzler, D.T. Colbert, G.E. Scuseria, D. Tománek, J.E. Fischer, R.E. Smalley, Crystalline ropes of metallic carbon nanotubes, Sci. 273 (1996) 483–487. doi:10.1126/science.273.5274.483.

[31] E. Muñoz, W.K. Maser, A.M. Benito, G.F. de la Fuente, M.T. Martínez, Single-walled carbon nanotubes produced by laser ablation under different inert atmospheres, Synth. Met. 103 (1999) 2490–2491. doi:10.1016/S0379-6779(98)01082-0.

[32] R. Hirlekar, M. Yamagar, H. Garse, V. Mohit, V. Kadam, Carbon nanotubes and its applications: A review, Asian J. Pharm. Clin. Res. 2 (2009) 17–27.

[33] G. Dresselhaus, M.S. Dresselhaus, R. Saito, Physical Properties of Carbon Nanotubes, World Scientific, London (1998).

[34] T. Yamaguchi, S. Bandow, S. Iijima, Synthesis of carbon nanohorn particles by simple pulsed arc discharge ignited between pre-heated carbon rods, Chem. Phys. Lett. 389 (2004) 181–185. doi:10.1016/j.cplett.2004.03.068.

[35] H. Wang, M. Chhowalla, N. Sano, S. Jia, G.A.J. Amaratunga, Large-scale synthesis of single-walled carbon nanohorns by submerged arc, Nanotechnol. 15 (2004) 546.

[36] K. Anazawa, K. Shimotani, C. Manabe, H. Watanabe, M. Shimizu, High-purity carbon nanotubes synthesis method by an arc discharging in magnetic field, Appl. Phys. Lett. 81 (2002) 739–741.

[37] M. Wang, X. Zhao, M. Ohkohchi, Y. Ando, Carbon nanotubes grown on the surface of cathode deposit by arc discharge, Fuller. Sci. Technol. 4 (1996) 1027–1039.

[38] R.L. Vander Wal, T.M. Ticich, Flame and furnace synthesis of single-walled and multi-walled carbon nanotubes and nanofibers, J. Phys. Chem. B. 105 (2001) 10249–10256.

[39] J. Chen, X. Gao, Recent advances in the flame synthesis of carbon nanotubes, Am. J. Mater. Synth. Process. 2 (2017) 71–89.

[40] W. Merchan-Merchan, A. V Saveliev, L. Kennedy, W.C. Jimenez, Combustion synthesis of carbon nanotubes and related nanostructures, Prog. Energy Combust. Sci. 36 (2010) 696–727.

[41] Z. Xu, H. Zhao, Simultaneous measurement of internal and external properties of nanoparticles in flame based on thermophoresis, Combust. Flame. 162 (2015) 2200–2213.

[42] M.S. Digge, R.S. Moon, S.G. Gattani, Applications of carbon nanotubes in drug delivery: A review, Int. J. PharmTech Res. 4 (2012) 839–847.

[43] T.W. Ebbesen, Carbon Nanotubes: Preparation and Properties, CRC Press, Boca Raton (1996).

[44] A. Bougrine, A. Naji, J. Ghanbaja, D. Billaud, Purification and structural characterization of single-walled carbon nanotubes, Synth. Met. 103 (1999) 2480–2481. doi:10.1016/S0379-6779(98)01064-9.

[45] L. Vaisman, H.D. Wagner, G. Marom, The role of surfactants in dispersion of carbon nanotubes, Adv. Colloid Interface Sci. 128–130 (2006) 37–46. doi:10.1016/j.cis.2006.11.007.

[46] K. MacKenzie, O. Dunens, A.T. Harris, A review of carbon nanotube purification by microwave assisted acid digestion, Sep. Purif. Technol. 66 (2009) 209–222. doi:10.1016/j.seppur.2009.01.017.

[47] M. Ghaedi, S. Hajati, M. Zaree, Y. Shajaripour, A. Asfaram, M.K. Purkait, Removal of methyl orange by multiwall carbon nanotube accelerated by ultrasound devise: Optimized experimental design, Adv. Powder Technol. 26 (2015) 1087–1093. doi:10.1016/j.apt.2015.05.002.

[48] S. Bandow, A.M. Rao, K.A. Williams, A. Thess, R.E. Smalley, P.C. Eklund, Purification of single-wall carbon nanotubes by microfiltration, J. Phys. Chem. B. 101 (1997) 8839–8842. doi:10.1021/jp972026r.

[49] R. Singh, V. Volli, L. Lohani, M.K. Purkait, Synthesis of carbon nanotubes from indus-
     trial wastes following alkali activation and film casting method, Waste Biomass Valori.
     11 (2020) 4957–4966. doi:10.1007/s12649-019-00827-2.

[50] R. Singh, V. Volli, L. Lohani, M.K. Purkait, Polymeric ultrafiltration membranes mod-
     ified with fly ash based carbon nanotubes for thermal stability and protein separation,
     Case Stud. Chem. Environ. Eng. 4 (2021) 100155. doi:10.1016/j.cscee.2021.100155.

[51] E. Borowiak-Palen, T. Pichler, X. Liu, M. Knupfer, A. Graff, O. Jost, W. Pompe,
     R. Kalenczuk, J. Fink, Reduced diameter distribution of single-wall carbon nano-
     tubes by selective oxidation, Chem. Phys. Lett. 363 (2002) 567–572. doi:10.1016/
     S0009-2614(02)01253-8.

[52] E. Farkas, M. Elizabeth Anderson, Z. Chen, A.G. Rinzler, Length sorting cut single wall
     carbon nanotubes by high performance liquid chromatography, Chem. Phys. Lett. 363
     (2002) 111–116. doi:10.1016/S0009-2614(02)01203-4.

[53] K.A. Shiral Fernando, Y. Lin, Y.-P. Sun, High aqueous solubility of functionalized
     single-walled carbon nanotubes, Langmuir. 20 (2004) 4777–4778. doi:10.1021/la036217z.

[54] W. Yang, P. Thordarson, J.J. Gooding, S.P. Ringer, F. Braet, Carbon nanotubes for bio-
     logical and biomedical applications, Nanotechnol. 18 (2007) 412001.

[55] V. Georgakilas, K. Kordatos, M. Prato, D.M. Guldi, M. Holzinger, A. Hirsch, Organic
     functionalization of carbon nanotubes, J. Am. Chem. Soc. 124 (2002) 760–761.
     doi:10.1021/ja016954m.

[56] J.-H. Kim, B.-G. Min, Functionalization of multi-walled carbon nanotube by treatment
     with dry ozone gas for the enhanced dispersion and adhesion in polymeric composites,
     Carbon Lett. 11 (2010) 298–303. doi:10.5714/cl.2010.11.4.298.

[57] S. Mallakpour, S. Soltanian, Surface functionalization of carbon nanotubes: Fabrication
     and applications, RSC Adv. 6 (2016) 109916–109935. doi:10.1039/c6ra24522f.

[58] Z. Chen, W. Thiel, A. Hirsch, Reactivity of the convex and concave surfaces of single-walled
     carbon nanotubes (SWCNTs) towards addition reactions: Dependence on the carbon-atom
     pyramidalization, ChemPhysChem. 4 (2003) 93–97. doi:10.1002/cphc.200390015.

[59] J. Tour, J. Hudson, C. Dyke, J. Stephenson, Functionalization of Carbon Nanotubes in
     Acidic Media, U.S. Patent Application, 2007/0280876 (2007).

[60] L. Zeng, L.B. Alemany, C.L. Edwards, A.R. Barron, Demonstration of covalent sidewall
     functionalization of single wall carbon nanotubes by NMR spectroscopy: Side chain
     length dependence on the observation of the sidewall sp3 carbons, Nano Res. 1 (2008)
     72–88. doi:10.1007/s12274-008-8004-9.

[61] M.L. Schipper, N. Nakayama-Ratchford, C.R. Davis, N.W.S. Kam, P. Chu, Z. Liu, X.
     Sun, H. Dai, S.S. Gambhir, A pilot toxicology study of single-walled carbon nano-
     tubes in a small sample of mice, Nat. Nanotechnol. 3 (2008) 216–221. doi:10.1038/
     nnano.2008.68.

[62] N.K. Mehra, N.K. Jain, Multifunctional hybrid-carbon nanotubes: New horizon in
     drug delivery and targeting, J. Drug Target. 24 (2016) 294–308. doi:10.3109/10611
     86X.2015.1055571.

[63] V. Khabashesku, E. Barrera, D. McIntosh, L. Para-Pena, Carbon Nanotube Reinforced
     Thermoplastic Polymer Composites Achieved Through Benzoyl Peroxide Initiated
     Interfacial Bonding to Polymer Matrices, U.S. Patent Application, 2007/0099792
     A (2007).

[64] K.M. Lee, L. Li, L. Dai, Asymmetric end-functionalization of multi-walled carbon
     nanotubes, J. Am. Chem. Soc. 127 (2005) 4122–4123. doi:10.1021/ja0423670.

[65] M.J. Moghaddam, S. Taylor, M. Gao, S. Huang, L. Dai, M.J. McCall, Highly efficient
     binding of DNA on the sidewalls and tips of carbon nanotubes using photochemistry,
     Nano Lett. 4 (2004) 89–93. doi:10.1021/nl034915y.

[66] N. Tagmatarchis, M. Prato, Functionalization of carbon nanotubes via 1,3-dipolar
     cycloadditions, J. Mater. Chem. (2004) 437–439. doi:10.1039/b314039c.

[67] N.G. Sahoo, S. Rana, J.W. Cho, L. Li, S.H. Chan, Polymer nanocomposites based on functionalized carbon nanotubes, Prog. Polym. Sci. 35 (2010) 837–867. doi:10.1016/j. progpolymsci.2010.03.002.

[68] W.T. Ford, S. Qin, Polymers Grafted to Carbon Nanotubes, US 7.414,088 B1 (2008). https://hdl.handle.net/11244/15399.

[69] E.V. Barrera, R. Wilkins, M. Shofner, M.X. Pulikkathara, R. Vaidyanathan, Functionalized Carbon Nanotube-Polymer Composites and Interactions with Radiation, 8,809,979 B2 (2014). https://hdl.handle.net/1911/80164.

[70] A.M. Díez-Pascual, Chemical functionalization of carbon nanotubes with polymers: A brief overview, Macromol. 1 (2021) 64–83. doi:10.3390/macromol1020006.

[71] Y. Zhang, Q. Li, W. Wang, A. Guo, J. Li, H. Li, Efficient and robust reactions for polyethylene covalently grafted carbon nanotubes, Macromol. Chem. Phys. 218 (2017) 1600449. doi:10.1002/macp.201600449.

[72] D. Baskaran, J.R. Dunlap, J.W. Mays, M.S. Bratcher, Grafting efficiency of hydroxy-terminated poly(methyl methacrylate) with multiwalled carbon nanotubes, Macromol. Rapid Commun. 26 (2005) 481–486. doi:10.1002/marc.200400546.

[73] R. Lucente-Schultz, V. Moore, A. Leonard, K. Price, D. Kosynkin, M. Lu, R. Partha, J. Conyers, J. Tour, Antioxidant single walled carbon nanotubes: Departments of chemistry and mechanical engineering and materials science, Smalley Inst. Nanoscale Sci. Technol. 131 (2009).

[74] J. Zhu, M. Yudasaka, M. Zhang, S. Iijima, Dispersing carbon nanotubes in water: A noncovalent and nonorganic way, J. Phys. Chem. B. 108 (2004) 11317–11320. doi:10.1021/ jp0494032.

[75] V. Georgakilas, V. Tzitzios, D. Gournis, D. Petridis, Attachment of magnetic nanoparticles on carbon nanotubes and their soluble derivatives, Chem. Mater. 17 (2005) 1613–1617. doi:10.1021/cm0483590.

[76] A. Hirsch, Functionalization of single-walled carbon nanotubes, Angew. Chemie Int. Ed. 41 (2002) 1853. doi:10.1002/1521-3773(20020603)41:11<853::AID-ANIE1853> 3.0.CO;2-N.

[77] P. Bilalis, D. Katsigiannopoulos, A. Avgeropoulos, G. Sakellariou, Non-covalent functionalization of carbon nanotubes with polymers, RSC Adv. 4 (2014) 2911–2934. doi:10.1039/c3ra44906h.

[78] M.I. Sajid, U. Jamshaid, T. Jamshaid, N. Zafar, H. Fessi, A. Elaissari, Carbon nanotubes from synthesis to in vivo biomedical applications, Int. J. Pharm. 501 (2016) 278–299. doi:10.1016/j.ijpharm.2016.01.064.

[79] M. Foldvari, M. Bagonluri, Carbon nanotubes as functional excipients for nanomedicines: I. Pharmaceutical properties, Nanomed. Nanotechnol. Biol. Med. 4 (2008) 173–182. doi:10.1016/j.nano.2008.04.002.

[80] H.K. Moon, C. Il Chang, D.-K. Lee, H.C. Choi, Effect of nucleases on the cellular internalization of fluorescent labeled DNA-functionalized single-walled carbon nanotubes, Nano Res. 1 (2008) 351–360. doi:10.1007/s12274-008-8038-z.

[81] C.A. Mitchell, J.L. Bahr, S. Arepalli, J.M. Tour, R. Krishnamoorti, Dispersion of functionalized carbon nanotubes in polystyrene, Macromol. 35 (2002) 8825–8830. doi:10.1021/ma020890y.

[82] V.C. Moore, M.S. Strano, E.H. Haroz, R.H. Hauge, R.E. Smalley, J. Schmidt, Y. Talmon, Individually suspended single-walled carbon nanotubes in various surfactants, Nano Lett. 3 (2003) 1379–1382. doi:10.1021/nl034524j.

[83] M.J. O'Connell, S.M. Bachilo, C.B. Huffman, V.C. Moore, M.S. Strano, E.H. Haroz, K.L. Rialon, P.J. Boul, W.H. Noon, C. Kittrell, J. Ma, R.H. Hauge, R.B. Weisman, R.E. Smalley, Band gap fluorescence from individual single-walled carbon nanotubes, Sci. 297 (2002) 593–596. doi:10.1126/science.1072631.

[84] Z. Liu, K. Chen, C. Davis, S. Sherlock, Q. Cao, X. Chen, H. Dai, Drug delivery with carbon nanotubes for in vivo cancer treatment, Cancer Res. 68 (2008) 6652–6660. doi:10.1158/0008-5472.CAN-08-1468.

[85] K. Welsher, Z. Liu, D. Daranciang, H. Dai, Selective probing and imaging of cells with single walled carbon nanotubes as near-infrared fluorescent molecules, Nano Lett. 8 (2008) 586–590. doi:10.1021/nl072949q.

[86] A. Figarol, J. Pourchez, D. Boudard, V. Forest, J.M. Tulliani, J.P. Lecompte, M. Cottier, D. Bernache-Assollant, P. Grosseau, Biological response to purification and acid functionalization of carbon nanotubes, J. Nanoparticle Res. 16 (2014). doi:10.1007/s11051-014-2507-y.

[87] J. Chen, H. Liu, W.A. Weimer, M.D. Halls, D.H. Waldeck, G.C. Walker, Noncovalent engineering of carbon nanotube surfaces by rigid, functional conjugated polymers, J. Am. Chem. Soc. 124 (2002) 9034–9035. doi:10.1021/ja026104m.

[88] D. Ghosh, A.F. Bagley, Y.J. Na, M.J. Birrer, S.N. Bhatia, A.M. Belcher, Deep, noninvasive imaging and surgical guidance of submillimeter tumors using targeted M13-stabilized single-walled carbon nanotubes, Proc. Natl. Acad. Sci. 111 (2014) 13948–13953. doi:10.1073/pnas.1400821111.

[89] K. Welsher, Z. Liu, S.P. Sherlock, J.T. Robinson, Z. Chen, D. Daranciang, H. Dai, A route to brightly fluorescent carbon nanotubes for near-infrared imaging in mice, Nat. Nanotechnol. 4 (2009) 773–780. doi:10.1038/nnano.2009.294.

[90] Z. Liu, S. Tabakman, K. Welsher, H. Dai, Carbon nanotubes in biology and medicine: In vitro and in vivo detection, imaging and drug delivery, Nano Res. 2 (2009) 85–120. doi:10.1007/s12274-009-9009-8.

[91] S. Sekiyama, M. Umezawa, Y. Iizumi, T. Ube, T. Okazaki, M. Kamimura, K. Soga, Delayed increase in near-infrared fluorescence in cultured murine cancer cells labeled with oxygen-doped single-walled carbon nanotubes, Langmuir. 35 (2019) 831–837. doi:10.1021/acs.langmuir.8b03789.

[92] L. Tang, Q. Xiao, Y. Mei, S. He, Z. Zhang, R. Wang, W. Wang, Insights on functionalized carbon nanotubes for cancer theranostics, J. Nanobiotechnol. 19 (2021) 423. doi:10.1186/s12951-021-01174-y.

[93] Y. Hwang, S.-H. Park, J. Lee, Applications of functionalized carbon nanotubes for the therapy and diagnosis of cancer, Polymers (Basel). 9 (2017) 13. doi:10.3390/polym9010013.

[94] Y. Zhou, K. Vinothini, F. Dou, Y. Jing, A.A. Chuturgoon, T. Arumugam, M. Rajan, Hyper-branched multifunctional carbon nanotubes carrier for targeted liver cancer therapy, Arab. J. Chem. 15 (2022) 103649. doi:10.1016/j.arabjc.2021.103649.

[95] B. Yu, L. Tan, R. Zheng, H. Tan, L. Zheng, Targeted delivery and controlled release of Paclitaxel for the treatment of lung cancer using single-walled carbon nanotubes, Mater. Sci. Eng. C. 68 (2016) 579–584. doi:10.1016/j.msec.2016.06.025.

[96] D. Wang, Y. Ren, Y. Shao, D. Yu, L. Meng, Facile preparation of doxorubicin-loaded and folic acid-conjugated carbon nanotubes@Poly(N-vinyl pyrrole) for targeted synergistic chemo–photothermal cancer treatment, Bioconjug. Chem. 28 (2017) 2815–2822. doi:10.1021/acs.bioconjchem.7b00515.

[97] J.M. González-Domínguez, L. Grasa, J. Frontiñán-Rubio, E. Abás, A. Domínguez-Alfaro, J.E. Mesonero, A. Criado, A. Ansón-Casaos, Intrinsic and selective activity of functionalized carbon nanotube/nanocellulose platforms against colon cancer cells, Colloids Surf. B Biointerfaces. 212 (2022) 112363. doi:10.1016/j.colsurfb.2022.112363.

[98] M.R.M. Radzi, N.A. Johari, W.F.A.W.M. Zawawi, N.A. Zawawi, N.A. Latiff, N.A.N.N. Malek, A.A. Wahab, M.I. Salim, K. Jemon, In vivo evaluation of oxidized multiwalled-carbon nanotubes-mediated hyperthermia treatment for breast cancer, Biomater. Adv. 134 (2022) 112586. doi:10.1016/j.msec.2021.112586.

[99] C. Xiang, Y. Zhang, W. Guo, X.-J. Liang, Biomimetic carbon nanotubes for neurologi-
      cal disease therapeutics as inherent medication, Acta Pharm. Sin. B. 10 (2020) 239–248.
      doi:10.1016/j.apsb.2019.11.003.

[100] Q. Guo, H. You, X. Yang, B. Lin, Z. Zhu, Z. Lu, X. Li, Y. Zhao, L. Mao, S. Shen, H.
      Cheng, J. Zhang, L. Deng, J. Fan, Z. Xi, R. Li, C.M. Li, Functional single-walled carbon
      nanotubes 'CAR' for targeting dopamine delivery into the brain of parkinsonian mice,
      Nanoscale. 9 (2017) 10832–10845. doi:10.1039/C7NR02682J.

[101] J. Cummings, P.S. Aisen, B. DuBois, L. Frölich, C.R. Jack, R.W. Jones, J.C. Morris, J.
      Raskin, S.A. Dowsett, P. Scheltens, Drug development in Alzheimer's disease: The path
      to 2025, Alzheimers. Res. Ther. 8 (2016) 39. doi:10.1186/s13195-016-0207-9.

[102] S. Lohan, K. Raza, S.K. Mehta, G.K. Bhatti, S. Saini, B. Singh, Anti-Alzheimer's poten-
      tial of berberine using surface decorated multi-walled carbon nanotubes: A preclinical
      evidence, Int. J. Pharm. 530 (2017) 263–278. doi:10.1016/j.ijpharm.2017.07.080.

[103] H.J. Lee, J. Park, O.J. Yoon, H.W. Kim, D.Y. Lee, D.H. Kim, W.B. Lee, N.-E. Lee, J. V.
      Bonventre, S.S. Kim, Amine-modified single-walled carbon nanotubes protect neurons
      from injury in a rat stroke model, Nat. Nanotechnol. 6 (2011) 121–125. doi:10.1038/
      nnano.2010.281.

[104] T.J. Webster, Lee, Khang, Kim, Moon, Kim, Bokara, Carbon nanotubes impregnated
      with subventricular zone neural progenitor cells promotes recovery from stroke, Int. J.
      Nanomed. 7 (2012) 2751. doi:10.2147/IJN.S30273.

[105] J. Lee, M.M. Farag, E.K. Park, J. Lim, H. Yun, A simultaneous process of 3D mag-
      nesium phosphate scaffold fabrication and bioactive substance loading for hard tissue
      regeneration, Mater. Sci. Eng. C. 36 (2014) 252–260. doi:10.1016/j.msec.2013.12.007.

[106] B. Huang, Carbon nanotubes and their polymeric composites: The applications in tissue
      engineering, Biomanufacturing Rev. 5 (2020) 1–26. doi:10.1007/s40898-020-00009-x.

[107] M. Tanaka, Y. Sato, H. Haniu, H. Nomura, S. Kobayashi, S. Takanashi, M. Okamoto,
      T. Takizawa, K. Aoki, Y. Usui, A. Oishi, H. Kato, N. Saito, A three-dimensional block
      structure consisting exclusively of carbon nanotubes serving as bone regeneration scaf-
      fold and as bone defect filler, PLoS One. 12 (2017) e0172601. doi:10.1371/journal.
      pone.0172601.

[108] M. Tanaka, Y. Sato, M. Zhang, H. Haniu, M. Okamoto, K. Aoki, T. Takizawa, K.
      Yoshida, A. Sobajima, T. Kamanaka, H. Kato, N. Saito, In vitro and in vivo evaluation
      of a three-dimensional porous multi-walled carbon nanotube scaffold for bone regener-
      ation, Nanomaterials. 7 (2017) 1–17. doi:10.3390/nano7020046.

[109] P. Khalid, M. Hussain, P. Rekha, A. Arun, Carbon nanotube-reinforced hydroxyapatite
      composite and their interaction with human osteoblast in vitro, Hum. Exp. Toxicol. 34
      (2015) 548–556. doi:10.1177/0960327114550883.

[110] Z. Jing, Y. Wu, W. Su, M. Tian, W. Jiang, L. Cao, L. Zhao, Z. Zhao, Carbon nanotube
      reinforced collagen/hydroxyapatite scaffolds improve bone tissue formation in vitro and
      in vivo, Ann. Biomed. Eng. 45 (2017) 2075–2087. doi:10.1007/s10439-017-1866-9.

[111] H. Sun, H. Lü, S. Lü, X.-X. Jiang, X. Li, H. Li, Q. Lin, Y. Mou, Y. Zhao, Y. Han, J. Zhou, C.
      Wang, Carbon nanotubes enhance intercalated disc assembly in cardiac myocytes via
      the β1-integrin-mediated signaling pathway, Biomat. 55 (2015) 84–95. doi:10.1016/j.
      biomaterials.2015.03.030.

[112] S.R. Shin, S.M. Jung, M. Zalabany, K. Kim, P. Zorlutuna, S. Bok Kim, M. Nikkhah, M.
      Khabiry, M. Azize, J. Kong, K. Wan, T. Palacios, M.R. Dokmeci, H. Bae, X. (Shirley)
      Tang, A. Khademhosseini, Carbon-nanotube-embedded hydrogel sheets for engineer-
      ing cardiac constructs and bioactuators, ACS Nano. 7 (2013) 2369–2380. doi:10.1021/
      nn305559j.

[113] S. Mombini, J. Mohammadnejad, B. Bakhshandeh, A. Narmani, J. Nourmohammadi, S. Vahdat, S. Zirak, Chitosan-PVA-CNT nanofibers as electrically conductive scaffolds for cardiovascular tissue engineering, Int. J. Biol. Macromol. 140 (2019) 278–287. doi:10.1016/j.ijbiomac.2019.08.046.

[114] A. Rhazouani, H. Gamrani, M. El Achaby, K. Aziz, L. Gebrati, M.S. Uddin, F. Aziz, Synthesis and toxicity of graphene oxide nanoparticles: A literature review of in vitro and in vivo studies, Biomed Res. Int. 2021 (2021) 1–19. doi:10.1155/2021/5518999.

[115] X. Zhang, W. Hu, J. Li, L. Tao, Y. Wei, A comparative study of cellular uptake and cytotoxicity of multi-walled carbon nanotubes, graphene oxide, and nanodiamond, Toxicol. Res. (Camb). 1 (2012) 62–68. doi:10.1039/c2tx20006f.

[116] J. Yuan, H. Gao, C.B. Ching, Comparative protein profile of human hepatoma HepG2 cells treated with graphene and single-walled carbon nanotubes: An iTRAQ-coupled 2D LC–MS/MS proteome analysis, Toxicol. Lett. 207 (2011) 213–221. doi:10.1016/j.toxlet.2011.09.014.

[117] Z. Liu, W. Cai, L. He, N. Nakayama, K. Chen, X. Sun, X. Chen, H. Dai, In vivo biodistribution and highly efficient tumour targeting of carbon nanotubes in mice, Nat. Nanotechnol. 2 (2007) 47–52. doi:10.1038/nnano.2006.170.

[118] X. Xue, J.-Y. Yang, Y. He, L.-R. Wang, P. Liu, L.-S. Yu, G.-H. Bi, M.-M. Zhu, Y.-Y. Liu, R.-W. Xiang, X.-T. Yang, X.-Y. Fan, X.-M. Wang, J. Qi, H.-J. Zhang, T. Wei, W. Cui, G.-L. Ge, Z.-X. Xi, C.-F. Wu, X.-J. Liang, Aggregated single-walled carbon nanotubes attenuate the behavioural and neurochemical effects of methamphetamine in mice, Nat. Nanotechnol. 11 (2016) 613–620. doi:10.1038/nnano.2016.23.

6 Graphene Quantum Dots for Drug Delivery

6.1 GRAPHENE QUANTUM DOTS (GQDS): AN OVERVIEW

The fields of energy, the environment, electronics, optics, and biomedicine all hold great promise for the use of carbon nanomaterials. Graphene is a 2D nanomaterial made of one layer of sp^2 hybridized carbon atoms that has drawn a lot of interest due to its distinct physicochemical characteristics. It has superior mechanical, electrical, thermal, optical, and chemical properties, which makes it suitable for various real-world applications [1,2]. Graphene possesses good mechanical strength with Young's modulus of 1 ± 0.1 TPa and ultimate tensile stress of 130 GPa, which delivers superior structural strength to its nanocomposites and significant potential for their application in automobile, aerospace industries, and tissue engineering [2,3]. Similarly, graphene with higher electric conductivity (10^4–10^5 S/m) and surface area (~2630 m^2/g) presents higher charge carrier mobility, which can be further used for sensing applications alongside health care and motion detection equipment [2,4,5]. The higher electrical and thermal conductivity (5300–5800 W/mK) of graphene delivers its potential for energy-storage devices like solar cells [6,7]. This is extremely encouraging and alluring for research in chemistry, physics, and materials science fields. Nevertheless, the zero-band gap semiconductor nature of graphene restricts its use in electronic and optoelectronic devices. In pristine graphene, there is no luminescence because there is no band gap. Fortunately, with the edge effects and quantum confinement in the derivatives of graphene, such as graphene nanorib-bons (GNRs) and graphene quantum dots (GQDs), an energy band gap can be initiated [8–10].

GQDs, a class of zero-dimensional (0D) nanomaterials of less than 20 nm size, have recently been recognized as a new and emerging material across all graphene derivatives. These exhibit distinctive quantum confinement and edge effects, which expand their potential for use in nanoscale optoelectronics [8]. Additionally, GQDs have encouraged the scientific community for their application in nanotechnology via numerous and remarkable properties such as biocompatibility, photo-stability, controllable photoluminescence, multicolored emission, truly outstanding dispersibility, aqueous solubility, and ease of surface functionalization [10–13]. Furthermore, the edge-functionalized GQDs include hydroxyl, carboxyl, epoxy, and carbonyl groups that can engage with a variety of biological molecules, including enzymes, proteins, and antibodies. To create high-sensitivity diagnostic nanodevices, GQDs have been effectively cross-linked to DNA molecules and antibodies through amidation [14]. As a result, high-quality colloidal GQDs have a ton of potential applications in the areas of biolabeling and bioimaging, biomolecule sensing, electrocatalysis, and light-emitting diodes [8]. Likewise, GQDs photoluminescent has drawn a lot of

DOI: 10.1201/9781003358114-6

interest because of their environmental friendliness, less toxicity, excellent biocompatibility, and higher photosensitivity [15].

In the novel drug delivery systems (DDSs), numerous nanocarriers have been explored to enhance the water solubility and targeted delivery of drugs. Multifunctional GQDs, which can be employed in the treatment of cancer, typically act as targeted cellular imaging and drug carriers at the same time. To understand cellular uptake, drug delivery systems (DDSs) may be observed utilizing organic fluorophores and semiconductor quantum dots. Additionally, owing to the inherent fluorescence of GQDs, it is easy to monitor cell movement instantaneously without the use of dyes [16]. Wang et al. (2014) demonstrated the ligand-modified GQDs to enable concurrent targeted delivery of drugs, real-time monitoring of cellular uptake and cell labeling. The folic acid ligands were successfully impregnated to the GQDs and further loaded with the anticancer agent, doxorubicin (DOX). The created nano assembly can effectively deliver the drug to the target cells and can indisputably distinguish cancer cells from normal cells. The intrinsic steady fluorescence of GQDs allows for real-time monitoring of the release of the drug and cellular uptake of the DOX-GQD-FA nano assembly. Using receptor-mediated cellular uptake, HeLa cells quickly internalize the nano assembly while DOX release and accretion get extended. According to records on *in-vitro* toxicity, the DOX-GQD-FA nano assembly may target HeLa cells differently and effectively, even though it demonstrates noticeably less cytotoxicity on normal cells [17]. Due to their significantly greater biocompatibility and reduced cytotoxicity in comparison to other QDs, GQDs have drawn great interest in nano and biomedicines. GQDs have the same optical characteristics as QDs and have been shown to be able to cross the blood-brain barrier (BBB). Because of this, GQDs are now being used to expand our understanding of neuroscience diagnostics and therapeutics. With their small size and surface chemistry, they are ideal drug delivery systems through the bloodstream, across the BBB, and up to the brain. Previously, the GQD-based neuroimaging methods and theranostic applications, including photothermal and photodynamic treatment alone or in conjunction with chemotherapy, have been developed effectively [18].

Considering the superior surface characteristics of GQDs, the present chapter describes recent developments in the field of GQDs for their applications in drug delivery and other biomedical fields. This chapter also discusses the details and advances in top-down and bottom-up approaches for synthesizing GQDs. Recommendations have been made to overcome the difficulties regarding the synthesis and functionalization of GQDs. The present chapter also highlights the recent advancements in the application of GQDs related to gene therapy, photodynamic therapy, and drug administration for cancer and neurological diseases.

6.2 SIGNIFICANCE OF GRAPHENE QUANTUM DOTS IN DRUG DELIVERY

Graphene and its variants have sparked intense attention since its discovery in 2004 because of its remarkable physicochemical features. A conventional graphene sheet is a few microns thick. Its zero band gap may be widened by lowering the size of the graphene sheet and via regulated doping of hetero-atom. By lowering the lateral size of a graphene sheet, its dimensionality may be lowered from 2D to 0D. A graphene sheet with a thickness smaller than 10 nm is commonly described as a GQD [19]. Not just graphene, but GQDs are a prominent emphasis of academic and industrial research seeing as to their adjustable energy band gap, charge transport selectivity, size, and fluorescent properties. Furthermore, GQDs have the ability to bond with a significant number of biomolecules by means of non-covalent interactions, as well as adequate aqueous solubility, high biocompatibility, and lower toxicity. The wide band gap of GQDs, as well as their ability to tailor their band gap across a diverse spectrum and carrier selectivity, plays an important role in catalysis, energy, and biomedical applications [20–22].

GQDs, with their exceptional surface characteristics, have been extensively employed for drug delivery, photothermal treatments, and gene therapy. As drug delivery carriers, GQDs are much more prevalent for enlightening the therapeutic efficacy of anticancer agents like DOX by speeding up their nuclear intake and endorsing their activity for DNA cleavage [23]. Because of the abundance of several reactive groups on the surface of GQDs, numerous drugs, requisite polymers, and targeting ligands may be attached in several ways to increase their pharmacological characteristics both *in-vitro* and *in-vivo* [24]. Additionally, the drug nanocarriers can be readily detected in real-time, and their cellular uptake and mobility could be supervised by exploiting the GQDs' built-in fluorescence features [17]. Despite the remarkable characteristics of GQDs, the hydrophobic nature caused by their carbon network is one of the primary obstacles to overcome for its application in DDSs. Previously, several approaches, including chemical PEGylation, oxidation, QD size reduction, and other techniques, have been researched to mitigate hydrophobic surface interactions and increase the biocompatibility of GQDs [21]. The details are provided in the subsequent sections.

6.3   SYNTHESIS OF GRAPHENE QUANTUM DOTS

GQDs can be synthesized using various techniques, which may well be divided into two categories: top-down and bottom-up approaches (**Figure 6.1**) [25]. A macroscopic/bulk method is used in the top-down approach, wherein the parent materials are reduced or fragmented into the required nanoscale size via diverse physical, chemical, and electrochemical techniques [26]. The top-down methods use a variety of processes, notably electrochemical oxidation, ultrasound/microwave-driven preparation methods, hydrothermal methods, and chemical oxidation to convert carbon-based nanomaterials like graphene, graphene oxide (GO), carbon nanotubes (CNTs), and fullerenes into the GQDs [27–29]. On the other hand, bottom-up methods exploit atomic or molecule constituents to produce nanostructures. The two most popular approaches, carbonization of precursors and controlled chemical fusing of the source molecules, are used to fabricate GQDs via bottom-up strategies from the aromatic, conjugated, and non-conjugated molecules. Similar to top-down methods, bottom-up methods may also be used to produce GQDs via employing a variety of physical and chemical approaches [10,25]. Alongside, biomass-based green synthesis techniques to produce GQD are becoming much more popular with traditional chemical methods due to their abundant availability, lower price, and ease of

Top-down

Carbon resource

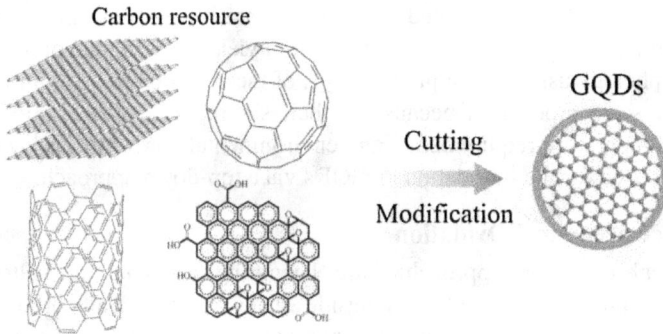

Bottom-up

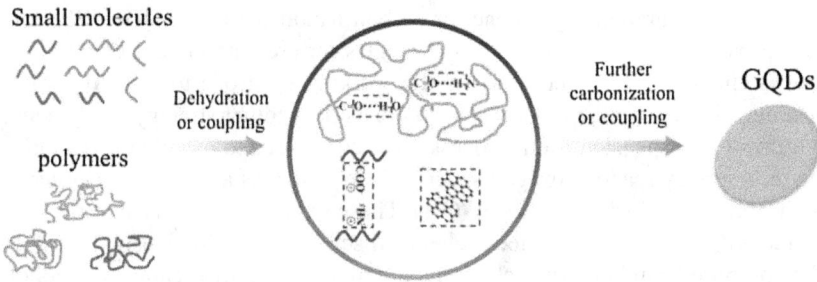

FIGURE 6.1 Schematic Representation of the Mechanism of the Top-Down and Bottom-Up Approaches Used for the Synthesis of Graphene Quantum Dots (GQDs). [Reproduced with permission from *Zhu et al. (2017)*] [25].

production along with environmental friendliness [30]. Additionally, supplementing GQDs with various metal and non-metal species results in remarkable optical, electrical, and biological features. As a result, doped GQD production techniques are crucial for a variety of applications. The recent developments in relation to the GQDs synthesis methods are described subsequently.

6.3.1 TOP-DOWN APPROACH

GQDs have indeed been synthesized using the "top-down" approach by slicing sp^2 or sp^3 carbon allotropes of graphene, carbon fiber, GO, and carbon black using acidic oxidation, micro fluidization, hydrothermal process, exfoliation, and electrochemical oxidation. These methods benefit from having large availability of raw materials, easy-to-follow procedures, and huge-scale manufacturing of bulk reagents and precursors. Additionally, top-down approaches for GQD synthesis frequently result in oxygenated groups on the surface; as a result, edge-functionalized GQDs exhibit good water solubility and surface passivation. Meanwhile, the disadvantages of the top-down approach comprise the need for specialized equipment, a precise reaction environment, and a nonselective breakdown of the aromatic carbon structure. These cause the development of fragmented and flawed assemblies and nanomaterials of inferior crystallinity. GQDs obtained are in aggregated forms with different sizes (3–25 nm) and have very low luminescent quantum yields. It is challenging to regulate their morphology using this approach. Most of these approaches are impractical for their large-scale production because of their significant expense, poor adaptability, high-temperature requirements, and environmental concerns. Following are some methods used for the fabrication of GQDs via a top-down approach.

6.3.1.1 Electrochemical Oxidation

Electrochemical oxidation approaches are becoming a viable and alternative approach for the production of GQDs, alongside all existing chemical methods. Electrochemical oxidation is a more promising approach as it can produce monodisperse GQDs by employing fewer chemicals, has greater control over the synthesis process, and is a facile process. This technique uses a redox potential of around 1.5 to 3 V to oxidatively split graphite, graphene, or carbon nanotubes into GQDs. When using this approach, there are two primary strategies for creating GQDs. One technique involves employing the precursors as the working electrode to directly and electrochemically oxidize the carbon-carbon bonds. In another strategy, the precursors are utilized in suspension. Both processes are considered to include the oxidation of the precursors by reactive oxygen species (ROS), such as an in-situ generated oxygen radical (O.) or hydroxyl radical (OH). These oxidizing radicals split the precursors into GQDs by acting as electrochemical scissors [10]. Previously, Huang et al. (2018) proposed a unique weak electrolyte (ammonia) electrochemical methodology to speed up the oxidation process and effectively produce the crystalline GQDs with significant yield in aqueous environments. The af-GQDs were synthesized in an electrochemical cell by employing Pt as the cathode and a circular graphene paper as the anode with an ammonia solution as the electrolyte, which was maintained in a steady voltage mode (30 V) for two hours (**Figure 6.2**) [31]. GQDs obtained were of 3–8 nm in size and also had a yield of 28%, that indicated about 28 times higher as compared to the strong electrolytes (such as NaOH solution). Simultaneously, GQDs demonstrated considerably higher crystallinity than bottom-up GQDs [31].

Similarly, Li et al. (2012) demonstrated an efficient electrochemical method using a graphene sheet as an electrode of dimension 5 mm × 10 mm to produce highly water-soluble GQDs. The electrolyte was 0.1 M phosphate buffer solution (PBS), and the CV scan rate was 0.5 V s^{-1} within ± 3.0 V. As reference and counter electrodes, Ag/AgCl and Pt wire were employed. The nitrogen-doped GQDs were extracted and filtered via a cellulose ester dialysis bag. The methodology consisted of extremely steady GQDs of 1 to 2 nm thickness with a size distribution of 3 to 5 nm in diameter, yielding green luminescence with a photoconversion efficiency of 1.28% [32]. Overall, it was observed that the electrochemical oxidation process could produce a stable GQDs solution; however, pretreatment and purification processes of raw materials and obtained GQDs take an elongated period, with relatively lower quantum yield, making large-scale GQD synthesis more challenging. These difficulties can be overcome by employing suitable pretreatment and purification processes such as solvent treatment.

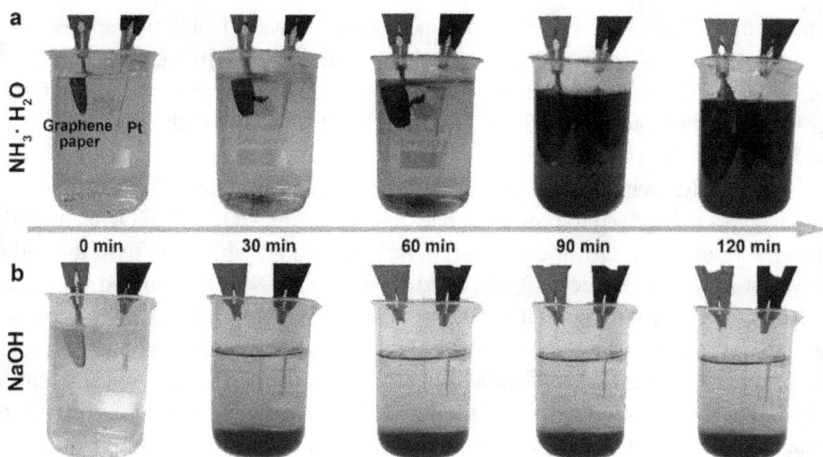

FIGURE 6.2 The Electrochemical Oxidation of Graphene Paper in (a) Ammonia (Weak Electrolyte) and (b) NaOH Solutions (Strong Electrolyte) at Variable Reaction Times. [Reprinted with permission from *Huang et al. (2018)*] [31].

6.3.1.2 Ultrasound/Microwave-Driven Preparation Methods

Ultrasonication treatment is one of the widely used approaches for the synthesis of numerous nanomaterials and nanocomposites, including GQDs. The tiny bubbles that emerged in the solution due to ultrasonic action further develop mechanical force via acoustic bubble cavitation and break the carbon-carbon bonds, slicing through GQDs [27,33]. Gao et al. (2017) have successfully synthesized three types of GQDs, namely, pristine GQDs, expanded GQDs, and graphene oxide quantum dots (GOQDs) from naturally expanded graphite and graphite oxide in a supercritical CO_2/H_2O system aided by ultrasonication treatment. The findings of the experiments suggest that this approach is a low-cost, environmentally friendly, faster, and large-scale approach for the synthesis of GQDs that can present an environmentally acceptable pathway for the fabrication of various GQDs, particularly the pristine graphene quantum dots (GQDs) [34].

The microwave approach considerably reduces the time required to synthesize GQDs, which could be produced in a matter of minutes and may be doped with multiple elements for enriching the varieties of GQDs and expanding their functionalities [11]. Zhang et al. (2016) have effectively produced GQDs using a microwave-assisted decomposition of aspartic acid (Asp) and NH_4HCO_3. The synthesized GQDs fluoresced intensely blue and had a high quantum yield of up to 14%. The robust fluorescence emission impact of Fe^{3+} on GQDs was exploited to discover its great selectivity among other metal ions. The probe showed a broader linear response concentration range (0–50 M) to Fe^{3+}, with a computed limit of detection (LOD) of 0.26 M. Furthermore, GQDs obtained via microwave-assisted method have displayed their sensitivity to pH (2 to 12) with higher prospective as optical pH sensors. More significantly, the GQDs have minimal cellular toxicity and good photostability, allowing them to be employed directly as fluorescent probes for cell imaging

[35]. Similarly, Shin et al. (2014) demonstrated a microwave irradiation approach for the large-scale fabrication of GQDs by using graphite flakes. In their study, beneath acidic and oxidative environments, natural graphite flakes were bombarded with high-powered microwaves (300 and 600 W) to obtain GQDs with size ranges from 2 to 5 nm and 70% yield [36].

Moreover, in combination treatment, the microwave and ultrasonic-assisted approach was being used to produce white-light-emitting GQDs (WGQDs). Initially, ultrasonication and microwave irradiation on oxidized graphite were used to synthesize yellow-green fluorescent GQDs. Further, the WGQDs were obtained via microwave irradiation of obtained GQDs in an alkaline solution (pH = 13) for 12 hours. The size of obtained GQDs was confirmed by TEM investigation to be in the region of 2–5 nm. A wide emission peak at 445 nm was detected in the colloidal solution of WGQDs. Those WGQDs were employed to deliver white-light-emitting diode devices [37]. Both these ultrasound and microwave-assisted methods may affect the aqueous stability of the GQDs by reducing the oxygenated functional entities. In addition, these methods are highly energy intensive, which enhances their operating cost and limits their large-scale applications. Meanwhile, optimizing process parameters and using green synthesis methods may overcome the shortcomings of ultrasound and microwave-assisted methods for synthesizing GQDs.

6.3.1.3   Chemical Oxidation

A chemical oxidation approach, commonly referred to as the oxidation cutting process, is frequently used in which the carbon bonds of graphene, GO, or CNTs are often disrupted by strong oxidants such as H_2SO_4 and HNO_3. Previously, Shen et al. (2011) revealed that GQDs could be readily obtained using an oxidative cutting method. Initially, synthesized GO by the modified Hummers method was further oxidized in HNO_3 to reduce the size of GO nanosheets. The resulting nanosheets were pretreated with an oligomeric PEG diamine that works as a passivating agent. PEG-treated GO sheets were further chemically reduced using hydrazine hydrate. Finally, the surface passivated GQDs with good fluorescence, and up-conversion characteristics are produced with a yield of 7.4 % and a size of 5–15 nm [38].

Similarly, GQDs can be synthesized using other carbon sources, such as CNTs and carbon nanofibers [21]. Peng et al. (2012) have prepared GQDs of size-tunable PL characteristics by oxidative cleavage of conventional pitch-based carbon fibers. Initially, these carbon fibers were sonicated, followed by oxidation by means of a strong combination of H_2SO_4 and HNO_3. After stirring for 24 h at diverse temperatures (80, 100, and 120 °C), the solution was diluted with deionized water. Further dialysis was employed to purify the resulting GQDs solution. This approach yielded scalable quantities of GQDs that varied in size from 1 to 4 nm with a zigzag edge shape. In addition, the resulting GQDs have demonstrated steady luminescence and excellent biocompatibility, with solubility in water along with other polar solvents, which make them suitable for therapeutic applications [39]. The chemical oxidation process is not particularly safe since it uses potent oxidants like H_2SO_4 and HNO_3, and also, the residual chemicals that are produced are likely to contaminate the surroundings. In line with this, Lu et al. (2017) described a more facile, green approach by avoiding concentrated acids and post-treatment processes while introducing metal impurities to the GOQDs. GOQDs were produced from black carbon as the substrate and hydrogen peroxide (H_2O_2) as the oxidant without any subsequent post-treatment processes. The entire process just requires 90 minutes, and the end product GOQDs exhibited a size of 3.0–4.5 nm with outstanding biocompatibility, salt tolerance, low toxicity, and strong light stability. It is a shorter and greener technique for the synthesis of GQDs as compared to several other methods that have been described [40].

6.3.1.4 Solvothermal/Hydrothermal Method

The GQDs can be extensively, rapidly, and simply synthesized via a hydrothermal approach. A variety of macromolecules or small molecules may be used as parent material to synthesize GQDs under elevated temperature and pressure. The basic principle behind the use of hydrothermal/solvothermal methods is to break down the bonds between carbon compounds for the synthesis of GQDs at elevated temperatures and higher pressure. Through a one-step solvothermal process, Tian et al. (2016) produced GQDs in a medium of N, N-dimethylformamide (DMF). Throughout the synthesis process, strong oxidants like sulfuric and nitric acid were totally avoided for the treatment of raw materials; also, no contaminants were introduced. In addition, without the use of dialysis, high-purity GQDs have been produced through evaporation, re-dissolution, and filtration. The outcomes suggested that the diameter and thickness of GQDs were primarily scattered between 20 and 40 nm and 1 and 1.5 nm, correspondingly, with a quantum yield (QY) of 15% under neutral circumstances. The PL signal demonstrated high stability under various pH levels, indicating their wide range of potential applications in various environments. This approach displayed several benefits, including low-cost, higher quantum yield, no need for purification or dialysis, and straightforward experimental conditions [41].

Furthermore, Zhang et al. (2017) developed an effective hydrothermal-assisted method for synthesizing reduced graphene oxide quantum dots (rGOQDs). In this process, GO was synthesized via a modified Hummers method by oxidation of parent material, graphite. The obtained GO was further treated with DMF in Teflon coated autoclave at 200 °C. The quantum yield of the process was 24.62%, while nitrogen (N) derived from DMF was used as surface doping. Additionally, they also investigated zebrafish via rGOQDs, which served as an important benchmark for the *in-vivo* biocompatibility of bio-probe [42]. Meanwhile, numerous elements or groups may be doped on GQDs using the hydrothermal process. Additionally, different GQDs may be prepared using a combination of the hydrothermal approach and chemical oxidation technique. However, due to the high temperature and pressure, it suffers from a safety concern, and it also often takes an extended time, at least five hours. Recently, researchers are also working on the use of other carbonaceous materials, such as biomass resources, for the synthesis of GQDs via the hydrothermal method to cut down the cost of raw materials. Wang et al. (2016) demonstrated a hydrothermal technique to synthesize high-quality GQDs with a yield of 15% from rice husk. The synthesized GQDs displayed bright and controllable photoluminescence and good water dispersibility. A cell viability test demonstrated that the obtained GQDs exhibited superior biocompatibility and may be effortlessly adapted for cell imaging by a simple translocation into the cytoplasm. It is important to note that mesoporous silica nanoparticles were also produced as a by-product when GQDs were being produced [43]. Such approaches have described a better use of biomass resources with enormous advantages for the environment as well as the economy.

6.3.2 BOTTOM-UP APPROACH

The bottom-up method entails developing GQDs from tiny molecular building blocks by condensing benzene derivatives into larger entities with well-defined shape, size, and desired characteristics. These techniques, however, demand complicated and stepwise synthesis approaches that necessitate unique reagents and conditions. Following are some bottom-up approaches employed for the synthesis of GQDs.

6.3.2.1 Chemical Vapor Deposition

Research communities throughout the world have documented an escalating number of preparation strategies based on well-known methods, such as chemical vapor deposition (CVD), because of the distinctive structure and exceptional characteristics of GQDs. CVD uses one or more gaseous components or elemental compounds to fabricate nanomaterials by chemical reaction on the surface of substrates. Previously, the CVD approach has been utilized for the synthesis of high-quality GQDs [44,45]. Deka et al. (2017) employed CVD to develop a PL sensor relying on the hydrophobic graphene quantum dots (h-GQDs) that can differentiate among aromatic and nonaromatic amino acids. Initially, using a customized CVD method, the researchers produced graphene on a Cu substrate, which was further transferred straight to n-hexane. Further, the reaction mixture was treated by ultrasonication for 8 h to produce h-GQDs. This was the first study for the straightforward production of CVD-assisted h-GQDs, which were capable of forming extremely stable dispersions in organic solvents without any functionalization, doping, or molecule-to-molecule interaction [46]. Recently, Kumar et al. (2018) described a straightforward, environmentally friendly, and rapid method for developing nitrogen-doped graphene quantum dots (N-GQDs) on copper foil using CVD, which utilizes only chitosan, a low-cost and compatible biopolymer, as the parent material for the carbon and nitrogen atoms. The synthesized GQDs exhibited a size of 10–15 nm with 2–5 nm thickness and highest nitrogen concentration of 4.2% [47]. It was observed that the CVD approach is able to synthesize the high-quality GQDs with well-controlled size and shape; however, it must be explored for large-scale synthesis. As CVD is considered an expensive technique for the synthesis of nanomaterials on a larger scale, a detailed cost analysis of the method is required.

6.3.2.2 Carbonization

The synthesis of GQDs through controlled carbonization or pyrolysis is an easy and environmentally friendly process. Its basic concept is to employ compatible organic compounds or polymers to dehydrate and carbonize further. Recently, Kashani et al. (2019) demonstrated a green synthesis method for GQDs by employing a novel one-pot "bottom-up" pyrolysis while eliminating the need for water and chemical reagents during the process. To synthesize His-GQDs, a label-free and selective probe, citric acid was employed as the carbon source and histidine as the amino-functionalized agent, both in optimum ratios. The obtained His-GQDs probe displayed a higher quantum yield of 62.8%, chemical stability, ultra-small size, biocompatibility, and outstanding optical characteristics. The His-GQDs were further employed for cellular imaging of human ACHN cell lines, which consist of graphene sheets with a normal size of 2.0 nm [48]. Bayat et al. (2017) demonstrated a high-yield and low-cost approach for the synthesis of green photoluminescent single-layer graphene quantum dots (SLGQDs) using glucose as a substrate and DI water as a solvent. The synthesized SLGQDs had a size distribution of around 8 nm and were evenly dispersed without evident aggregation. The peak emission wavelength of the obtained GQDs was 540 nm. The mechanism behind the synthesis of SLGQDs was divided into three steps as follows. The first step describes the glucose dehydration to produce the C=C and fundamental building block of the graphene structure. While the second step revealed that the hydroxyl group of a nearby glucose molecule and the hydrogen atoms of glucose interacted to form the water molecule, the third step showed the covalent interaction of carbon atoms to produce GQDs [49]. Xu et al. (2013) synthesized greatly fluorescent GQDs with the use of a simplistic heating mantle device. This process involves the one-step decomposition of the natural amino acid L-glutamic acid. When exposed to ultraviolet, blue, and green light, respectively, the produced GQDs have displayed intense blue, green, and red luminosity. In addition, the GQDs fluoresced in the near-infrared (NIR) region between 800–850 nm in a luminescence manner. With a considerable Stokes shift of 455 nm, this NIR fluorescence offers a major benefit for the precise identification and imaging of biological specimens. The fluorescence quantum yield (QY) of the GQDs, which was as high as 54.5%, was examined along with other fluorescence parameters, including fluorescence life periods and photo-stability [50].

Similarly, Dong et al. (2012) developed an easier bottom-up approach to synthesize GQDs of better photoluminescent characteristics by tuning the degree of carbonization of citric acid. The obtained GQDs are nanosheets with a thickness of 0.5 to 2.0 nm and a width of around 15 nm. It exhibits an excitation-independent PL emission activity and a PL quantum yield that is comparatively substantial (9.0%). The GO nanostructures, in comparison, are made up of sheets with a height of only one nanometer and a width of hundreds of nanometers. It shows an excitation-dependent PL emission activity and a modest (2.2%) PL quantum yield [51].

6.3.2.3 Electron Beam Irradiation Method

It is important to consider that the electron beam irradiation (EBI) approach has not been extensively employed since it needs expensive specialist equipment and poses a radiation risk. Wang et al. (2017) reported an ambient temperature synthesis approach for single-crystal fluorescent GQDs by employing the EBI method. In their study, initially, the hydrazine hydrate was dissolved with 1,3,6-trinitropyrene. Afterward, the mixture was stirred, sealed, and exposed to radiation under a dynamitron electron accelerator's titanium window. Following irradiation, the specimen was dialyzed for two days using a 0.22 mm microporous membrane filter and a dialysis bag, finally yielding GQDs with 32% quantum yield [52]. Under similar circumstances, other small compounds, including 1-Nitropyrene, urea, and CA, can also be employed as precursors to produce GQDs [11].

6.4 FUNCTIONALIZATION OF GRAPHENE QUANTUM DOTS

The science world is currently concentrating on GQDs due to their inherent surface characteristics, which make them suitable for various biomedical and photovoltaic applications. The characteristics of GQDs may be tuned by adjusting the size, shape, surface chemistry, edge orientations, and chemical functionalization. GQDs are well adaptable for their functionalization, which significantly contributes to various biomedical applications such as drug delivery, biosensing, phototherapy, bioimaging, and gene delivery [53]. The chemical adsorption of molecules avoids the breakdown of the carbon skeleton without interstitial contaminants, rendering the functionalization process in GQDs a potential strategy. Functionalization within the GQDs is much more significant since it assists in tuning their surface characteristics, which is favorable for various applications, including biomedical. The surface functionalization process also contributed to altering the optical, catalytic, and biological characteristics of GQDs by promoting electron transfer and the existence of functional entities such as carboxyl, amine, hydroxyl, and other biological receptors targeted groups. The existence of these functional entities on the surface as well as on the edge of GQDs has broadened the field of study [54]. Through selecting raw substrates that have the desired functional entities, functionalization can take place throughout the synthesis process of GQDs or by post-synthesis via molecular attachment. Qian et al. (2013), during their theoretical and experimental study of the surface chemistry of functionalized GQDs, found that the diamines had the highest potential to govern the optical characteristics or quantum yield of GQDs due to their extraordinary protonation phenomena **(Figure 6.3)** [55].

In some instances, cross-linking with alkylamines such as polyethylene glycol-amine (PEG-amine) and poly-ethylenimine (PEI) and amino compounds cause a red and blue shift in the PL of GQDs. For example, Jin et al. (2013) examined both the experimental and theoretical evidence to demonstrate that the band gap is lowered by the charge transport out from surface functional entities to GQDs as a result of the higher electron density and the induced red-shifted PL [56]. To investigate the biocompatibility of functionalized GQDs, Yuan et al. (2014) have compared the cytotoxic effects of three GQDs tailored via various functional groups (NH_2, COOH, and CO-N $(CH_3)_2$, respectively) on the distribution of the cells in A549 and C6 cells. The results obtained after the cytotoxicity study indicated that even at a concentration of 200 µg/mL, there was no upsurge in apoptosis or necrosis, which demonstrates that even after being modified with distinct functional entities, GQDs were able to maintain their outstanding biocompatibility. Such an exclusive characteristic of GQDs can significantly enhance their adaptability in numerous biomedical applications [57]. Markovic et al. (2012) investigated the molecular pathways of GQD-mediated photodynamic cytotoxicity, discovering that the development of oxidative stress resulted in *in-vitro* photodynamic cytotoxicity, with consequent activation of both the apoptosis and autophagy have programmed cell death [58]. However, investigations on human breast cancer have demonstrated that GQDs may quickly enter the cytoplasm and do not obstruct cell growth, as they are not harmful substances. These cytotoxicity research findings at the cellular level support the use of GQDs in biological applications. But as a warning, greater emphasis must be placed on the efficacy of GQDs

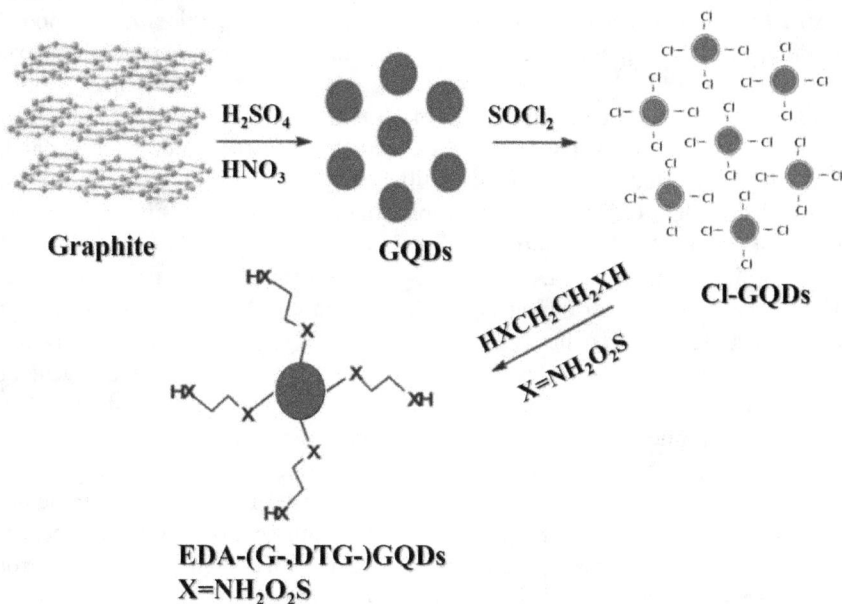

FIGURE 6.3 Schematic Representation of Synthesis of Functionalized GQDs with Specified Diamines, Glycols, and Dithioglycols. [Reproduced with permission from *Qian et al. (2013)*] [55].

by researching their cellular absorption processes and intracellular and *in-vivo* metabolic routes of toxicity [59].

6.5 APPLICATION OF GRAPHENE QUANTUM DOT-BASED NANOCARRIERS

GQDs have been used extensively for several years for their applications in the biomedical field due to their favorable cytotoxicity, numerous receptors, facile surface modification, and superior biocompatibility. In several instances, GQDs have demonstrated certain exceptional abilities that enable them to take the place of the conventional nanomaterials presently used across this field. Researchers are constantly investigating the prospects of GQDs for various cutting-edge medical applications owing to the intriguing and encouraging results. This section primarily focuses on the most current developments in the utilization of GQDs in the fields of drug delivery, gene delivery, and photodynamic therapy.

6.5.1 DRUG DELIVERY

GQDs have drawn much attention for applications in drug administration because of their intriguing physicochemical and biological characteristics. Numerous functional groups found on the edges of GQDs offer effective binding sites for therapeutics, drugs, and targeted ligands. Additionally, the occurrence of sp^2 carbon in the structure of GQDs enables the attachment of chemotherapeutic drug compounds that often involve aromatic rings to the surface of GQDs, boosting the drug loading efficiency [22,60]. Moreover, owing to the poor water solubility of chemotherapy, drugs like doxorubicin (DOX) and methotrexate (MTX) cannot be efficiently transported to a particular tissue in the body. Such chemotherapeutic agents can be efficiently transported through a hydrophilic carrier of a higher surface-to-volume ratio, such as GQDs. GQDs provide multiple binding sites for the liking of drug molecules through π-π stacking onto the basal plane. According to Nahain et al. (2013), the use of hyaluronic acid (HA) (GQD-HA) as a targeting mediator allows for the effective and precise distribution of graphene quantum dots (GQDs). Their study has demonstrated that HA has been attached to a GQD that admits the intriguing adhesive characteristics of the catechol moiety dopamine hydrochloride attached to HA **(Figure 6.4a)** [61]. The fluorescence spectra showed substantial fluorescence intensity despite the attachment of HA, and the transmission electron microscopy determined that the particles were around 20 nm in size. *In-vivo* bioavailability analysis showed that the tumor tissue emitted more intense fluorescence when the produced GQD-HA was administered to CD44 receptor highly expressed tumor-bearing female mice (Balb/c). *In-vitro* cellular imaging revealed high fluorescence from CD44 overexpressed A549 cells. Outcomes from both *in-vivo* and *in-vitro* experiments demonstrated the benefit of employing HA as a targeting agent. The kinetic study on the loading and release behavior of the hydrophobic drug DOX from a GQD under moderately acidic circumstances demonstrated that a GQD might be believed to be a novel drug carrier. In addition, the MTT assay greatly endorsed the designation of GQD-HA as a biocompatible conjugate [61].

Further, Wang et al. (2013) demonstrate that the unique structural characteristics of GQDs provide an excellent potential for drug distribution and an upsurge in anticancer effectiveness despite prior premodification **(Figure 6.4b)** [23]. Employing the DOX/GQD conjugates, they might effectively distribute DOX to the nucleus since the nanoconjugates follow distinct cellular and nuclear internalization routes than free DOX. Additionally, the nanoconjugates might significantly increase DOX's DNA cleavage activity. This improvement greatly increased DOX's cytotoxicity when coupled with effective nuclear delivery. Moreover, the DOX/GQD conjugates could upgrade the chemotherapeutic efficacy of anticancer agents whose effectiveness is subpar owing to drug resistance by increasing the nuclear absorption and cytotoxicity of DOX to drug-resistant cancer cells [23].

Recently, Nasrollahi et al. (2020) have used ferritin protein nanocages to incorporate GQDs in order to establish multifunctional platforms for cancer treatment and multimodal imaging. It was anticipated that encapsulating ultra-small GQDs would improve overall bioimaging performance while slowing down their rapid elimination from the body. GQDs and iron are encased within the core of AfFtn-AA to increase the usefulness of protein nanostructure as multimodal imaging nanoprobes, which are proficient for both fluorescence and magnetic resonance imaging (MRI). The AfFtn-AA is an artificial ferritin nanocage made from Archaeoglobus fulgidus, an archaeon. The development of the GQD-iron complex in the ferritin nanocages ((GQDs/Fe)AA) is accomplished by iron-mediated self-assembly of ferritin dimers that results in the co-encapsulation. The (GQDs/Fe)AA

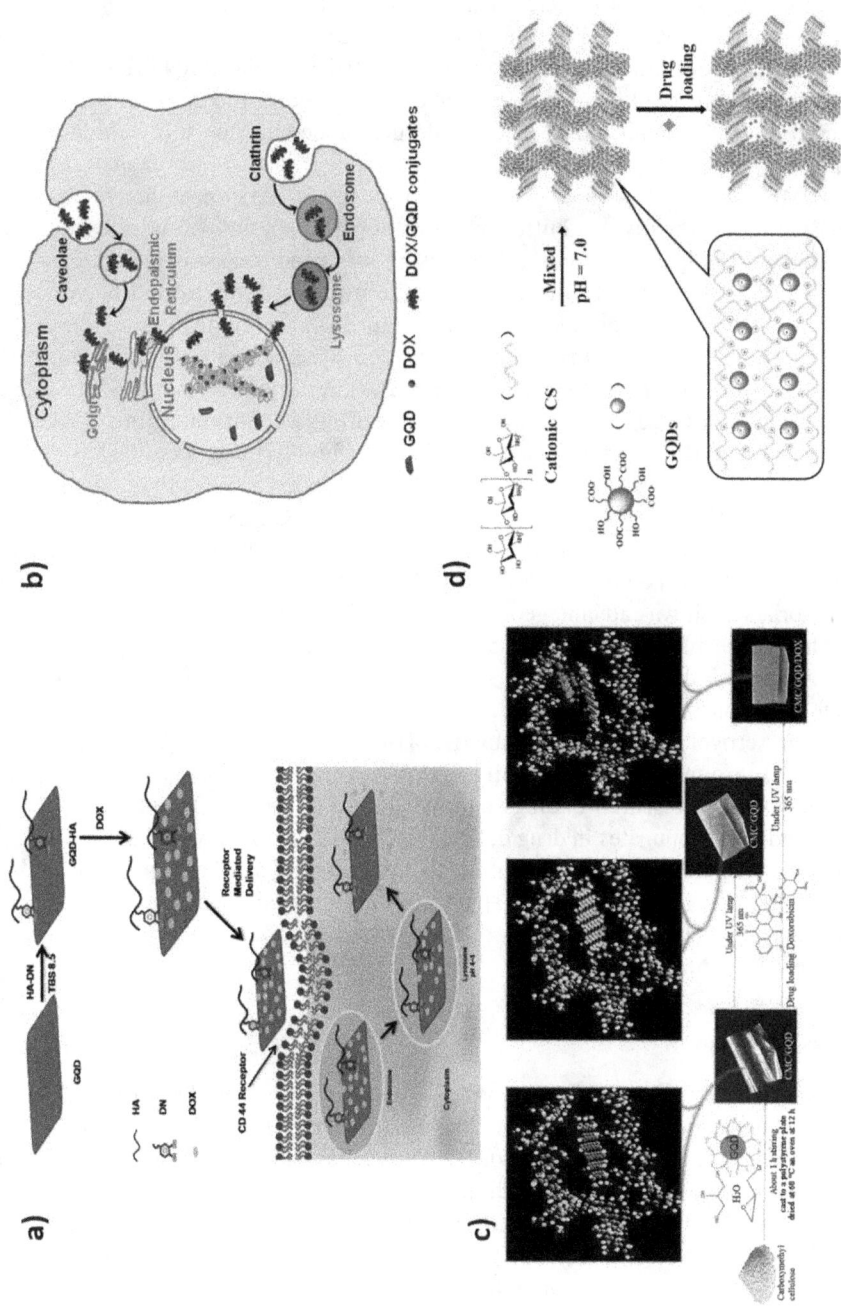

FIGURE 6.4 (a) Hyaluronic Acid (HA)–Based Target Delivery of GQDs and Subsequent Drug Release from the GQD's Surface in a Habitat of Cancer Cells. [Reproduced with permission from *Nahain et al. (2013)* [61], (b) Mechanism for the Delivery of DOX from GQD/DOX Nanoconjugate. Reproduced with permission form *Wang et al. (2013)* [23], (c) Schematic Representation of Synthesis of CMC/GQD Hydrogel for the Loading and Release of DOX from the DOX-Loaded CMC/GQD Nanocomposite. [Reprinted with permission from *Javanbakht et al. (2018)* [63], (d) Formation of the Drug-Loaded GQDs–CS Hybrid Xerogel. [Reproduced with permission from *Lv et al. (2016)* [64].

demonstrates excellent pH-sensitive fluorescence with excellent relaxivities on MDA-MB-231 cells as well as substantial relaxivities in MRI. (GQDs/Fe)AA displays minimal cytotoxicity on the cells with higher loading efficiency (35%) for DOX as a drug carrier as well as an imaging agent. Overall, the pH-responsive fluorophore, MRI agent, and drug nanocarrier properties of the (GQDs/Fe)AA demonstrate intriguing implications in cancer diagnostics and therapeutics [62]. Javanbakht et al. (2018) synthesized a new hydrogel nanocomposite film exhibiting antitumor capabilities by employing GQD as a nanoparticle in carboxymethyl cellulose (CMC) hydrogel with DOX of broad-spectrum anticancer activities **(Figure 6.4c)** [63]. Three distinct buffer solutions of pH 7.4, 7, and 4.5 were used for drug release investigations, and the MTT assay was used to assess the effectiveness of DOX-loaded CMC/GQD nanocomposite hydrogel films toward blood cancer cell lines (K562). The produced hydrogel films displayed improved *in-vitro* swelling, breakdown, permeability, and pH-sensitive drug delivery capabilities while being nontoxic to blood cancer cells (K562). The acquired findings support the application of these nanocomposite hydrogel films as antitumor films and DDS [63]. Lv et al. (2016) established the synthesis of highly fluorescent GQDs-chitosan (CS) hybrid xerogels. The proposed method provided a space to regulate the morphology of the xerogels by altering the amount of GQDs in the xerogel **(Figure 6.4d)** [64]. It was observed that when the GQDs concentration in the xerogel approached 43% (wt%), the GQDs-CS displayed a porous and three-dimensional (3D) framework, which was advantageous for the loading as well as the sustained release of drug molecules. The GQDs-CS may be used for *in-vivo* imaging in its as-prepared state as it demonstrated robust blue, green, and red fluorescence upon stimulation at various wavelengths. Additionally, the pH-dependent drug release behavior of the xerogel can be mediated by the pH-tempted protonation/deprotonation of the $-NH_2$ groups on chitosan chains [64].

Similarly, numerous research findings have advocated the application of GQDs and GQD-based nanoconjugates in drug delivery. However, the toxicity of these formulations is still demanding improvement for their large-scale synthesis and commercial use. The use of green synthesis approaches and natural chemotherapeutic agents can improve the biocompatibility of GQD-based nanoformulations, which must be explored for their applicability.

6.5.2 GENE THERAPY

Despite most studies focusing on drug delivery to tumors, GQDs have demonstrated significant potency for the distribution of various substances, including DNA and peptides. Delivering nucleic acids (DNA or RNA) to cells with the goal of increasing or restoring gene expression to treat disease is a crucial aspect of gene therapy. GQDs' capacity to penetrate the blood-brain barrier (BBB) and transport nucleic acid cargo to cell cytosols and nuclei is due to their small size. GQDs are a great possibility for gene carriers due to their minimal toxicity, strong solubility, and luminescent features that make it simple to monitor drug release.

Recently, Ghafary et al. (2017) developed a novel nanoconjugate with gene delivery and real-time tracking and capabilities, which is made up of GQDs, the chimeric peptide MPG-2H1, and plasmid DNA (pDNA) **(Figure 6.5)** [65]. Through non-covalent interactions among each component, the nanoconjugate was developed. In comparison to the standard peptide-pDNA combination, the improved complex has achieved transfection efficiency that was almost eight times higher. The findings of this work indicate that GQDs may be an effective transfection vector for applications involving gene delivery. GQDs offer increased drug loading relative to certain other nanomaterials drug carrier systems because of the substantial existence of the sp^2 domain and the potential for π-π stacking. Unfortunately, the active sites on the edge of GQDs are likely to be confined to ligands, which makes it unlikely that they will be used in gene delivery applications as these biomolecules must be covalently attached to the edge groups [65].

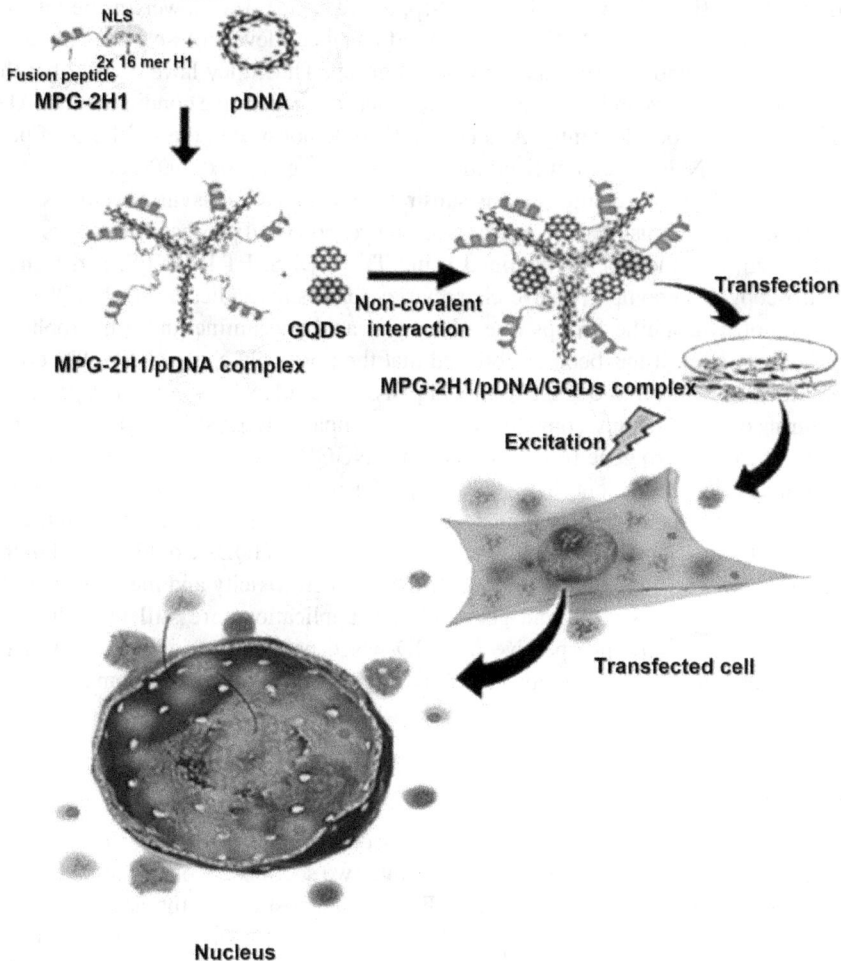

FIGURE 6.5 Assembling of MPG-2H1/pDNA/GQDs Complexes by Non-covalent Interactions, Transfection into Cells, and Excitation. [Reprinted with permission from *Ghafary et al. (2017)*] [65].

Additionally, novel nanoconjugates were designed by Xiao et al. (2016), in which the GQDs were coupled with neuroprotective peptide glycine-proline-glutamate (GQDG) and given to APP/PS1 transgenic mice. It was demonstrated that GQDs and GQDG might prevent the agglomeration of Aβ_{1-42} fibrils *in-vitro* tests using ThT and CD. To test the memory and learning abilities of APP/PS1 transgenic mice, a Morris water maze was used. In comparison to the Tg control groups, the surface area of Aβ plaque deposition decreased in the GQDG group. Likewise, immunohistochemistry testing was performed on freshly formed neural precursor cells and neurons. Moreover, neurons were gene-gun-impregnated with DiI to display a dendritic spine. The findings of this study displayed an improvement in memory and learning function, and more dendritic spines were detected. ELISA and suspension array were used to test amyloid-β (Aβ) and inflammation factors, respectively.

As compared to the control group, the levels of many pro-inflammatory cytokines (IL-1α, IL-1β, IL-6, IL-33, IL-17α, MIP-1β, and TNF-α) were lower in the GQDG group. In contrast, the GQDG group showed advanced levels of anti-inflammatory cytokines (IL-4 and IL-10) than the Control group. Thus, they have shown that the GQDG is an effective medication for treating neurodegenerative conditions like Alzheimer's disease [66]. Recently, Ahn et al. (2021) demonstrated the synthesis of positively charged NGQDs and utilized them to transport genes like pDNA and mRNA. PEI and citric acid were employed as substrates for the NGQD synthesis to result in positive charges. By using microwave-assisted hydrothermal processes, NGQDs were synthesized, and they were examined using TEM, DLS, FT-IR, XPS, and Raman spectroscopy. The comprehensive characterization results indicate that NGQDs are made up of hydrophilic groups like carboxylic acid and amine and a hydrophobic graphene domain. It has been established that the positively charged NGQDs effectively transfect cells and engage to model pDNA and mRNA, which are representative forms of gene therapy constituents. When compared to Lipofectamine, the "gold standard" for *in-vitro* gene transfection agents, NGQDs' gene transfection efficiency was found to be equivalent. The NGQDs performed better against Lipofectamine, even in the instance of mRNA transfection. Given the past research on the intracellular distribution of NGQDs, they have anticipated that NGQDs would be used in the therapeutic setting by following more research on their toxicity and metabolism [67].

Although GQD research and gene delivery applications are still in their early stages, the remarkable prospective of GQD-based nanocarriers has recently been demonstrated, and we have good cause to think that this innovative nanomaterial can give more types of medications.

6.5.3 PHOTOTHERAPY

Phototherapy is a nonintrusive therapeutic procedure that utilizes fluorescent light to address a variety of diseases. It is separated into two sections: photodynamic therapy (PDT) and photothermal therapy (PTT). During diagnostics, the therapeutic agent is supplied to the ailment site (tumors), which is further photoexcited via exposure to light of a certain wavelength. Cells are destroyed in PTT by the photothermal agent (PT), which absorbs near-infrared (NIR) light and produces heat. Contrarily, PDT uses photosensitizers (PSs), which, when triggered by light, produce ROS that, in response, induces cell damage. **Figure 6.6** illustrates the phototherapy mechanism

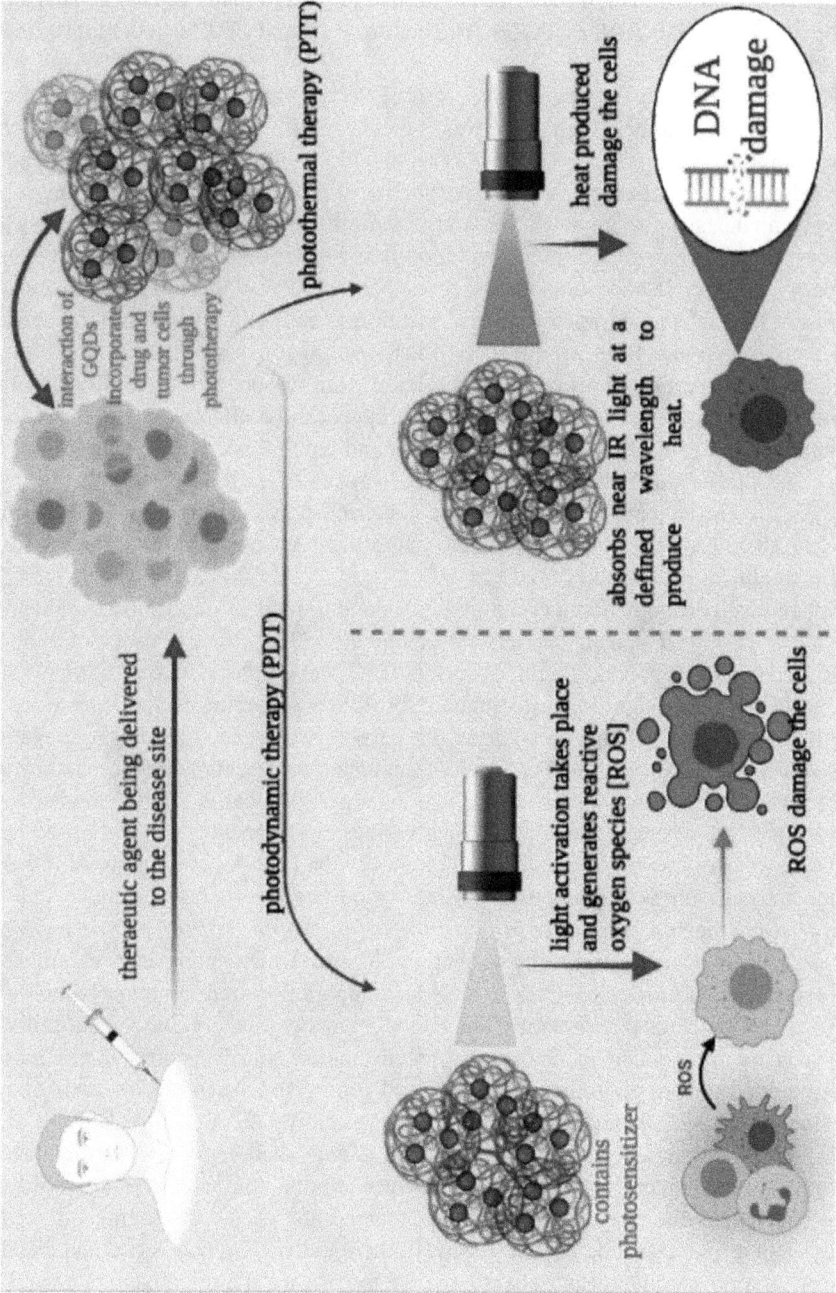

FIGURE 6.6 Schematic Representation of the Phototherapy Mechanism of GQDs. [Reproduced with permission from *Kumar et al. (2022)*] [21].

of GQDs. The upsurge in the systemic adverse effects when standard radio and chemotherapies are used to treat tumors is the biggest concern [21,68]. Due to their exceptional features, much more effective treatment behavior, and negligible adverse effects, nanomaterials such as GQDs designed for PTT and PDT have demonstrated remarkable prospects.

The development of therapeutic agents of the next generation indicates that phototherapy will be the best method of treating cancers. In addition to killing cancer cells, phototherapy treatments can also assist in making other therapeutic treatments like radiation, gene therapy, and chemotherapy more effective [21]. PTT, in particular, enhances the therapeutic impact of radiotherapy and chemotherapy. PTT induces hypothermia, which increases blood flow inside tumors and boosts oxygen delivery to tumors. In addition, enhancing the permeability of the cell membranes at the tumor locations may improve drug absorption as well as a release into the cells. In a similar manner, ROS produced by PDT encourages drug distribution at the location of the tumor and prevents drug release from tumors to increase the effectiveness of chemotherapeutic drugs. Phototherapies can be effectively enhanced by the application of different photothermal (PT) and photosensitizer (PS) substances. These substances might be, among other derivatives of carbon, metal nanostructures, 2D oxide nanoparticles, and semiconducting polymer quantum dots. Such nanoparticles were employed as possible phototherapeutic agents, particularly for cancer treatment [21,69].

In contrast, carbon nanomaterials with adequate dimensions and substantial surface areas work well as drug carriers for therapeutics. The effective usage of nanostructured materials in phototherapies such as CNT and graphene with its derivatives are ascribed to their significant instinctual absorption properties in the wide wavelength range (750–1700 nm). In addition, the carbon-based nanomaterials aggregate specifically in tumor locations as a result of their superior retention and permeability characteristics. Because of their small size, nanoparticles can attain these characteristics and offer perfect contenders for a variety of therapeutic applications. The GQDs have also drawn the greatest attention over the past decade among all other carbon nanostructures because they possess good characteristics that make them ideal phototherapeutic agents [70,71].

Due to their comparatively tiny diameters (20 nm), which enable easy clearance and excretion via kidneys, GQDs exhibit biocompatibility and nontoxic behavior. They can be used for phototherapy due to their low cytotoxicity, biocompatibility, and capacity to produce ROS during photoexcitation. Furthermore, GQDs may transport electrons to photothermal agents and conjugated drugs, which could also improve their chemotherapeutic efficacy synergistically [72]. Recently, Choi et al. (2017) described the fabrication and utilization of core-shell nanoparticles that have a graphene oxide quantum dot (GOQD) for the shell and an upconversion nanoparticle (UCNP) for the core. The UCNP was created and used for imaging-directed upconversion luminescence investigations. In their study, GOQD was produced and utilized as a prospective drug delivery vehicle to enhance the effectiveness of anticancer therapy. A unique nanostructure was made by combining the special qualities of UCNPs and GOQDs to provide desirable drug administration and cell imaging functionality.

Additionally, GOQDs were loaded with Hypocrellin A (HA) for photodynamic treatment (PDT). GOQD was coupled with HA by a π-π interaction and loaded on PEGylated UCNP without a complex synthetic procedure that may have broken the structure of HA. These core-shell nanoparticles were employed in the MTT assay to reveal that the GOQDs shells with UCNPs-loaded with the HA might be the ideal candidates for multifunctional agents for cell imaging, drug administration, and cell therapies [73]. The effects of γ-irradiation on the photoluminescent characteristics of GQDs have been studied by Jovanovic et al. (2015). The key result indicates that low-dose γ-irradiated GQDs are viable contenders for PDT because they perform as superior photo generators when exposed to lower doses of γ-irradiation compared to elevated doses of γ-irradiation [74]. Wang et al. (2015) designed targeted therapeutic and diagnostic GQDs that were linked to the aptamer AS1411. GQDs are able to target tumor cells with excellent selectivity and demolish cells despite low dosages owing to the employment of aptamers. Due to their superior qualities, including size, fluorescence, cytocompatibility, and NIR sensitivity, GQDs are a perfect companion to the aptamer when it comes to targeting tumors [75]. When targeting tumor cells in PDT, photosensitizer solubility is a challenge. The hydrophobic properties of compounds like verteporfin and Ce6 (derivatives of porphyrins) discourage their usage as photosensitizers [21]. By combining the photosensitizers with PEG, these solubility challenges can be fixed, and GQDs will consequently be sequestered inside the conjugated PEG shells. Therefore, PDT may be redox-triggered on synthesized PEGylated GQDs. Additionally, photosensitizer adhesion increases their hydrophilicity without reducing PDT efficiency, preventing quick discharge from the circulation, and improving their hydrophilicity. Overall, the PEGylated GQDs have greatly improved bioimaging and biocompatibility, and they have produced excellent therapeutic efficacy during PDT [76].

Li et al. (2017) revealed the GQDs-FA nanostructures' ability to load the theragnostic drug IR780 after functionalizing GQDs using folic acid. The IR780 offers concurrent fluorescence and phototherapeutic imaging. The presence of carboxyl groups around the margin of an undamaged sp^2 domain was believed to be the cause of the GQDs-FA ability. The significant π-π stacking interactions between IR780 and GQDs-FA have been made possible. The interfacial carboxyl units increase the solubility of IR780 in water by a factor of approximately 2400. This molecular configuration significantly increased the tumor targeting and photo-stability and provided 87.9% of the photothermal conversion efficacy of IR780/GQDs-FA. When tumor cells are exposed to an 808 nm laser, these properties enable significant hyperthermia over cells and totally eliminate them [77]. Tian et al. (2017) developed a multifunctional system for simultaneous chemo and photothermal treatment by using a straightforward one-pot process, which consists of implanted GQDs as localized photothermal seeds and zeolitic imidazolate framework-8 (ZIF-8), which serves as drug carriers. The ZIF-8/GQD nanoparticles' structure, drug release behavior, photothermal impact, and simultaneous therapeutic efficacy were all thoroughly examined. The findings demonstrated that the narrow size distribution of ZIF-8/ GQD nanoparticles of particle size 50–100 nm have encapsulated DOX throughout the production process and triggered DOX release under acidic circumstances. The near-infrared (NIR) radiation could be effectively transformed into heat by the

DOX-loaded ZIF-8/GQD nanoparticles, raising the temperature further. More crucially, the outcomes demonstrated that the combination of chemo- and photothermal treatment with DOX-ZIF-8/GQD nanoparticles had a notable interdependent effect using breast cancer 4T1 cells as a model cellular system. Relative to chemotherapy and photothermal treatment separately, the combined impact has a better efficacy in eradicating cancer cells. As flexible nanocarriers for combinatorial cancer treatment, ZIF-8/GQD nanoparticles are therefore expected to show promise [78].

The GQDs have displayed inherent photothermal and photodynamic characteristics and applicability toward drug delivery. However, further investigations are required in the area of combined therapies to improve the loading efficiency and pH-responsive release behavior of chemotherapeutic agents.

6.6 SUMMARY

The present chapter summarizes the recent developments in the synthesis of GQDs via top-down and bottom-up approaches with various functionalization strategies to improve their surface and physicochemical characteristics. It was observed that the diversity in the size, structure, and functionalized form of GQDs results in a number of modifications to their physical, biological, chemical, optical, and electrical characteristics. Both the top-down and bottom-up approaches for the synthesis of GQDs have affected the aqueous stability of the GQDs by reducing the oxygenated functional entities. In addition, some of these methods, such as microwave, ultrasound, and hydrothermal methods, are considered highly energy intensive, which enhances their operating cost and limits their large-scale application. Meanwhile, the optimization of process parameters and the use of green synthesis methods may overcome these shortcomings. Also, specifically, the bottom-up approaches suffer from low quantum yield, which is a major drawback of these methods.

Herein, the recent developments related to the application of GQDs in the field of drug delivery, gene therapy, and phototherapy have also been discussed. It was observed that GQDs, with their small size, low toxicity, and aqueous stability, have provided significant advantages for drug delivery. However, for their large-scale manufacturing and commercial usage, these formulations' toxicity still has to be improved. The biocompatibility of GQD-based nanoformulations can be improved by using green manufacturing techniques and natural chemotherapeutic agents, which need to be investigated for their application. For the further application of GQDs in the biomedical field, the functionalization approaches must be adapted using various biopolymers to improve their dispersion stability. It is not necessary to use a lot of GQDs for drug delivery applications, but their regulated size and purity must be considered. Overall, GQDs have displayed significant potential for drug delivery-related applications, specifically in anticancer therapeutics.

REFERENCES

[1] J. Douda, C.R. González Vargas, E.V. Basiuk, A.I. Díaz Cano, J.A. Fuentes García, X.A. Hernández Contreras, Optical properties of amine-functionalized graphene oxide, Appl. Nanosci. 9 (2019) 567–578. doi:10.1007/s13204-019-00956-z.

[2] M. Dahiya, S.A. Bansal, Graphene-reinforced nanocomposites: Synthesis, microme-chanics models, analysis and applications—a review, Proc. Inst. Mech. Eng. Part C J. Mech. Eng. Sci. 236 (2022) 9218–9240. doi:10.1177/09544062221091773.

[3] C. Lee, X. Wei, J.W. Kysar, J. Hone, Measurement of the elastic properties and intrinsic strength of monolayer graphene, Sci. 321 (2008) 385–388. doi:10.1126/science.1157996.

[4] C. Fang, J. Zhang, X. Chen, G.J. Weng, Calculating the electrical conductivity of graphene nanoplatelet polymer composites by a Monte Carlo method, Nanomat. 10 (2020) 1129. doi:10.3390/nano10061129.

[5] M.S. Iyer, W. Fu-Ming, I. Rajangam, Electrochemical detection of CA125 using thionine and gold nanoparticles supported on heteroatom-doped graphene nanocomposites, Appl. Nanosci. 11 (2021) 2167–2180. doi:10.1007/s13204-021-01966-6.

[6] E.-C. Cho, J.-H. Huang, C.-P. Li, C.-W. Chang-Jian, K.-C. Lee, Y.-S. Hsiao, J.-H. Huang, Graphene-based thermoplastic composites and their application for LED thermal man-agement, Carbon N. Y. 102 (2016) 66–73. doi:10.1016/j.carbon.2016.01.097.

[7] A.A. Balandin, S. Ghosh, W. Bao, I. Calizo, D. Teweldebrhan, F. Miao, C.N. Lau, Superior thermal conductivity of single-layer graphene, Nano Lett. 8 (2008) 902–907. doi:10.1021/nl0731872.

[8] A. Kalluri, D. Debnath, B. Dharmadhikari, P. Patra, Graphene quantum dots: Synthe-sis and applications, in: E. Kumar (Ed.), Enzyme Nanoarchitectures Enzyme Armored with Graphene, Academic Press, New York (2018): pp. 335–354. doi:10.1016/bs.mie.2018.07.002.

[9] N.S. Samanta, S. Banerjee, P. Mondal, Anweshan, U. Bora, M.K. Purkait, Preparation and characterization of zeolite from waste Linz-Donawitz (LD) process slag of steel industry for removal of Fe3+ from drinking water, Adv. Powder Technol. 32 (2021) 3372–3387. doi:10.1016/j.apt.2021.07.023.

[10] M.C. Biswas, M.T. Islam, P.K. Nandy, M.M. Hossain, Graphene quantum dots (GQDs) for bioimaging and drug delivery applications: A review, ACS Mater. Lett. 3 (2021) 889–911. doi:10.1021/acsmaterialslett.0c00550.

[11] C. Zhao, X. Song, Y. Liu, Y. Fu, L. Ye, N. Wang, F. Wang, L. Li, M. Mohammadniaei, M. Zhang, Q. Zhang, J. Liu, Synthesis of graphene quantum dots and their applications in drug delivery, J. Nanobiotechnol. 18 (2020) 142. doi:10.1186/s12951-020-00698-z.

[12] M. Bacon, S.J. Bradley, T. Nann, Graphene quantum dots, Part. Part. Syst. Charact. 31 (2014) 415–428. doi:10.1002/ppsc.201300252.

[13] Z. Farka, T. Juřík, D. Kovář, L. Trnková, P. Skládal, Nanoparticle-based immunochem-ical biosensors and assays: Recent advances and challenges, Chem. Rev. 117 (2017) 9973–10042. doi:10.1021/acs.chemrev.7b00037.

[14] J.K. Kim, M.J. Park, S.J. Kim, D.H. Wang, S.P. Cho, S. Bae, J.H. Park, B.H. Hong, Balancing light absorptivity and carrier conductivity of graphene quantum dots for high-efficiency bulk heterojunction solar cells, ACS Nano. 7 (2013) 7207–7212. doi:10.1021/nn402606v.

[15] H. Wang, P. Agarwal, S. Zhao, J. Yu, X. Lu, X. He, A biomimetic hybrid nanoplatform for encapsulation and precisely controlled delivery of theranostic agents, Nat. Commun. 6 (2015). doi:10.1038/ncomms10081.

[16] F. Chen, W. Gao, X. Qiu, H. Zhang, L. Liu, P. Liao, W. Fu, Y. Luo, Graphene quantum dots in biomedical applications: Recent advances and future challenges, Front. Lab. Med. 1 (2017) 192–199. doi:10.1016/j.flm.2017.12.006.

[17] X. Wang, X. Sun, J. Lao, H. He, T. Cheng, M. Wang, S. Wang, F. Huang, Multifunctional graphene quantum dots for simultaneous targeted cellular imaging and drug delivery, Colloids Surf. B Biointerfaces. 122 (2014) 638–644. doi:10.1016/j.colsurfb.2014.07.043.

[18] G. Perini, V. Palmieri, G. Ciasca, M. De Spirito, M. Papi, Unravelling the potential of graphene quantum dots in biomedicine and neuroscience, Int. J. Mol. Sci. 21 (2020) 3712. doi:10.3390/ijms21103712.

[19] Z. Zeng, S. Chen, T.T.Y. Tan, F.-X. Xiao, Graphene quantum dots (GQDs) and its derivatives for multifarious photocatalysis and photoelectrocatalysis, Catal. Today. 315 (2018) 171–183. doi:10.1016/j.cattod.2018.01.005.

[20] Y. Wang, J. Li, X. Li, J. Shi, Z. Jiang, C.Y. Zhang, Graphene-based nanomaterials for cancer therapy and anti-infections, Bioact. Mater. 14 (2022) 335–349. doi:10.1016/j.bioactmat.2022.01.045.

[21] P. Kumar, C. Dhand, N. Dwivedi, S. Singh, R. Khan, S. Verma, A. Singh, M.K. Gupta, S. Kumar, R. Kumar, A.K. Srivastava, Graphene quantum dots: A contemporary perspective on scope, opportunities, and sustainability, Renew. Sustain. Energy Rev. 157 (2022) 111993. doi:10.1016/j.rser.2021.111993.

[22] S. Kumbhar, M. De, Carbon quantum dots modified Bi_2WO_6 nanosheets for photo-oxidation of glycerol to value-added product, Mater. Today Proc. (2022). doi:10.1016/j.matpr.2022.11.230.

[23] C. Wang, C. Wu, X. Zhou, T. Han, X. Xin, J. Wu, J. Zhang, S. Guo, Enhancing cell nucleus accumulation and DNA cleavage activity of anti-cancer drug via graphene quantum dots, Sci. Rep. 3 (2013) 2852. doi:10.1038/srep02852.

[24] D. Iannazzo, A. Pistone, M. Salamò, S. Galvagno, R. Romeo, S. V. Giofré, C. Branca, G. Visalli, A. Di Pietro, Graphene quantum dots for cancer targeted drug delivery, Int. J. Pharm. 518 (2017) 185–192. doi:10.1016/j.ijpharm.2016.12.060.

[25] S. Zhu, Y. Song, J. Wang, H. Wan, Y. Zhang, Y. Ning, B. Yang, Photoluminescence mechanism in graphene quantum dots: Quantum confinement effect and surface/edge state, Nano Today. 13 (2017) 10–14. doi:10.1016/j.nantod.2016.12.006.

[26] J. Shen, Y. Zhu, X. Yang, C. Li, Graphene quantum dots: Emergent nanolights for bio-imaging, sensors, catalysis and photovoltaic devices, Chem. Commun. 48 (2012) 3686. doi:10.1039/c2cc00110a.

[27] A.D. Sontakke, M.K. Purkait, Fabrication of ultrasound-mediated tunable graphene oxide nanoscrolls, Ultrason. Sonochem. 63 (2020) 104976. doi:10.1016/j.ultsonch.2020.104976.

[28] A.D. Sontakke, R. Fopase, L.M. Pandey, M.K. Purkait, Development of graphene oxide nanoscrolls imparted nano-delivery system for the sustained release of gallic acid, Appl. Nanosci. (2022). doi:10.1007/s13204-022-02582-8.

[29] A.D. Sontakke, M.K. Purkait, A brief review on graphene oxide nanoscrolls: Structure, Synthesis, characterization and scope of applications, Chem. Eng. J. 420 (2021) 129914. doi:10.1016/j.cej.2021.129914.

[30] P. Mondal, A. Anweshan, M.K. Purkait, Green synthesis and environmental application of iron-based nanomaterials and nanocomposite: A review, Chemosphere. 259 (2020) 127509. doi:10.1016/j.chemosphere.2020.127509.

[31] H. Huang, S. Yang, Q. Li, Y. Yang, G. Wang, X. You, B. Mao, H. Wang, Y. Ma, P. He, Z. Liu, G. Ding, X. Xie, Electrochemical cutting in weak aqueous electrolytes: The strategy for efficient and controllable preparation of graphene quantum dots, Langmuir. 34 (2018) 250–258. doi:10.1021/acs.langmuir.7b03425.

[32] Y. Li, Y. Zhao, H. Cheng, Y. Hu, G. Shi, L. Dai, L. Qu, Nitrogen-doped graphene quantum dots with oxygen-rich functional groups, J. Am. Chem. Soc. 134 (2012) 15–18. doi:10.1021/ja206030c.

[33] D. Huang, L. Yin, X. Lu, S. Lin, Z. Niu, J. Niu, Directional electron transfer mechanisms with graphene quantum dots as the electron donor for photodecomposition of perfluorooctane sulfonate, Chem. Eng. J. 323 (2017) 406–414. doi:10.1016/j.cej.2017.04.124.

[34] H. Gao, C. Xue, G. Hu, K. Zhu, Production of graphene quantum dots by ultrasound-assisted exfoliation in supercritical CO_2/H_2O medium, Ultrason. Sonochem. 37 (2017) 120–127. doi:10.1016/j.ultsonch.2017.01.001.

[35] C. Zhang, Y. Cui, L. Song, X. Liu, Z. Hu, Microwave assisted one-pot synthesis of graphene quantum dots as highly sensitive fluorescent probes for detection of iron ions and pH value, Talanta. 150 (2016) 54–60. doi:10.1016/j.talanta.2015.12.015.

[36] Y. Shin, J. Lee, J. Yang, J. Park, K. Lee, S. Kim, Y. Park, H. Lee, Mass production of graphene quantum dots by one-pot synthesis directly from graphite in high yield, Small. 10 (2014) 866–870. doi:10.1002/smll.201302286.

[37] Z. Luo, G. Qi, K. Chen, M. Zou, L. Yuwen, X. Zhang, W. Huang, L. Wang, Microwave-assisted preparation of white fluorescent graphene quantum dots as a novel phosphor for enhanced white-light-emitting diodes, Adv. Funct. Mater. 26 (2016) 2739–2744. doi:10.1002/adfm.201505044.

[38] J. Shen, Y. Zhu, C. Chen, X. Yang, C. Li, Facile preparation and upconversion luminescence of graphene quantum dots, Chem. Commun. 47 (2011) 2580–2582. doi:10.1039/C0CC04812G.

[39] J. Peng, W. Gao, B.K. Gupta, Z. Liu, R. Romero-Aburto, L. Ge, L. Song, L.B. Alemany, X. Zhan, G. Gao, S.A. Vithayathil, B.A. Kaipparettu, A.A. Marti, T. Hayashi, J.-J. Zhu, P.M. Ajayan, Graphene quantum dots derived from carbon fibers, Nano Lett. 12 (2012) 844–849. doi:10.1021/nl2038979.

[40] Q. Lu, C. Wu, D. Liu, H. Wang, W. Su, H. Li, Y. Zhang, S. Yao, A facile and simple method for synthesis of graphene oxide quantum dots from black carbon, Green Chem. 19 (2017) 900–904. doi:10.1039/C6GC03092K.

[41] R. Tian, S. Zhong, J. Wu, W. Jiang, Y. Shen, W. Jiang, T. Wang, Solvothermal method to prepare graphene quantum dots by hydrogen peroxide, Opt. Mater. (Amst). 60 (2016) 204–208. doi:10.1016/j.optmat.2016.07.032.

[42] J.-H. Zhang, T. Sun, A. Niu, Y.-M. Tang, S. Deng, W. Luo, Q. Xu, D. Wei, D.-S. Pei, Perturbation effect of reduced graphene oxide quantum dots (rGOQDs) on aryl hydrocarbon receptor (AhR) pathway in zebrafish, Biomaterials. 133 (2017) 49–59. doi:10.1016/j.biomaterials.2017.04.026.

[43] Z. Wang, J. Yu, X. Zhang, N. Li, B. Liu, Y. Li, Y. Wang, W. Wang, Y. Li, L. Zhang, S. Dissanayake, S.L. Suib, L. Sun, Large-scale and controllable synthesis of graphene quantum dots from rice husk biomass: A comprehensive utilization strategy, ACS Appl. Mater. Interfaces. 8 (2016) 1434–1439. doi:10.1021/acsami.5b10660.

[44] D. Liu, X. Chen, Y. Hu, T. Sun, Z. Song, Y. Zheng, Y. Cao, Z. Cai, M. Cao, L. Peng, Y. Huang, L. Du, W. Yang, G. Chen, D. Wei, A.T.S. Wee, D. Wei, Raman enhancement on ultra-clean graphene quantum dots produced by quasi-equilibrium plasma-enhanced chemical vapor deposition, Nat. Commun. 9 (2018) 193. doi:10.1038/s41467-017-02627-5.

[45] J. Lee, K. Kim, W.I. Park, B.-H. Kim, J.H. Park, T.-H. Kim, S. Bong, C.-H. Kim, G. Chae, M. Jun, Y. Hwang, Y.S. Jung, S. Jeon, Uniform graphene quantum dots patterned from self-assembled silica nanodots, Nano Lett. 12 (2012) 6078–6083. doi:10.1021/nl302520m.

[46] M.J. Deka, D. Chowdhury, CVD assisted hydrophobic graphene quantum dots: Fluorescence sensor for aromatic amino acids, ChemistrySelect. 2 (2017) 1999–2005. doi:10.1002/slct.201601737.

[47] S. Kumar, S.T. Aziz, O. Girshevitz, G.D. Nessim, One-step synthesis of N-doped graphene quantum dots from chitosan as a sole precursor using chemical vapor deposition, J. Phys. Chem. C. 122 (2018) 2343–2349. doi:10.1021/acs.jpcc.7b05494.

[48] H.M. Kashani, T. Madrakian, A. Afkhami, F. Mahjoubi, M.A. Moosavi, Bottom-up and green-synthesis route of amino functionalized graphene quantum dot as a novel biocompatible and label-free fluorescence probe for in vitro cellular imaging of human ACHN cell lines, Mater. Sci. Eng. B. 251 (2019) 114452. doi:10.1016/j.mseb.2019.114452.

[49] A. Bayat, E. Saievar-Iranizad, Synthesis of green-photoluminescent single layer graphene quantum dots: Determination of HOMO and LUMO energy states, J. Lumin. 192 (2017) 180–183. doi:10.1016/j.jlumin.2017.06.055.

[50] X. Wu, F. Tian, W. Wang, J. Chen, M. Wu, J.X. Zhao, Fabrication of highly fluorescent graphene quantum dots using l-glutamic acid for in vitro/in vivo imaging and sensing, J. Mater. Chem. C. 1 (2013) 4676. doi:10.1039/c3tc30820k.

[51] Y. Dong, J. Shao, C. Chen, H. Li, R. Wang, Y. Chi, X. Lin, G. Chen, Blue luminescent graphene quantum dots and graphene oxide prepared by tuning the carbonization degree of citric acid, Carbon N. Y. 50 (2012) 4738–4743. doi:10.1016/j.carbon.2012.06.002.

[52] L. Wang, W. Li, B. Wu, Z. Li, D. Pan, M. Wu, Room-temperature synthesis of graphene quantum dots via electron-beam irradiation and their application in cell imaging, Chem. Eng. J. 309 (2017) 374–380. doi:10.1016/j.cej.2016.10.022.

[53] R. Rabeya, S. Mahalingam, K.S. Lau, A. Manap, M. Satgunam, C.H. Chia, M. Akhtaruzzaman, Hydrothermal functionalization of graphene quantum dots extracted from cellulose, Chem. Phys. Lett. 795 (2022) 139520. doi:10.1016/j.cplett.2022.139520.

[54] S. Kadian, S.K. Sethi, G. Manik, Recent advancements in synthesis and property control of graphene quantum dots for biomedical and optoelectronic applications, Mater. Chem. Front. 5 (2021) 627–658. doi:10.1039/D0QM00550A.

[55] Z. Qian, J. Ma, X. Shan, L. Shao, J. Zhou, J. Chen, H. Feng, Surface functionalization of graphene quantum dots with small organic molecules from photoluminescence modulation to bioimaging applications: An experimental and theoretical investigation, RSC Adv. 3 (2013) 14571. doi:10.1039/c3ra42066c.

[56] S.H. Jin, D.H. Kim, G.H. Jun, S.H. Hong, S. Jeon, Tuning the photoluminescence of graphene quantum dots through the charge transfer effect of functional groups, ACS Nano. 7 (2013) 1239–1245. doi:10.1021/nn304675g.

[57] X. Yuan, Z. Liu, Z. Guo, Y. Ji, M. Jin, X. Wang, Cellular distribution and cytotoxicity of graphene quantum dots with different functional groups, Nanoscale Res. Lett. 9 (2014) 108. doi:10.1186/1556-276X-9-108.

[58] Z.M. Markovic, B.Z. Ristic, K.M. Arsikin, D.G. Klisic, L.M. Harhaji-Trajkovic, B.M. Todorovic-Markovic, D.P. Kepic, T.K. Kravic-Stevovic, S.P. Jovanovic, M.M. Milenkovic, D.D. Milivojevic, V.Z. Bumbasirevic, M.D. Dramicanin, V.S. Trajkovic, Graphene quantum dots as autophagy-inducing photodynamic agents, Biomaterials. 33 (2012) 7084–7092. doi:10.1016/j.biomaterials.2012.06.060.

[59] C. Luo, Y. Li, L. Guo, F. Zhang, H. Liu, J. Zhang, J. Zheng, J. Zhang, S. Guo, Graphene quantum dots downregulate multiple multidrug-resistant genes via interacting with their C-rich promoters, Adv. Healthc. Mater. 6 (2017) 1700328. doi:10.1002/adhm.201700328.

[60] S. Tiwari, A.D. Sontakke, K. Baruah, M.K. Purkait, Development of graphene oxide-based nano-delivery system for natural chemotherapeutic agent (Caffeic Acid), Mater. Today Proc. (2022). doi:10.1016/j.matpr.2022.11.373.

[61] A.A. Nahain, J.-E. Lee, I. In, H. Lee, K.D. Lee, J.H. Jeong, S.Y. Park, Target delivery and cell imaging using hyaluronic acid-functionalized graphene quantum dots, Mol. Pharm. 10 (2013) 3736–3744. doi:10.1021/mp400219u.

[62] F. Nasrollahi, B. Sana, D. Paramelle, S. Ahadian, A. Khademhosseini, S. Lim, Incorporation of graphene quantum dots, iron, and doxorubicin in/on ferritin nanocages for bimodal imaging and drug delivery, Adv. Ther. 3 (2020) 1900183. doi:10.1002/adtp.201900183.

[63] S. Javanbakht, H. Namazi, Doxorubicin loaded carboxymethyl cellulose/graphene quantum dot nanocomposite hydrogel films as a potential anticancer drug delivery system, Mater. Sci. Eng. C. 87 (2018) 50–59. doi:10.1016/j.msec.2018.02.010.

[64] O. Lv, Y. Tao, Y. Qin, C. Chen, Y. Pan, L. Deng, L. Liu, Y. Kong, Highly fluorescent and morphology-controllable graphene quantum dots-chitosan hybrid xerogels for in vivo imaging and pH-sensitive drug carrier, Mater. Sci. Eng. C. 67 (2016) 478–485. doi:10.1016/j.msec.2016.05.031.

[65] S.M. Ghafary, M. Nikkhah, S. Hatamie, S. Hosseinkhani, Simultaneous gene delivery and tracking through preparation of photo-luminescent nanoparticles based on graphene quantum dots and chimeric peptides, Sci. Rep. 7 (2017) 1–14. doi:10.1038/s41598-017-09890-y.

[66] S. Xiao, D. Zhou, P. Luan, B. Gu, L. Feng, S. Fan, W. Liao, W. Fang, L. Yang, E. Tao, R. Guo, J. Liu, Graphene quantum dots conjugated neuroprotective peptide improve learning and memory capability, Biomaterials. 106 (2016) 98–110. doi:10.1016/j. biomaterials.2016.08.021.

[67] M. Ahn, J. Song, B.H. Hong, Facile synthesis of N-doped graphene quantum dots as novel transfection agents for mRNA and pDNA, Nanomaterials. 11 (2021) 2816. doi:10.3390/ nano11112816.

[68] H. Zhu, Y. Fang, Q. Miao, X. Qi, D. Ding, P. Chen, K. Pu, Regulating near-infrared pho-todynamic properties of semiconducting polymer nanotheranostics for optimized cancer therapy, ACS Nano. 11 (2017) 8998–9009. doi:10.1021/acsnano.7b03507.

[69] A.D. Sontakke, A. Bhattacharjee, R. Fopase, L.M. Pandey, M.K. Purkait, One-pot, sus-tainable and room temperature synthesis of graphene oxide-impregnated iron-based metal-organic framework (GO/MIL-100(Fe)) nanocarriers for anticancer drug delivery systems, J. Mater. Sci. (2022). doi:10.1007/s10853-022-07773-w.

[70] T.A. Tabish, S. Zhang, Graphene quantum dots: Syntheses, properties, and biolog-ical applications, Compr. Nanosci. Nanotechnol. (2016) 171–192. doi:10.1016/ B978-0-12-803581-8.04133-3.

[71] L. Cheng, X. Wang, F. Gong, T. Liu, Z. Liu, 2D nanomaterials for cancer theranostic applications, Adv. Mater. 32 (2020) 1902333. doi:10.1002/adma.201902333.

[72] Y. Cao, H. Dong, Z. Yang, X. Zhong, Y. Chen, W. Dai, X. Zhang, Aptamer-conjugated graphene quantum dots/porphyrin derivative theranostic agent for intracellular cancer-related microRNA detection and fluorescence-guided photothermal/photodynamic synergetic therapy, ACS Appl. Mater. Interfaces. 9 (2017) 159–166. doi:10.1021/acsami. 6b13150.

[73] S.Y. Choi, S.H. Baek, S.-J. Chang, Y. Song, R. Rafique, K.T. Lee, T.J. Park, Synthesis of upconversion nanoparticles conjugated with graphene oxide quantum dots and their use against cancer cell imaging and photodynamic therapy, Biosens. Bioelectron. 93 (2017) 267–273. doi:10.1016/j.bios.2016.08.094.

[74] S.P. Jovanović, Z. Syrgiannis, Z.M. Marković, A. Bonasera, D.P. Kepić, M.D. Budimir, D.D. Milivojević, V.D. Spasojević, M.D. Dramićanin, V.B. Pavlović, B.M. Todorović Marković, Modification of structural and luminescence properties of graphene quantum dots by gamma irradiation and their application in a photodynamic therapy, ACS Appl. Mater. Interfaces. 7 (2015) 25865–25874. doi:10.1021/acsami.5b08226.

[75] X. Wang, X. Sun, H. He, H. Yang, J. Lao, Y. Song, Y. Xia, H. Xu, X. Zhang, F. Huang, A two-component active targeting theranostic agent based on graphene quantum dots, J. Mater. Chem. B. 3 (2015) 3583–3590. doi:10.1039/C5TB00211G.

[76] D. Dong, Z. Wu, J. Wang, G. Fu, Y. Tang, Recent progress in Co_9S_8-based materials for hydrogen and oxygen electrocatalysis, J. Mater. Chem. A. 7 (2019) 16068–16088. doi:10.1039/C9TA04972J.

[77] S. Li, S. Zhou, Y. Li, X. Li, J. Zhu, L. Fan, S. Yang, Exceptionally high payload of the IR780 iodide on folic acid-functionalized graphene quantum dots for targeted pho-tothermal therapy, ACS Appl. Mater. Interfaces. 9 (2017) 22332–22341. doi:10.1021/ acsami.7b07267.

[78] Z. Tian, X. Yao, K. Ma, X. Niu, J. Grothe, Q. Xu, L. Liu, S. Kaskel, Y. Zhu, Metal–organic framework/graphene quantum dot nanoparticles used for synergistic chemo- and photo-thermal therapy, ACS Omega. 2 (2017) 1249–1258. doi:10.1021/acsomega.6b00385.

7 Fullerene-Based Drug Delivery System

7.1 INTRODUCTION TO FULLERENE

Carbon, the most prevalent element in organic molecules, has been shown to occur in two allotropes: diamond and graphite. Fullerenes, a third kind of carbon, were discovered in 1985. Smalley, Kroto, and Curl headed a group of scientists that sought to mimic the environment wherein carbon nucleates in the atmospheres of red giant stars. In their study, a portion of solid graphite was evaporated into plasma comprising ions and atoms by irradiating it with a laser. Because of the interaction with the helium atoms, the unbound ions and atoms were cooled. Clusters with varying quantities of carbon atoms were synthesized because of the collision. When the compounds were analyzed using a mass spectrometer, it was discovered that clusters between 60 and 70 carbon atoms predominate and that 60 atoms were present in the majority of clusters [1]. At the outset, the researchers faced difficulties in synthesizing a sufficient quantity of fullerenes. They barely managed to prepare around 10–15 g. Nonetheless, it took five years for Krätschmer and Huffman (1990) [2] and Kroto et al. (1991) [3] to establish alternative higher-yield sample preparation methodologies for fullerenes. The freshly discovered particle was given the architect Richard Buckminster Fuller's title since he designed the dome in 1967, which has the same form as the carbon clusters [4].

The three researchers who invented fullerenes were awarded with the 1996 Nobel Prize in Chemistry because fullerenes sparked such fascination and enthusiasm among scientists and researchers. Eventually, it was discovered that fullerenes naturally occur in both interstellar dust and earthly geological formations, however, only within the ppm range. Given that there are no substantial changes during the interaction, fullerene is a good candidate for electron transfer processes. As a result, C_{60} has the ability to effectively slow down charge carrier recombination. Additionally, fullerene exhibits moderate reactions in the visible spectrum as well as substantial absorption of U.V. radiation [5]. As a result, it may also function as a suitable sensitizer to emit electrons when paired with a semiconductor photocatalyst after the irradiation of a visible light source. Fullerene, on the other hand, lacks active areas on the cages for direct catalytic uses. Significantly, fullerene cages have a high degree of hydrophobicity and are inaccessible in polar solvents such as water. Numerous studies have described adding hydroxyl functional groups to the exterior of fullerene to integrate it into a polar environment [5].

The present chapter deals with the various structural attributes and physicochemical characteristics of fullerene, along with its significance and prospects as a nanocarrier for drug delivery. The methods for synthesizing fullerene, such as arc discharge, gas-phase, and wet-chemical processes, have been illustrated with

DOI: 10.1201/9781003358114-7

their advancements. Furthermore, the functionalization strategies are highlighted to enhance the surface characteristics of fullerene. The recent advancements in the applications of fullerene for nucleic acid delivery, chemotherapeutics, and neurodegenerative diseases have been elucidated in the last section.

7.2 STRUCTURAL FEATURES AND PHYSICOCHEMICAL PROPERTIES OF FULLERENE

The first fullerene, C_{60}, was discovered in 1985, but the family of fullerenes also comprises a large variety of other carbon-based compounds with various symmetries and atom counts. The most prevalent fullerene, also known as "Buckminsterfullerene," is made up of 60 carbon atoms organized in 20 hexagons and 12 pentagons, giving it the shape of a hollow sphere (**Figure 7.1**) [6]. The extremely stable and symmetrical structure of C_{60} garnered a lot of attention. Zero-dimensional fullerenes are thought to have highly intriguing chemical and physical characteristics for medical and technological purposes [7].

Fullerenes satisfy Euler's theorem, which states that exactly 12 pentagons must be present in a closed construction made of hexagons and pentagons. According to this criterion, the smallest robust fullerene is C_{60}, with the most rigid form due to the absence of two adjacent pentagons. The great uniformity of the C_{60} structure is a significant characteristic. The structure is mapped onto itself by 120 symmetrical functions, including rotation along the axis and reflection in a plane. As a result, C_{60} is the most symmetrical molecule [8]. The fullerene has two different bond lengths: C_5-C_5 single bonds in pentagons and C_5-C_6 double bonds in hexagons, both of which measure 1.45 ± 0.015 Å and 1.40 ± 0.015 Å, correspondingly [9].

Through sp^2 hybridization, each of the carbon atoms in fullerene joins three other nearby atoms. The collection of orbitals is oriented in the xy-plane and is organized at 120-degree inclinations. Hence, through resonance, such delocalized pi electrons maintain the spheroid structure [10]. The diameter of a C_{60} molecule, sometimes referred to as a Buckyball or Buckminsterfullerene, is around 7 Å. A solid composed of loosely linked C_{60} molecules is synthesized during condensation. Fullerites are this type of crystal structure. This solid is cubic, weakly bound, electrically insulating, and has a lattice constant of 14.71. It appears as a yellow powder that, when

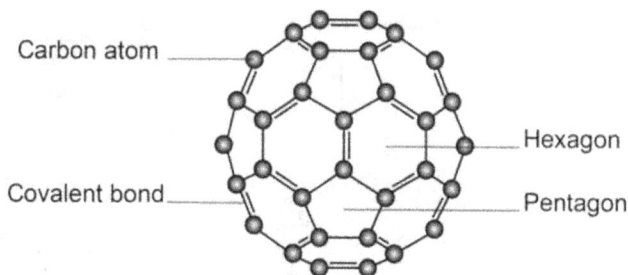

FIGURE 7.1 Structure of Fullerene C_{60} Molecule. [Reprinted with permission from *Rondags et al., (2017)*] [6].

dissolving in toluene, becomes pink [4]. The Buckyballs polymerize when exposed to intense UV light, responsible for binding between nearby balls. C_{60} does not dissolve in toluene after it has polymerized [11]. The free rotation has been seen at normal temperatures in NMR investigations of C_{60} benzene solvates. The balls are in their crystalline orientations and spinning freely at around -13° [4]. Their motions start to become restricted to particular directions at lower temperatures. The balls subsequently get fully struck below 183° [12]. Chemically, the molecule is highly stable; temperatures exceeding 1000 °C are needed to split the balls. Fullerenes may be converted to graphite by roasting them to 1500 °C in the absence of air. In addition to C_{60}, fullerenes can include between 30 and 980 carbon atoms, generating various configurations with various characteristics and application areas.

The fundamental soccer ball configuration starts to lose roundness when hexagons are introduced or subtracted. C_{70}, which comprises 25 hexagons, has a rugby ball-like form. The form of giant fullerenes is pentagonal. Asteroids resemble smaller fullerenes. Loss of stability results from the loss of roundness, with C_{60} proving to be the most stable of all. In addition to C_{60} and C_{70}, C_{76}, C_{78}, C_{84}, and C_{86} have all been isolated and thoroughly researched. Diamond has a higher density than fullerenes (3.51 g/cc against 1.65 g/cc). Fullerenes are water-insoluble. Toluene, o-dichlorobenzene, xylene, and carbon disulfide are effective solvents [13,14]. Yellow to yellowish-green colors can be seen in thin layers of fullerenes.

Several chemical variations of fullerenes were identified soon after their discovery (**Figure 7.2**) [4]. The following are a few notable fullerene species.

7.2.1 ALKALI-DOPED FULLERENES

Being extremely electronegative, fullerene molecules easily combine with elements that provide electrons, most frequently alkali metals [15]. By filling up the gap

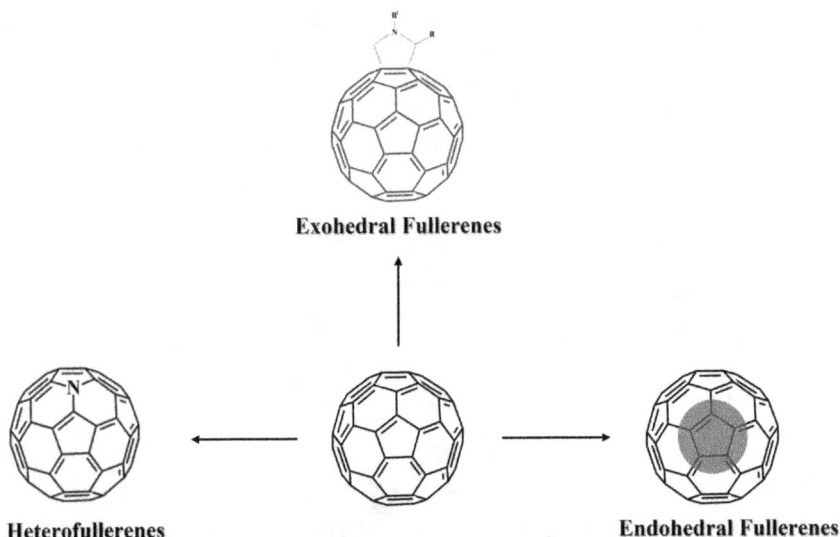

Exohedral Fullerenes

Heterofullerenes   **Endohedral Fullerenes**

FIGURE 7.2 Chemical Modifications of Fullerene [4].

among Buckyballs and giving the nearby C_{60} molecule a valence electron, alkali metal atoms from this reaction produce an intriguing family of compounds known as alkali-doped fullerides. When potassium or rubidium make up the alkali atoms, the resulting compounds—such as K_3C_{60} and Rb_3C_{60}—are known as superconductors because they conduct electricity even without resistance at temperatures below 20–40 K [16].

7.2.2 ENDOHEDRAL FULLERENES

It is feasible to contain another atom inside of fullerenes since they have a hollow interior and a closed shell of carbon atoms. This subclass of fullerene derivatives is called endohedral fullerenes. They are called metallofullerenes once the entrapped element is a metal [17]. Even though C_{60} is the most prevalent fullerene, only a tiny number of endohedral compounds have indeed been developed utilizing C_{60} as the framework. C_{82}, C_{84}, or even higher fullerenes are used to make the majority of endohedral materials. In addition to a few of the noble gases, lanthanum, yttrium, scandium, and other elements can combine to produce stable endohedral compounds [18]. Endohedral material should be formed concurrently with the construction of the cage since it is extremely hard to break up carbon cage molecules to encapsulate a foreign atom inside of them [19].

7.2.3 EXOHEDRAL FULLERENES

Exohedral fullerenes, also known as fullerene derivatives, are compounds produced by a chemical interaction between fullerenes and perhaps other chemical groups. They are the most significant and useful of all fullerene species.

The term "functionalized fullerenes" also refers to fullerene derivatives. As a consequence of the conjugated π-system of electrons that fullerenes have, there are two basic chemical transformations that may occur on their surface: addition reactions and redox reactions, which result in covalent exohedral adducts and salts, respectively [20]. Many fullerene derivatives have been developed with enhanced solubility profiles since fullerenes are insoluble in water.

7.2.4 HETEROFULLERENES

A further important class of altered fullerenes is the heterofullerenes. These are hetero-analogs of fullerenes with carbon counts of 60 and more; one or more carbon atoms in the cages are replaced with heteroatoms, such as trivalent nitrogen or boron atoms. Aza (60) fullerene $C_{59}N$ and its dimer $(C_{59}N)_2$ are the most basic nitrogen fullerene derivatives [21].

7.3 FULLERENE AS A DRUG CARRIER: SIGNIFICANCE AND PROSPECTS

Fullerenes are chemically inert, hollow, and infinitely adjustable. They are not digested when given orally in the water-soluble form, but when given as an intravenous injection, they are quickly disseminated to numerous bodily regions and unalterably eliminated by the kidney [4]. Water-soluble fullerenes were discovered to have very low acute toxicity [22]. Fullerenes may be used in biology and medicinal chemistry due to all these intriguing features, which indicate a promising future for them as pharmaceuticals. Nevertheless, there is a considerable obstacle to this potential, namely fullerenes' inherent anisotropy toward the water. Several approaches are being explored to get over this restriction. Among them involve the development of fullerene derivatives with altered solubility profiles, the embedding of C_{60} in cyclodextrins or calixarenes, or formulations in aqueous suspension. Fullerene derivatives have been produced in large quantities.

Fullerenes have been the subject of several inventions, and the fullerene patent repository is expanding quickly. As fullerenes and their derivatives showed early signs of potential activity in numerous medicinal fields, such as nucleic acid delivery, chemotherapeutics, and neurodegenerative diseases, they are currently the subject of extensive research.

The primary function of fullerenes is to serve as a photosensitizer for the photoproduction of singlet oxygen ($^1O_2$) ROS; as a result, they are used in photodynamic treatment (PDT) and blood sterilization [23–25]. Regrettably, the dispersibility of fullerene is a substantial hurdle to its use in nanomedicine. The main problem is their inability to dissolve in many solvents, notably water, where singlet oxygen has a lengthy lifetime. A variety of approaches have been developed to functionalize fullerenes with hydrophilic groups in order to improve their solubility in water [26,27]. The ability of fullerene to scavenge free radicals like reactive oxygen species (ROS) and reactive nitrogen species (RNS) and serve as an antioxidant has boosted its adoption in biological applications. Cells can be shielded against nitric oxide-induced apoptosis with the use of derivatives of glutathione C_{60} [28].

When pre-incubated with C_{60}, the IgE-dependent mediators generated by human mast cells (hMCs) and peripheral blood basophils were significantly inhibited, supporting the role of fullerenes as a strong allergen inhibitor [29]. Fullerenes may have the capacity to serve as photosensitizers. They may absorb photons in the visible and UV range depending on the polarity of the medium, leading to the production of photo-excited fullerene molecules in the triplet state and, in certain situations, singlet oxygen or ROS. Additionally, fullerenes might be used with light-harvesting antennas to increase the quantum yield (QY) of ROS formation. So, the use of fullerenes in PDT can be utilized to treat cancer and get rid of germs. The cage-like nanoscale structure of fullerenes enables the development of molecular or particulate structures, including one or even more organic chemicals covalently bonded to the fullerene cage surface in a geometrically controlled manner. For the purpose of inhibiting cellular and enzymatic activity, targeted drug transport through biological membranes and receptor ligands are acceptable. The liposome encapsulation technique is a different way of developing fullerenes to be utilized in pharmaceutical applications with better dispersion, absorption, and delivery efficiency [30].

Although significant scientific advances have been achieved in the realm of fullerene treatments, the failure of clinical studies results from worries regarding the long-term safety and toxicity of fullerene. Yet since fullerene-based cosmetics have been used for a long time in human skin care and have passed clinical testing, it is safe to apply them externally at most [31,32]. The sturdy cage-like structure of fullerenes allows for enough room for the encapsulation of atoms, drug molecules, and particles. For instance, highly reliable water-soluble gadolinium metallofullerenes (gadofullerenes) are incredibly fascinating MRI contrast agents. Fullerenes may self-assemble into fullerosomes, which are multivalent drug delivery systems (DDSs) with the potential for diverse targeting properties [33].

7.4 METHODS FOR THE SYNTHESIS OF FULLERENE

For decades, carbon clusters have piqued the interest of researchers in numerous fields. Researchers from a variety of backgrounds, including chemists and engineers, are always looking for new ways to use their findings in areas such as catalysis and combustion. Little carbon clusters have been detected in carbon stars and comet tails, and astrophysicists are trying to figure out what role they play. Moreover, the discovery of C_{60} buckminsterfullerene may be traced back to the earliest investigations into carbon cluster production. Keep in mind that the accidental synthesis of fullerenes may be traced back to basic science. Carbon-cage clusters, their genesis, fundamental science, and application development continue to pique researchers' interests today. Graphite and diamond are two allotropes of carbon that have been known for ages. The fullerene timeline, in contrast, did not progress until the 1980s, when many significant investigations were conducted. Fullerenes were first made experimentally and found during this decade [34].

The investigation conducted by Krätschmer and Huffman was pioneering for the synthesis of fullerenes in 1990 and marked a turning point in the production of cageless molecules [35]. Some contemporary laboratories continue to rely on the electric arc approach, which vastly improves the accessibility of C_{60} and C_{70} fullerene samples. Due to the abundance of pure C_{60} available to scientists throughout the 1990s, the number of fullerene-related investigations surged considerably. Numerous long-awaited fullerene research is now feasible due to a shift in emphasis from laser vaporization to electric arc. It took another five years (1990) for electric arc synthesis, invented by Krätschmer and Huffman, to replace the microgram quantities previously produced by the laser vaporization technique (1985) [35,36]. This electric arc method ultimately becomes the most important method for mass-producing kilogram quantities of fullerene soot. The arc reactor generated gram-scale quantities of purified and widely dispersed C_{60} in the 1990s and beyond. Early in the 1990s, a fundamental question is posed. Both lasers and electric arcs have been utilized in the production of fullerenes. Intuitively, one may consider various methods for evaporating a carbon source in a low-pressure environment containing helium or argon. Numerous attempts to produce fullerenes between 1990 and 2022 are reported and will be briefly discussed next. Solar energy, a radio-frequency furnace, chemical vapor deposition (CVD), and combustion are some of the more unusual techniques that may be utilized to make them.

7.4.1 GAS-PHASE METHOD

In 1991, researchers at the Massachusetts Institute of Technology evaluated the possibility of producing fullerene in soot-laden flames. In their ground-breaking study,

Howard et al. show the synthesis of C_{60} and C_{70} fullerenes utilizing a flame technique [37]. The authors describe how pressure (20 torrs), temperature (1800 K), carbon-to-oxygen ratio (0.995), and flame residence time impact the combustion and condensation of hydrocarbons. When these factors are tuned, one kilogram of carbon fuel yields three kilograms of fullerenes [37]. This unique combustion technique using flames indicates promise as early as 1991, just one year after the K-H electric arc synthesis was introduced [35,38]. The operator may change the ratio of C_{70} to C_{60} fullerenes, which is one of the flame method's less-discussed attributes. The ratio C_{70}/C_{60} may be altered from 0.26 to 5.70 by modifying the experimental conditions. Controlling the formation of fullerenes is a significant finding about their origin. The authors also observe and examine how the development of fullerenes differs from that of soot [37]. For example, the sootiest flames do not always create the most fullerene. In fact, fullerene yield increases with either 1. decreased pressure or 2. increased temperature [37]. The MIT group in 1996 released another significant study on the combustion technique employing benzene, oxygen, and argon flames [39]. This later attempt aims to examine higher fullerenes, which represents a significant shift from the first. The HPLC techniques used to generate, extract, and separate them are of tremendous interest. Beyond C_{60} and C_{70}, all fullerenes are sought. C_{76}, C_{78}, C_{84}, C_{90}, and C_{96} are merely a few of the larger cage constructions that are being considered for production and isolation [39]. They emphasize the importance of solvent selection while attempting to extract this lesser-known, higher fullerenes. To remove soot efficiently, they designed a method of advanced extraction using several solvents [39].

In 1991, Howard et al. first introduced the notion of employing a bigger flame for industrial-scale fullerene manufacturing. Due to industry investment, their commercial production became a reality 13 years later, confirming that their prediction was accurate [37]. The combustion synthesis was developed by TDA Research and Frontier Carbon Corporation (formed in Japan as a joint venture by Mitsubishi in December 2001) to produce fullerenes on an unprecedented scale of tons per year [40]. The transition of fullerene production from university laboratories to the industrial setting has reduced the ten-year reliance on solitary academic groups for sample collaborations. Instead, they would be made and sold inexpensively by a business. By doing so, the sample availability issue that has plagued the business for decades would be resolved (1985–2004). Its commercialization constitutes a major scientific advancement in the realms of flame-based technology, low-cost hydrocarbons, and continuous-flame synthesis [40]. When experiments are improved, soot collected by the flame method has the potential to contain as much as 20% fullerene. In addition to the cost of raw materials, the authors emphasize the importance of other industrial processes [40].

7.4.2 Arc Discharge Method

From 1985 to 1990, evidence of the presence of fullerenes increased. Several laboratories undertook independent, repeatable synthesis and mass spectrometry-based identification of their presence [41]. During this period, scientists intended to increase fullerene production from micrograms to milligrams. Due to the exceedingly low yield of soot and fullerenes that could be removed, the laser extraction technique of the 1980s was problematic. Despite increased interest in soot and fullerenes, researchers needed a more efficient way of generating these substances. Without huge amounts of pure C_{60} and C_{70} samples, a paradigm shift in fullerene manufacturing was required for several planned experiments. From this perspective, it is simple to understand why Huffman's technique of creating fullerenes made such a stir and had such a deep impact [35,38,41]. Their electric arc synthesis has made it possible for the first time to produce soot and fullerenes in the gram range. They may apply their arc approach with any chamber design without incurring excessive costs. With this electric arc process, it is also feasible to create nanotubes, endohedral metallofullerenes, and empty-cage fullerenes. In 1990, Krätschmer and Huffman's research team published two essential studies [35,38]. They discovered that graphite rods could be vaporized by resistive heating in the presence of a quenching gas. The collected carbon smoke particles are then studied further. The authors provided experimental evidence for an all-carbon, icosahedral C_{60} molecule by comparing the infrared and ultraviolet absorption spectra of C-12 and C-13 tagged samples resulting from their arc synthesis [38]. The observed number of bands was consistent with theory, confirming the symmetric, soccer-ball-shaped C_{60} structure. Remember that the foreshadowing would come in the last sentence of their report. They anticipated that their K-H arc approach would enable the extraction of huge quantities of fullerenes from soot [38]. Time validated their concluding assertion. In the year 2020, 30 years and a global pandemic later, their electric arc technology is still extensively used to manufacture carbon nanomaterials. In September 1990, *Nature* published "Solid C_{60}: a unique form of carbon" by Krätschmer and Huffman as their second article [35]. Macroscopic quantities of isolated C_{60} were produced, separated, and characterized, illuminating the methods involved. This research described the unique electric arc method experimentally. Resultantly heated carbon rods were vaporized at 100 torrs of He buffer gas. Gram quantities of fullerenes were extracted from soot using an aromatic solvent (benzene). Adding solvents like carbon disulfide or carbon tetrachloride may also dissolve and extract fullerenes from the soot matrix. Krätschmer and Huffman proposed sublimation as an alternative to solvent extraction for extracting fullerenes from soot and producing thin layers of C_{60}-coated surfaces [35]. In actuality, IR and UV-Vis spectroscopy was employed to characterize these coatings. This is largely recognized as the first source chronicling the evolution of the electric arc approach for producing fullerenes. This research comprises some of the initial experimental characterizations of C_{60}. The arc process facilitated the synthesis of substantial quantities of pure C_{60}, which made this achievement feasible [35]. In addition, Krätschmer and Huffman were able to isolate 100 mg of C_{60} in just one day, an achievement that goes back 30 years to this influential article. In the concluding portion of this second research, the authors predicted the effects of their electric arc discovery, as they did in their investigation [35,38]. Krätschmer and Huffman's electric arc approach for synthesizing fullerene is well-known among researchers working with carbon nanomaterials today. In current times, the pioneering characterization investigations that empirically verified C_{60}'s I_h structure are rarely accorded the respect they deserve [35]. In December 1990, Haufler et al. successfully extracted grams of C_{60} using an electric arc reactor [42]. Evident are the best parameters for its synthesis. The reactor was pressurized to 100 torrs, the bleed rate was 1 sccm, the current was between 100 and 200 amps, and the RMS voltage was between 10 and 20 volts [42]. This system generated 10 g/h of soot. While doing the extraction, the authors selected a process unique from that of Krätschmer and Huffman. Instead, Smalley's team produced around 10% extractable fullerenes from soot by boiling toluene for three hours in a Soxhlet extraction [43]. In terms of the ratio of fullerene to soot, their performance is comparable to that of a number of commercially marketed electric arc reactors. The first experimental reactions with C_{60} were also documented. In 1990, electrochemical approaches were added to the ever-expanding palette of conclusive methods for characterizing C_{60}. The Birch reduction was employed to produce $C_{60}H_{36}$, and the DDQ reagent was then used to remove the hydrogen, leaving pure C_{60} [42]. In doing so, they created a reversible reaction with C_{60}. The chemistry of functionalizing the surfaces of fullerene cages has begun. Haufler foresaw the importance of their reactivity discoveries, predicting a chemically derivatized rich outer surface of fullerenes, and theorized that metal atoms could be utilized inside the cavity to fine-tune the fullerene's electrical and optical properties [42]. Exohedral functionalization and endohedral encapsulation, two prospective study subjects, have witnessed the publication of tens of thousands [41]. In another study, the authors improved their reactor parameters (current, rod diameter, graphite supply, helium pressure, and soot extraction technique) to increase the extractable yield of soluble fullerene to 14% [44,45].

7.4.3 Microwave-Based Process

In addition to the well-known methods outlined before, there exist technologies that synthesize fullerene using microwaves. In 1995, Ikeda et al. reported successfully synthesizing fullerene using naphthalene and microwave-induced N_2 plasma in a cylindrical coaxial cavity at atmospheric pressure. In nitrogen plasma generated by microwaves, molecular species like benzene and naphthalene may be excited and ionized, and the plasma state can be easily regulated [46].

Recent research has investigated the prospect of utilizing microwaves to transform graphite powder into fullerenes, therefore creating a new route for fullerene production. As it evenly warms the precursors, the microwave technique offers advantages over more conventional heating methods. The amount of graphite powder utilized and the microwave power led to a higher yield of produced fullerene, but time and temperature had no influence on fullerene synthesis [47].

7.5 FUNCTIONALIZATION OF FULLERENE

Fullerene's distinct physical and chemical properties make it a promising candidate for use in biological and material chemistry applications, although the molecule is often functionalized before being put to such uses [48]. Fullerene C_{60} has many interesting features, but its insolubility in water and limited solubility in many organic solvents prevent it from being used in biological applications [49]. Functionalizing fullerene relies heavily on its double-bond structure. They may participate in additional reactions, allowing for modifying the carbon cage's outer sphere and synthesizing derivatives with a wide range of functional groups [50]. As pure fullerene lacks a hydrogen atom, it is unable to participate in substitution processes; nonetheless, fullerenes are oxidizing agents and may generate active oxygen forms when exposed to UV-visible light [48].

Fullerenes can be altered in two ways: 1. by covering up part of the fullerene surface with a solubilizing agent and 2. by chemically altering the fullerene by covalent functionalization [48]. The first group can benefit from inserting fullerene into artificial lipid membranes, inducing co-solvation with polyvinylpyrrolidone in organic solvents and attaching polymer chains to fullerene [48,51]. The hydrophilicity of fullerene and the range of its biological and pharmacological uses have been improved by a variety of functionalization techniques. The transformation of fullerene's carbon atoms from sp^2 to sp^3 hybridization is the driving force behind the reaction [52]. Molecules can be covalently conjugated to C_{60} by free-radical processes, cyclopropanation, or cycloaddition reactions such as [1 + 2], [2 + 2], [3 + 2], and [4 + 2] [52]. As a result of its electron-deficient state, fullerene reacts in a wide range of cycloaddition reactions, including [1 + 2], [4 + 2] (Diels-Alder reactions), [3 + 2], and [2 + 2]. Several cycloaddition procedures have been used to create a wide variety of fullerene derivatives [53]. The latter strategy, chemical modification, is a cutting-edge and efficient approach that yielded several fullerene derivatives with attached amine ($-NH_2$), hydroxyl ($-OH$), and/or carboxyl ($-COOH$) groups, including examples of some of the so-obtained derivatives.

Brettreich et al. used a dendrimeric approach to attaching carboxylic groups to fullerene, which increased the molecule's solubility in water and achieved excellent results among the many fullerene functionalizing approaches [54]. To improve fullerene solubility in aqueous and polar environments, Filippone et al. synthesized a (permethylated-cyclodextrin)-fullerene conjugate by covalently linking C_{60} and cyclodextrins. Fullerenols, which have a $C_{60}(OH)_n$ formula and include a hydroxyl group, are very soluble in water and have been used to neutralize oxygen-free radicals and protect neural tissue [55]. In addition, amyotrophic lateral sclerosis (ALS) patients have benefited from carboxy fullerenes in the therapy of neurodegeneration [56].

7.6 APPLICATIONS OF FULLERENE

Fullerenes are a family of carbon-based nanomaterials with distinctive structural and electrical features that make them desirable for a broad variety of applications, including medication administration. Its usage as a medication delivery system is one of the most promising uses of fullerenes. Fullerenes may be functionalized with hydroxyl, carboxylic acid, and amine groups, enabling their usage as nanocarriers for the delivery of drugs. Fullerenes' huge surface area gives adequate space for drug loading, while their unique physical and chemical characteristics allow for effective drug transport to target cells or tissues. Using fullerenes as medication delivery systems offer several benefits:

- Biocompatibility: it has been demonstrated that fullerenes are biocompatible and do not generate considerable toxicity, making them excellent for use in biomedical applications.

- Fullerenes can prevent the degradation of medicines, enhancing their stability and extending their half-life in the body.
- The functionalization of fullerenes with targeting moieties, such as antibodies or peptides, enables the selective delivery of medications to specific cells or organs.
- Fullerenes have unique optical and magnetic characteristics that can be utilized for biological imaging techniques like fluorescence and magnetic resonance imaging.
- Fullerenes may be functionalized with a variety of functional groups, enabling its usage in diverse applications, including medication administration and imaging.

Despite these benefits, the use of fullerenes as a drug delivery method is not without its drawbacks. For instance, fullerenes are rapidly eliminated from the body, which might reduce their effectiveness. Researchers have devised techniques to improve the stability and bioavailability of fullerenes, including encapsulation in liposomes and polymer nanoparticles. Fullerenes have demonstrated considerable potential as drug delivery systems owing to their biocompatibility, drug stability, targeted drug delivery, imaging capabilities, and multifunctionality, among other features. This section focuses on the use of fullerenes as a carrier for nucleic acid-based medicines, along with its prowess in cancer and neurodegenerative therapeutics. However, further study is required to enhance their design and increase their clinical effectiveness and safety.

7.6.1 Nucleic Acid Delivery

Fullerene and its functionalized derivatives have been researched for possible medicinal applications because of their distinctive characteristics. Theoretically, compounds from this class may serve as carefully regulated drug delivery systems. Fullerene and its functionalized derivatives are a relatively recent medicinal technique for nucleic acid delivery. The method entails targeted distribution in cells devoid of nucleic acids. The vast majority of approaches for targeting the transfer of DNA, RNA, siRNA, LNA, and plasmid DNA to specific cellular locations rely on viral delivery [57]. Small chemicals have been transported by nanoparticles, such as fullerenes, in a number of investigations because of their low cost, high efficiency, and absence of allergic reactions [58]. In a pH-balanced solution, a cationic tetra-amino fullerene and siRNA form nanoscale complexes. When these complexes agglutinate with plasma proteins in circulation, micrometer-sized particles are generated. After inhibiting the expression of certain cancer genes, the agglutinate is swiftly eliminated from the lung [59]. This is because it quickly clogs the capillaries in the lungs. Further research revealed that a certain amphiphilic skeleton of C_{60}-Dex-NH_2 may form micelle-like aggregation structures in water, therefore shielding siRNA against oxidative destruction. When exposed to visible light, C_{60}-Dex-NH_2 caused regulated ROS generation leading to lysosome membrane breakdown, enabling lysosomal escape, and enhancing the *in-vitro* and *in-vivo* efficiency of siRNA gene silencing. Both MDA-MB-231-EGFP cells and 4T1-GFP-Luc2 tumor-bearing mice showed a maximum gene silencing efficiency of 53%. According to the published research, conjugated nucleic acids supplied via fullerene-based systems significantly enhance the specificity of their effects on their intended targets. At the same time, healthy cells are considerably more resistant to adverse effects [60].

7.6.2 Chemotherapy

Causes of cancer include chemical or poisonous chemicals, ionizing radiation, viruses, and human genetics [60]. Cancer is the uncontrolled proliferation of aberrant cells in the body. Cancer treatments have historically used a wide variety of medications. The biggest issue with cancer treatment is the severe adverse effects of the medications, which need careful dosing [61]. Drug resistance is another problem in cancer treatment, forcing doctors to utilize combinations of medications with additive side effects.

Fullerene, a nanoparticle with promising structural properties for use in medication administration, is one example. Many of the negative effects of chemotherapy may be alleviated, thanks to fullerene, because it can transport a large number of drugs and deliver them precisely 22, 23. For instance, doxorubicin has the potential for conjugation with fullerene because of the cardiomyopathy-related adverse effects of this drug [62]. This conjugation was tested at various pH levels, and findings showed that drug release was maximized at a pH of 5.25. Based on the findings, such conjugation for selective medication delivery with minimal unwanted consequences can be employed. As fullerene is hydrophobic and doxorubicin is water-soluble, this strategy required the insertion of ethylene glycol spacers to improve the water solubility of the doxorubicin-methano-C_{60} conjugate [48]. Another study covered paclitaxel's hydrophilic surface by using Buckysomes, which are spherical nanostructures composed of amphiphilic fullerenes with hydrophobic areas. According to the results of this research, the suggested complex has the potential to significantly improve medication absorption [63].

By attaching a hydrophilic shell to the outer surface of the conjugation of doxorubicin and fullerene, researchers were able to create a new, unique drug delivery system based on an "on-off" drug delivery method. In its inactive ("off") form, this drug delivery system is relatively stable in physiological solutions, down to a pH of 5.5; in its active ("on") state, however, fullerene's ROS production leads to two distinct treatment modalities. The first is the production of oxygen radicals that kill cells (programmed cell death; PDT), and the second is the explosive release of doxorubicin (chemotherapy) by destroying the ROS-sensitive linkers [60]. Several nanomaterials have been investigated so far in the development of revolutionary techniques for cancer treatment; nevertheless, fullerene and fullerene-based systems are among the most promising alternatives due to their distinctive structures and features.

7.6.3 Neurodegenerative Diseases

Drug delivery to the CNS is complicated by the presence of the blood-brain barrier, a physical barrier formed of tight endothelial junctions that restrict paracellular permeability [60]. Nanomaterials with great potential for transporting medications into the brain include fullerene and its water-soluble derivatives. The research examined the effectiveness of a hexamethonium delivery method with and without a fullerene complex. According to the study, the sophisticated medication delivery method increased efficacy by a factor of 40. Water-soluble derivatives of C_{60} fullerene were synthesized in another work, this time using four different types of connections between the fullerene cage and the solubilizing added atoms [64]. The proliferation of neural stem cells (NSCs) was induced *in-vitro* by fullerene derivatives 1–6 (compounds 1–3 contain C–C bonds; compounds 4–5 contain C–S bonds; and compound 6 contains C–P bonds), and the function of the injured central nervous system in zebrafish was restored.

Interestingly, compound 3, which included phenyl butyric acid residues, dramatically increased NSC proliferation and brain repair through a shift in cellular metabolism that resulted in a decrease in reactive oxygen species (ROS) activity and an increase in adenosine triphosphate (ATP) activity. Compounds 7–9, which are fullerene derivatives, have been shown to limit the growth of glioblastoma cells in zebrafish. Compound 7, which included phenylalanine tails, dramatically slowed glioblastoma development and served as an anticancer agent. Metabolic alterations in the cells were linked to the aftereffects of increased ROS activity and decreased ATP activity [64]. The neurodegeneration associated with amyotrophic lateral sclerosis (ALS) has also been treated by means of carboxy fullerenes [65]. The brain's intricate anatomy inherently prevents any substance from crossing the blood-brain barrier. Despite this restriction, therapeutics can be delivered through the twisted structures of fullerene-based delivery systems.

Maintaining a healthy level of oxidation and antioxidant activity inside the body is crucial to the integrity of our biological system. Toxicities and illnesses induced by excess free radicals, such as cancer and atherosclerosis, necessitate the administration of exogenous antioxidants due to our insufficient endogenous antioxidant defense system and the huge free-radical synthesis by normal cellular metabolism and aberrant responses [60]. These nanoparticles are able to react with free radicals, including superoxide, hydroxyl radicals, and hydrogen peroxide, because of the presence of many double bonds in the fullerene cage [48]. Two types of fullerenes, C_{60} and C_{82}, were employed as antioxidants in a recent study. These fullerenes were conjugated with copper, silver, and gold. Results showed that fullerenes' antiradical ability was enhanced in the presence of the metals [66]. Fullerene's antioxidant properties have been used in anti-aging skincare and beauty products, according to previous studies [67]. A suspension of fullerene with an average size of 450 nm was created and injected into the hippocampi of Wistar rats, demonstrating its capacity to pass the blood-brain barrier. Although the results showed a decline in spatial memory and BDNF protein levels, the results also showed a decline in reactive oxygen species [68]. Fullerenols were examined for their antioxidant capabilities in oxidizing solutions, including luminescent bacteria and their enzymes. Catalytic activity was linked to the enhancement of biological processes, and the hormesis phenomenon was shown to be responsible for the effect on bacterial cells [69]. Oxidative stress is a leading cause of modern society's most pressing issues. The oxidative stress system may be brought into equilibrium using fullerene-based systems. Further research is needed to properly comprehend the significance of fullerene-based delivery methods in regulating oxidative stress.

Neurodegenerative illnesses like Alzheimer's and Parkinson's have been linked to the overproduction of oxygen species and the hyperactivation of N-methyl-d-aspartic acid or N-methyl-d-aspartate (NMDA) and glutamic receptors [60]. The major reasons fullerene derivatives were used in neurological illnesses were their radical scavenging capacity, their ability to activate reactive oxygen species, and their ability to bind with peptides [48]. Their peptide-interacting abilities have also been used in the fight against Alzheimer's disease. The major amyloid-forming component of yeast prion protein Sup35, the hydrophilic GNNQQNY peptide, was examined for its sensitivity to the hydrophobic fullerene C_{60} in an experiment [70]. In addition to blocking the inter-peptide interactions necessary for oligomerization and β-sheet formation, the results showed that fullerenes totally prohibit fibril-like bilayer β-sheets, generated by GNNQQNY peptides [70]. Oxygen species inhibited A-beta and reduced concomitant cytotoxicity when UCNP@C_{60}-pep was exposed to near-infrared light, resulting in ROS species. Antioxidant activity in fullerene and fullerenols has been quite impressive. It has been observed that they can inhibit glutamate receptors and thereby decrease apoptosis in cortical neurons [71]. Both hexa(sulfobutyl)-fullerenes and trimesic acid (TMA) fullerenes were shown to be effective in the treatment of neurodegenerative illnesses 55, 56, thanks to their capacity to trap free radicals. The neuronal degeneration caused by ROS has been shown to be mitigated by using water-soluble derivatives, such as fullerenols and malonic acid fullerenes [72]. The prevalence of neurodegenerative illnesses is increasing, and as a result, the physical and social aspects of people's lives suffer. This may be because people are living longer and thus developing a systemic insufficiency. By adopting delivery systems based on fullerenes, the criticalities of the issue can be surmounted.

7.7 SUMMARY

Carbon, the most prevalent element in organic molecules, has been shown to occur in two allotropes: diamond and graphite. Fullerenes, a third kind of carbon, were discovered in 1985 by Smalley, Kroto, and Curl. In their study, a portion of solid graphite was evaporated into plasma comprising ions and atoms by irradiating it with a laser. Clusters with varying quantities of carbon atoms were synthesized as a consequence of the collision. It was discovered that clusters between 60 and 70 carbon atoms predominate and that 60 atoms were present in the majority of clusters.

At the outset, the researchers faced difficulties in synthesizing a sufficient quantity of fullerenes, and it took five years for Krätschmer and Huffman (1990) and Kroto et al. (1991) to establish alternative higher-yield sample preparation methodologies. The freshly discovered particle was given the architect Richard Buckminster Fuller's title since he designed the dome in 1967, which has the same form as the carbon clusters.

The three researchers who invented fullerenes were awarded the 1996 Nobel Prize in Chemistry because they sparked such fascination and enthusiasm among scientists and researchers. The most prevalent fullerene, C_{60}, was discovered in 1985 and is made up of 60 carbon atoms organized in 20 hexagons and 12 pentagons, giving it the shape of a hollow sphere. It is a good candidate for electron transfer processes and exhibits moderate reactions in the visible spectrum as well as substantial absorption of UV radiation. However, it lacks active areas on the cages for direct catalytic uses and is inaccessible in polar solvents such as water.

This chapter discussed the various structural attributes and physicochemical characteristics of fullerene and its significance and prospects as a nanocarrier for drug delivery. It illustrated the methods with advancements for synthesizing fullerene and highlighted functionalization strategies to enhance the surface characteristics. The chapter also discussed recent advancements in fullerene for nucleic acid delivery, chemotherapeutics, and neurodegenerative diseases.

REFERENCES

[1] H.W. Kroto, J.R. Heath, S.C. O'Brien, R.F. Curl, R.E. Smalley, C60: Buckminsterfullerene, Nature. 318 (1985) 162–163. doi:10.1038/318162a0.

[2] W. Krätschmer, L.D. Lamb, K. Fostiropoulos, D.R. Huffman, Solid C60: A new form of carbon, Nature. 347 (1990) 354–358. doi:10.1038/347354a0.

[3] H.W. Kroto, A.W. Allaf, S.P. Balm, C60: Buckminsterfullerene, Chem. Rev. 91 (1991) 1213–1235. doi:10.1021/cr00006a005.

[4] S. Thakral, R. Mehta, Fullerenes: An introduction and overview of their biological properties, Indian J. Pharm. Sci. 68 (2006) 13. doi:10.4103/0250-474X.22957.

[5] J. Scaria, A. V Karim, G. Divyapriya, P.V. Nidheesh, M. Suresh Kumar, Carbon-supported semiconductor nanoparticles as effective photocatalysts for water and wastewater treatment, in: P. Singh, A. Borthakur, P.K. Mishra, E.P. Tiwary (Eds.), Nano-Materials as Photocatalysts for Degradation of Environmental Pollutants, Elsevier, Cambridge (2020): pp. 245–278. doi:10.1016/B978-0-12-818598-8.00013-4.

[6] A. Rondags, W.Y. Yuen, M.F. Jonkman, B. Horváth, Fullerene C 60 with cytoprotective and cytotoxic potential: Prospects as a novel treatment agent in dermatology? Exp. Dermatol. 26 (2017) 220–224. doi:10.1111/exd.13172.

[7] Y. Pan, X. Liu, W. Zhang, Z. Liu, G. Zeng, B. Shao, Q. Liang, Q. He, X. Yuan, D. Huang, M. Chen, Advances in photocatalysis based on fullerene C60 and its derivatives: Properties, mechanism, synthesis, and applications, Appl. Catal. B. 265 (2020) 118579. doi:10.1016/j.apcatb.2019.118579.

[8] R. Taylor, J.P. Hare, A.K. Abdul-Sada, H.W. Kroto, Isolation, separation and characterisation of the fullerenes C60 and C70: The third form of carbon, J. Chem. Soc. Chem. Commun. (1990) 1423. doi:10.1039/c39900001423.

[9] J.M. Hawkins, A. Meyer, T.A. Lewis, S. Loren, F.J. Hollander, Crystal structure of osmylated C 60: Confirmation of the soccer ball framework, Sci. 252 (1979, 1991) 312–313. doi:10.1126/science.252.5003.312.

[10] R.C. Haddon, L.E. Brus, K. Raghavachari, Rehybridization and π-orbital alignment: The key to the existence of spheroidal carbon clusters, Chem. Phys. Lett. 131 (1986) 165–169. doi:10.1016/0009-2614(86)80538-3.

[11] W. Kolodziejski, J. Klinowski, 13C → 1H → 13C cross-polarization NMR in toluene-solvated fullerene-70, Chem. Phys. Lett. 247 (1995) 507–509. doi:10.1016/S0009-2614(95)01272-9.

[12] M.F. Meidine, P.B. Hitchcock, H.W. Kroto, R. Taylor, D.R.M. Walton, Single crystal X-ray structure of benzene-solvated C60, J. Chem. Soc. Chem. Commun. (1992) 1534. doi:10.1039/c39920001534.

[13] N. Sivaraman, R. Dhamodaran, I. Kaliappan, T.G. Srinivasan, P.R.V. Rao, C.K. Mathews, Solubility of C60 in organic solvents, J. Org. Chem. 57 (1992) 6077–6079. doi:10.1021/jo00048a056.

[14] N. Sivaraman, R. Dhamodaran, I. Kaliappan, T.G. Srinivasan, P.R.P. Vasudeva Rao, C.K.C. Mathews, Solubility of C 70 in organic solvents, Fullerene Sci. Technol. 2 (1994) 233–246. doi:10.1080/15363839408009549.

[15] R.C. Haddon, A.F. Hebard, M.J. Rosseinsky, D.W. Murphy, S.J. Duclos, K.B. Lyons, B. Miller, J.M. Rosamilia, R.M. Fleming, A.R. Kortan, S.H. Glarum, A. V Makhija, A.J. Muller, R.H. Eick, S.M. Zahurak, R. Tycko, G. Dabbagh, F.A. Thiel, Conducting films of C60 and C70 by alkali-metal doping, Nature. 350 (1991) 320–322. doi:10.1038/350320a0.

[16] A.F. Hebard, M.J. Rosseinsky, R.C. Haddon, D.W. Murphy, S.H. Glarum, T.T.M. Palstra, A.P. Ramirez, A.R. Kortan, Superconductivity at 18 K in potassium-doped C60, Nature. 350 (1991) 600–601. doi:10.1038/350600a0.

[17] M. Saunders, H.A. Jimenez-Vazquez, R.J. Cross, S. Mroczkowski, M.L. Gross, D.E. Giblin, R.J. Poreda, Incorporation of helium, neon, argon, krypton, and xenon into fullerenes using high pressure, J. Am. Chem. Soc. 116 (1994) 2193–2194. doi:10.1021/ja00084a089.

[18] M. Saunders, R.J. Cross, H.A. Jiménez-Vázquez, R. Shimshi, A. Khong, Noble gas atoms inside fullerenes, Sci. 271 (1979, 1996) 1693–1697. doi:10.1126/science.271.5256.1693.

[19] H.M. Lee, M.M. Olmstead, T. Suetsuna, H. Shimotani, N. Dragoe, R.J. Cross, K. Kitazawa, A.L. Balch, Crystallographic characterization of Kr@C60 in (0.09Kr@C60/0.91C60)·{NiII(OEP)}·2C6H6, Chem. Comm. (2002) 1352–1353. doi:10.1039/b202925c.

[20] G.-W. Wang, M. Saunders, R.J. Cross, Reversible Diels–Alder addition to fullerenes: A study of equilibria using 3 He NMR spectroscopy, J. Am. Chem. Soc. 123 (2001) 256–259. doi:10.1021/ja001346c.

[21] A. Hirsch, B. Nuber, Nitrogen heterofullerenes, Acc. Chem. Res. 32 (1999) 795–804. doi:10.1021/ar980113b.

[22] S. Yamago, H. Tokuyama, E. Nakamura, K. Kikuchi, S. Kananishi, K. Sueki, H. Nakahara, S. Enomoto, F. Ambe, In vivo biological behavior of a water-miscible fullerene: 14C labeling, absorption, distribution, excretion and acute toxicity, Chem. Biol. 2 (1995) 385–389. doi:10.1016/1074-5521(95)90219-8.

[23] S.S. Lucky, K.C. Soo, Y. Zhang, Nanoparticles in photodynamic therapy, Chem. Rev. 115 (2015) 1990–2042. doi:10.1021/cr5004198.

[24] G. Accorsi, N. Armaroli, Taking advantage of the electronic excited states of [60]-fullerenes, J. Phys. Chemistry C. 114 (2010) 1385–1403. doi:10.1021/jp9092699.

[25] L. Yin, H. Zhou, L. Lian, S. Yan, W. Song, Effects of C 60 on the photochemical formation of reactive oxygen species from natural organic matter, Environ. Sci. Technol. 50 (2016) 11742–11751. doi:10.1021/acs.est.6b04488.

[26] Y. Fan, H. Liu, R. Han, L. Huang, H. Shi, Y. Sha, Y. Jiang, Extremely high brightness from polymer-encapsulated quantum dots for two-photon cellular and deep-tissue imaging, Sci. Rep. 5 (2015) 9908. doi:10.1038/srep09908.

[27] A. Herreros-López, M. Carini, T. Da Ros, T. Carofiglio, C. Marega, V. La Parola, V. Rapozzi, L.E. Xodo, A.A. Alshatwi, C. Hadad, M. Prato, Nanocrystalline cellulose-fullerene: Novel conjugates, Carbohydr. Polym. 164 (2017) 92–101. doi:10.1016/j.carbpol.2017.01.068.

[28] Z. Hu, C. Zhang, P. Tang, C. Li, Y. Yao, S. Sun, L. Zhang, Y. Huang, Protection of cells from nitric oxide-mediated apoptotic death by glutathione C 60 derivative, Cell Biol. Int. 36 (2012) 677–681. doi:10.1042/CBI20110566.

[29] J.J. Ryan, H.R. Bateman, A. Stover, G. Gomez, S.K. Norton, W. Zhao, L.B. Schwartz, R. Lenk, C.L. Kepley, Fullerene nanomaterials inhibit the allergic response, J. Immunol. 179 (2007) 665–672. doi:10.4049/jimmunol.179.1.665.

[30] K.D. Patel, R.K. Singh, H.W. Kim, Carbon-based nanomaterials as an emerging platform for theranostics, Mater. Horiz. 6 (2019) 434–469. doi:10.1039/c8mh00966j.

[31] T.M. Benn, P. Westerhoff, P. Herckes, Detection of fullerenes (C60 and C70) in commercial cosmetics, Environ. Pollut. 159 (2011) 1334–1342. doi:10.1016/j.envpol.2011.01.018.

[32] S.-R. Chae, E.M. Hotze, Y. Xiao, J. Rose, M.R. Wiesner, Comparison of methods for fullerene detection and measurements of reactive oxygen production in cosmetic products, Environ. Eng. Sci. 27 (2010) 797–804. doi:10.1089/ees.2010.0103.

[33] M. Wang, V. Nalla, S. Jeon, V. Mamidala, W. Ji, L.-S. Tan, T. Cooper, L.Y. Chiang, Large femtosecond two-photon absorption cross sections of fullerosome vesicle nanostructures derived from a highly photoresponsive amphiphilic C 60 -light-harvesting fluorene dyad, J. Phys. Chemistry C. 115 (2011) 18552–18559. doi:10.1021/jp207047k.

[34] S. Stevenson, Preparation, extraction/isolation from soot, and solubility of fullerenes, Handbook Fuller. Sci. Technol. (2022) 19–43. doi:10.1007/978-981-16-8994-9_20/COVER.

[35] W. Krätschmer, L.D. Lamb, K. Fostiropoulos, D.R. Huffman, Solid C60: A new form of carbon, Nature. 347 (1990) 354–358. doi:10.1038/347354A0.

[36] H.W. Kroto, J.R. Heath, S.C. O'Brien, R.F. Curl, R.E. Smalley, C60: Buckminsterfullerene, Nature. 318 (1985) 162–163. doi:10.1038/318162a0.

[37] J.B. Howard, J.T. McKinnon, Y. Makarovsky, A.L. Lafleur, M.E. Johnson, Fullerenes C60 and C70 in flames, Nature. 352 (1991) 139–141. doi:10.1038/352139A0.

[38] W. Krätschmer, K. Fostiropoulos, D.R. Huffman, The infrared and ultraviolet absorption spectra of laboratory-produced carbon dust: Evidence for the presence of the C60 molecule, Chem. Phys. Lett. 170 (1990) 167–170. doi:10.1016/0009-2614(90)87109-5.

[39] H. Richter, A.J. Labrocca, W.J. Grieco, K. Taghizadeh, A.L. Lafleur, J.B. Howard, Generation of higher fullerenes in flames, J. Phys. Chemistry B. 101 (1997) 1556–1560. doi:10.1021/JP962928C/ASSET/IMAGES/LARGE/JP962928CF00003.JPEG.

[40] H. Murayama, S. Tomonoh, J.M. Alford, M.E. Karpuk, Fullerene production in tons and more: from science to industry, Fuller. Nanotub. Carbon Nanostructures. 12 (2006) 1–9. doi:10.1081/FST-120027125.

[41] S. Stevenson, Preparation, extraction/isolation from soot, and solubility of fullerenes, in: X. Lu, T. Akasaka, Z. Slanina (Eds.), Handbook of Fullerene Science and Technology, Springer Nature, Singapore (2022): pp. 19–43. doi:10.1007/978-981-16-8994-9_20.

[42] R.E. Haufler, J. Conceicao, L.P.F. Chibante, Y. Chai, N.E. Byrne, S. Flanagan, M.M. Haley, S.C. O'Brien, C. Pan, Z. Xiao, W.E. Billups, M.A. Ciufolini, R.H. Hauge, J.L. Margrave, L.J. Wilson, R.F. Curl, R.E. Smalley, Efficient production of C60 (buckminsterfullerene), C60H36, and the solvated buckide ion, J. Phys. Chemistry. 94 (1990) 8634–8636. doi:10.1021/J100387A005.

[43] L.P.F. Chibante, A. Thess, J.M. Alford, M.D. Diener, R.E. Smalley, Solar generation of the fullerenes, J. Phys. Chemistry. 97 (1993) 8696–8700. doi:10.1021/J100136A007.

[44] H. Ajie, M.M. Alvarez, S.J. Anz, R.D. Beck, F. Diederich, K. Fostiropoulos, D.R. Huffman, W. Krätschmer, Y. Rubin, K.E. Schriver, D. Sensharma, R.L. Whetten, Characterization of the soluble all-carbon molecules C60 and C70, J. Phys. Chemistry. 94 (1990) 8630–8633. doi:10.1021/J100387A004.

[45] F. Diederich, R. Ettl, Y. Rubin, R.L. Whetten, R. Beck, M. Alvarez, S. Anz, D. Sensharma, F. Wudl, K.C. Khemani, A. Koch, The higher fullerenes: Isolation and characterization of C76, C84, C90, C94, and C70O, an oxide of D5h-C70, Sci. 252 (1979, 1991) 548–551. doi:10.1126/SCIENCE.252.5005.548.

[46] T. Ikeda, T. Kamo, M. Danno, New synthesis method of fullerenes using microwave-induced naphthalene-nitrogen plasma at atmospheric pressure, Appl. Phys. Lett. 67 (1998) 900. doi:10.1063/1.114688.

[47] R. Hetzel, T. Manning, D. Lovingood, G. Strouse, D. Phillips, Production of fullerenes by microwave synthesis, Fuller. Nanotub. Carbon Nanostructures. 20 (2011) 99–108. doi:10.1080/1536383X.2010.533300.

[48] S. Goodarzi, T. Da Ros, J. Conde, F. Sefat, M. Mozafari, Fullerene: Biomedical engineers get to revisit an old friend, Mater. Today. 20 (2017) 460–480. doi:10.1016/j.mattod.2017.03.017.

[49] E. Nakamura, H. Isobe, Functionalized fullerenes in water: The first 10 years of their chemistry, biology, and nanoscience, Acc. Chem. Res. 36 (2003) 807–815. doi:10.1021/ar030027y.

[50] O.D. Hendrickson, A. V Zherdev, I. V Gmoshinskii, B.B. Dzantiev, Fullerenes: In vivo studies of biodistribution, toxicity, and biological action, Nanotechnol. Russ. 9 (2014) 601–617. doi:10.1134/S199507801406010X.

[51] A. Ikeda, Y. Doi, M. Hashizume, J.I. Kikuchi, T. Konishi, An extremely effective DNA photocleavage utilizing functionalized liposomes with a fullerene-enriched lipid bilayer, J. Am. Chem. Soc. 129 (2007) 4140–4141. doi:10.1021/JA070243S.

[52] M. Prato, Fullerene materials, fullerenes and related structures, in: Topics in Current Chemistry, vol. 199. Springer, Berlin (1999): pp. 173–187. doi:10.1007/3-540-68117-5_5.

[53] A. Mateo-Alonso, D. Bonifazi, M. Prato, Functionalization and applications of[60]fullerene, C. Nanotechnol. (2006) 155–189. doi:10.1016/B978-044451855-2/50010-3.

[54] M. Brettreich, A. Hirsch, A highly water-soluble dendro[60]fullerene, Tetrahedron Lett. 39 (1998) 2731–2734. doi:10.1016/S0040-4039(98)00491-2.

[55] S. Filippone, F. Heimann, A. Rassat, A highly water-soluble 2:1 β-cyclodextrin–fullerene conjugate, Chem. Comm. 2 (2002) 1508–1509. doi:10.1039/B202410A.

[56] J.C. Lin, C.H. Wu, Surface characterization and platelet adhesion studies on polyurethane surface immobilized with C60, Biomater. 20 (1999) 1613–1620. doi:10.1016/S0142-9612(99)00068-X.

[57] K.F.A. Clancy, J.G. Hardy, Gene delivery with organic electronic biomaterials, Curr. Pharm. Des. 23 (2017). doi:10.2174/1381612823666170710124137.

[58] J. Wang, L. Xie, T. Wang, F. Wu, J. Meng, J. Liu, H. Xu, Visible light-switched cytosol release of siRNA by amphiphilic fullerene derivative to enhance RNAi efficacy in vitro and in vivo, Acta Biomater. 59 (2017) 158–169. doi:10.1016/j.actbio.2017.05.031.

[59] Y.S. Youn, D.S. Kwag, E.S. Lee, Multifunctional nano-sized fullerenes for advanced tumor therapy, J. Pharm. Investig. 47 (2017). doi:10.1007/S40005-016-0282-8.

[60] H. Kazemzadeh, M. Mozafari, Fullerene-based delivery systems, Drug Discov. Today. 24 (2019) 898–905. doi:10.1016/J.DRUDIS.2019.01.013.

[61] M. Torrice, Does nanomedicine have a delivery problem? ACS Cent. Sci. 2 (2016) 434–437. doi:10.1021/ACSCENTSCI.6B00190.

[62] M. Kepinska, R. Kizek, H. Milnerowicz, Fullerene as a doxorubicin nanotransporter for targeted breast cancer therapy: Capillary electrophoresis analysis, Electrophoresis. 39 (2018) 2370–2379. doi:10.1002/ELPS.201800148.

[63] M. Kumar, K. Raza, C60-fullerenes as drug delivery carriers for anticancer agents: Promises and hurdles, Pharm. Nanotechnol. 5 (2017). doi:10.2174/2211738505666170301142232.

[64] F.Y. Hsieh, A. V. Zhilenkov, I.I. Voronov, E.A. Khakina, D.V. Mischenko, P.A. Troshin, S.H. Hsu, Water-soluble fullerene derivatives as brain medicine: Surface chemistry determines if they are neuroprotective and antitumor, ACS Appl. Mater. Interfaces. 9 (2017) 11482–11492. doi:10.1021/ACSAMI.7B01077.

[65] A. Azhar, G.M. Ashraf, Q. Zia, S.A. Ansari, A. Perveen, A. Hafeez, M. Saeed, M.A. Kamal, A. Alexiou, M. Ganash, N.S. Yarla, S.S. Baeesa, M.M. Alfiky, O.S. Bajouh, Frontier view on nanotechnological strategies for neuro-therapy, Curr. Drug Metab. 19 (2018) 596–604. doi:10.2174/1389200219666180305144143.

[66] E.B. Andrade, A. Martínez, Free radical scavenger properties of metal-fullerenes: C60 and C82 with Cu, Ag and Au (atoms and tetramers), Comput. Theor. Chem. 1115 (2017) 127–135. doi:10.1016/j.comptc.2017.06.015.

[67] S.J. Sohn, J.M. Yu, E.Y. Lee, Y.J. Nam, J. Kim, S. Kang, D.H. Kim, A. Kim, S. Kang, Anti-aging properties of conditioned media of epidermal progenitor cells derived from mesenchymal stem cells, Dermatol. Ther. (Heidelb). 8 (2018) 229–244. doi:10.1007/s13555-018-0229-2.

[68] Â.B. Kraemer, G.M. Parfitt, D. da S. Acosta, G.E. Bruch, M.F. Cordeiro, L.F. Marins, J. Ventura-Lima, J.M. Monserrat, D.M. Barros, Fullerene (C60) particle size implications in neurotoxicity following infusion into the hippocampi of Wistar rats, Toxicol. Appl. Pharmacol. 338 (2018) 197–203. doi:10.1016/j.taap.2017.11.022.

[69] A.S. Sachkova, E.S. Kovel, G.N. Churilov, O.A. Guseynov, A.A. Bondar, I.A. Dubinina, N.S. Kudryasheva, On mechanism of antioxidant effect of fullerenols, Biochem. Biophys. Rep. 9 (2017) 1–8. doi:10.1016/j.bbrep.2016.10.011.

[70] J. Lei, R. Qi, L. Xie, W. Xi, G. Wei, Inhibitory effect of hydrophobic fullerenes on the β-sheet-rich oligomers of a hydrophilic GNNQQNY peptide revealed by atomistic simulations, RSC Adv. 7 (2017) 13947–13956. doi:10.1039/C6RA27608C.

[71] J. Leszek, G. Md Ashraf, W.H. Tse, J. Zhang, K. Gasiorowski, M.F. Avila-Rodriguez, V. V. Tarasov, G.E. Barreto, S.G. Klochkov, S.O. Bachurin, G. Aliev, Nanotechnology for Alzheimer disease, Curr. Alzheimer Res. 14 (2017). doi:10.2174/15672050146661 70203125008.

[72] J.I. Hardt, J.S. Perlmutter, C.J. Smith, K.L. Quick, L. Wei, S.K. Chakraborty, L.L. Dugan, Pharmacokinetics and toxicology of the neuroprotective e,e,e-methanofullerene(60)-63-tris malonic acid [C3] in mice and primates, Eur. J. Drug Metab Pharmacokinet. 43 (2018) 543–554. doi:10.1007/s13318-018-0464-z.

8 Carbon-Based Nanocomposites for Drug Delivery

8.1 INTRODUCTION TO CARBON NANOHYBRIDS

Researchers have grown interested in developing innovative drug delivery methods for various medical substances in recent years. In fact, many studies examine the design, synthesis, and characterization of new materials to be employed as delivery systems to improve the efficacy of a particular medication [1]. To maximize the therapeutic agent's efficacy and safety, the optimal drug delivery system (DDS) must carry the therapeutic agent in the appropriate quantity, at the correct rate, and to the right place in the body. This strategy can prolong the pharmacological impact, reduce unpleasant effects, and reduce administration frequency, enhancing patient compliance [2].

The demand for carriers for novel biological therapeutic agents, such as nucleic acids and proteins, and the pharmaceutical industry's interest in generating novel formulations due to looming patent expirations necessitate the adoption of innovative drug delivery systems. Biologics, polymers, silicon-based, carbon-based, metals, or mixes thereof are employed in alternative drug delivery techniques, and these substances can be organized in microscale or, more recently, nanoscale forms [3].

Nanomedicine is described as "the monitoring, repair, production, and control of human biological systems at the molecular level" using nanodevices and nanostructures [4]. It entails applying nanotechnology for disease detection, prevention, and treatment, and it acts as a valuable tool for understanding particular molecular mechanisms causing disease [2].

Nanomaterials have significant potential for the early detection and diagnosis of infectious and malignant diseases, as well as for the creation of drugs, the administration of medications, and the delivery of genes and proteins. Due to the extraordinary selectivity of their interactions with subcellular structures in the human body, these cutting-edge materials have the potential to be utilized in clinical settings as drug-targeting systems to reduce side effects [5]. Nanocarriers can carry the active chemical directly into cells by eliminating biological barriers and separating the problematic target tissue from the healthy tissue [6].

Using nanocomposites may be advantageous in various industries, including technology, medicine, biotechnology, pharmacy, polymeric materials, ceramics, textiles, paint, automobiles, food, and a great deal more. Nanocomposites fall into natural or artificial categories, depending on where the component phases originated. The discontinuous phase often comprises a smaller portion of the total than the continuous

DOI: 10.1201/9781003358114-8

phase. The continuous phase, which might be made of polymeric, metallic, ceramic, or a combination of these and other materials, is often chemically different from the nanoscale discontinuous phase. Here, we will look closely at natural nanocomposites. "In-situ," "mixed in solution," and "melt compounding" stand out as particularly beneficial among the several known production techniques. For both organic and inorganic discontinuous phases, dispersion is essential. Most of the time, superficially altering the discontinuous phase with a chemical similar to the continuous phases will result in better integration. Nanocomposites are materials that can have a variety of beneficial properties depending on their composition and compatibility with different organic and inorganic fillers and reinforcements. For instance, natural nanocomposites are a class of materials with a wide variety of potential applications in industries, including farming, food science, medicine, and pharmacology. Natural nanocomposites are desirable from an environmental perspective since they are derived from natural sources, may be regenerated, and disintegrate more quickly [7]. Nonetheless, they often have poor mechanical, chemical, and physical characteristics. From the original design through the use of renewable raw materials, clean energy, zero waste manufacturing, shorter processing times, etc., the notion of green chemistry, preventive is better than clean, is used throughout the whole process of developing natural nanocomposites [8].

Obtaining copper chitosan nanocomposites for use in tissue engineering has been the subject of numerous studies; these materials are produced using a solution-based mixing method assisted by ultrasonic energy and exhibit promising antimicrobial activity against common pathogens like Staphylococcus aureus [9]. In addition to chitosan, there are currently natural nanocomposites made from cellulose, nanocellulose, starch, polylactic acid (PLA), various polysaccharides derived from glucose, and cellulose with the addition of various nanoparticles, including single, double, or multiple walled carbon nanotubes, graphene, carbon nanofibers, and fullerenes.

8.2   TYPES OF CARBON NANOHYBRIDS

Natural nanocomposites are multi-phase compounds, i.e., having two or more phases, generated from natural sources such as plants, vegetables, trees, seeds, microorganisms, and animals [10]. At least one phase has a nanometric dimension (usually 100 nm). Research interest in this nanomaterial is growing due to its durability, affordability, low weight, high specific resistance, strong mechanical properties, and biodegradability [11]. Natural nanocomposites can be classed by source—plant, mineral, or animal. Animal nanocomposites are usually generated from animal waste or skins, mineral nanocomposites can be made naturally or chemically, and vegetable nanocomposites are made from leaves, stems, and roots, with cellulose as the main component [11,12].

A natural nanocomposite requires at least one natural component. Compared to synthetics and composite materials with typical padding, nanocomposites consisting of chitosan, chitin, starch, glucose, cotton, different polysaccharide derivatives, cellulose and derivatives, natural fibers, and natural rubber have remarkable mechanical and thermal qualities [13]. Natural nanocomposites are those materials made up of two or more phases, at least one of which has a nanometric scale (generally <100 nm) and which are also obtained from natural sources, such as plants, vegetables, trees, seeds, bacteria, etc. animals, among others [12]. At present, this type of nanomaterial has increased the interest of its research since it has multiple favorable properties such as durability, low cost, low weight, high specific resistance, good mechanical properties, and biodegradability.

There are different classifications of natural nanocomposites; one regarding their source, which can be animal, mineral, or vegetable. The nanocomposites extracted from animal sources are generally taken from the skins or waste produced by animals, those obtained from minerals can be obtained in a natural or modified way, and finally, the vegetables that are taken from their leaves, stems, and roots, cellulose being the main one [10]. According to Franco-Aguirre et al. in 2023 [7], nanocomposites can also be classified by their size and dimension, where we will find four different nanometric scales that are described in **Table 8.1** [7].

In recent years, natural polymer nanocomposites have been widely studied because the addition of nanometric fillers significantly increases the physicochemical properties, which is attractive for their application in different areas [14]. The union of two or more materials on a nanometric scale can occur in multiple combinations using various materials. However, to obtain a natural nanocomposite, the addition of at least one component of natural origin will be necessary. An example is nanocomposites based on chitosan, chitin, starch, glucose, cotton, different polysaccharide derivatives, cellulose and derivatives, natural fibers, and natural rubber, among others of great interest, thanks to their extraordinary mechanical and thermal properties concerning polymers—synthetics and composite materials with conventional padding [13].

8.2.1 GRAPHENE-BASED NANOHYBRIDS

Graphene (GN) is the term given to the atomically thin layer of graphite composed of carbon atoms organized in a honeycomb configuration in two dimensions. When nearby carbon atoms' sp^2 orbitals meet, three bonds are formed in the GN layer [15]. The remaining p_z orbitals then form the conduction and valance bands related to the full π and empty π^* orbitals. The unique honeycomb structure of carbon atoms and their sp^2-hybridized bonds give GN not only a high specific surface area but also

---

TABLE 8.1

Classification of Nanocomposites according to Their Size and Dimension. Reprinted with permission from *Franco-Aguirre et al. (2023)* [7]

Classification	Dimension	Examples
0D	Nanometer-scale from 1 to 50 nm	Fullerenes, nano clays, nanodiamonds, etc.
1D	Nanometer-scale from 1 to 100 nm	Nanotubes and nanofibers
2D	It is found on the nanometric scale and with another dimension on the micron scale	Graphene, nanofilms, and nanocoatings
3D	All dimensions are microscale	Nanostructure

exceptional mechanical (stiffness 1 TPa), thermal (conductivity 5000 W ml K1), optical (transparency 97.7% transmittance), and electronic (charge-carrier mobility 250,000 cm^2 V^{-1} s^{-1} at room temperature) properties [16–19]. Since GN lacks a band gap and is inert to chemical processes, it must be functionalized to enhance its dispersion and overcome restrictions in technical applications such as semiconductors and sensors [20,21].

Mechanical exfoliation, epitaxial growth, and thermal reduction of graphene oxide (GO) are the most common ways of producing graphene nanoribbons (GN); nevertheless, the latter two are preferred because they provide a large-scale synthesis of GN [19,20,22]. GO is produced by grafting epoxide, carbonyl, carboxyl, and hydroxyl groups onto the GN structure. GO's 2D layer structure is made of sp^2-hybridized carbon atoms organized in a hexagonal lattice and amorphous domains of sp^3 C-O bonds due to the inclusion of these oxygenated functional groups. The polar oxygen functional groups make GO hydrophilic, allowing for its dispersion in a range of solvents, and the included functional groups serve as anchor sites for further chemical functionalization of GO to tune its physicochemical properties [15]. Because of the simplicity with which GO may be disseminated and functionalized, a variety of graphene-based structures with tunable electrical, optical, mechanical, and transport characteristics can be fabricated. This permits its manufacture on a wide scale. Some applications, however, necessitate the reconstruction of certain GN features. The oxygenated functional groups of graphene oxide (GO) are removed chemically or thermally to produce reduced graphene oxide (RGO). Polymer-based nanocomposites supplemented with RGO by in-situ GO reduction via polymerization or melt process in a polymeric matrix are one of the potential strategies [23–25].

8.2.2 Carbon Nanotube-Based Nanohybrids

The hexagonal arrangement of sp^2-hybridized carbon atoms that make up carbon nanotubes (CNTs) has a C-C spacing of around 1.4 [26]. These may be seen as nanometer-sized cylindrical structures made of rolled-up graphite planes [27]. A hemisphere with a fullerene structure is often present on at least one end of the cylindrical nanotube [15]. Two different forms of CNTs depend on the production process: single-wall CNT (SWCNT) and multiwall CNT [18]. (MWCNT). Whereas MWCNTs comprise two or more concentric cylindrical shells of graphene sheets coaxially organized around a central hollow core with van der Waals forces operating between neighboring layers, SWCNTs comprise a single rolled layer of graphene. MWCNT has an average interlayer spacing of 0.34 nm for the graphene layers, with each layer creating a separate tube with an outside diameter of 2.5 to 100 nm, compared to a range of 0.6 to 2.4 nm for SWCNT [18].

CNTs have been used for numerous applications in the field of biotechnology, such as platforms for ultrasensitive antibody recognition, nucleic acid sequencers, bioseparators, biocatalysts, and ion channel blockers for accelerating biochemical reactions and biological processes [19,21–24,28,29]. They have been used in nanomedicine as carriers of contrast agent magnetic resonance imaging, scaffolds for neuronal and ligamentous tissue growth for regenerative interventions of the central nervous system and orthopedic sites, substrates for detecting antibodies associated with human autoimmune diseases with high specificity, and substrates for detecting antibodies associated with autoimmune diseases [15]. They have been demonstrated to be efficient substrates for gene sequencing and as gene and medication delivery vectors to challenge traditional viral and particle delivery methods when coated with nucleic acids (DNA or RNA), vaccines, and proteins [30,31].

It should be noted that the exceptional reactivity of CNTs—due to their enormous surface area and achieved by their infinitesimal size—serves as both their best and worst qualities, particularly when they enter the bodies of humans and other living things, even though the precise mechanisms governing their toxicity are still unknown [32,33].

The World Health Organization (WHO) defines CNT as having a fiber-like structure, and the physical resemblance to asbestos fibers is the primary cause for worry in terms of public health [34]. It has been established that when long MWNT, a nanotube that resembles asbestos, is exposed to the mesothelial lining of a mouse body cavity (used as a model for the mesothelial lining of the chest cavity), length-dependent pathogenic processes are seen. Inflammation and the development of granulomas are examples of these processes [35]. Moreover, it has been observed that CNTs have carcinogenic qualities and frequently result in mesothelioma in intact male rats [36].

As the CNT's water insolubility or near insolubility is the primary source of toxicological concerns, several investigations have been carried out to create highly functional CNT derivatives with less toxic effects [37]. The hydrophobic interactions between the sp^2 carbon tube shells of a CNT always result in aggregation or bundles that are securely linked in their purest form [38].

Covalent and non-covalent functionalization must be distinguished when discussing the functionalization of a CNT. Covalent functionalization is based on the covalent attachment of functional components to the carbon scaffold of the nanotube. It may be carried out at the tubes' termini or sidewalls. Direct covalent sidewall functionalization is connected to a shift from sp^2 to sp^3 hybridization and a concomitant loss of conjugation. Using previously existing defect sites to undergo chemical reactions is known as defect functionalization. Defect sites can include the irregular pentagon and heptagon shapes seen in the hexagonal graphene structure, as well as open ends and sidewall holes that are terminated, for instance, by carboxylic groups. Moreover, oxygenated sites created during oxidative purification must be seen as flaws [39,40].

Using different adsorption forces, such as van der Waals's and π-π stacking interactions, a non-covalent functionalization is primarily based on supramolecular complexation. These functionalizations are all derivatizations of exohedral structures. Endohedral functionalization of CNTs, or the filling of the tubes with atoms or tiny molecules, is a specific instance [41]. Covalent or non-covalent bonding (wrapping) of polymer molecules on the surface of the CNT is one surface modification method [42].

8.2.3 GRAPHENE OXIDE-BASED NANOHYBRIDS

The graphene analogs that are both oxidative and hydrophilic functional groups such as hydroxyl, carboxyl, and epoxy are highly concentrated in graphene oxide (GO) and reduced graphene oxide (rGO), enhancing their stability, water dispersibility, and ability to emit visible and infrared light [43]. Graphene and its derivative GO are now the topics of intensive study due to their intriguing potential for application in various biomedical engineering domains, such as drug delivery, biosensing, cancer treatments, and tissue engineering [44]. Managing flaws in graphene-based nanomaterials has direct relevance for a wide range of uses. Among the family of graphene-derived materials, GO and rGO are considered ubiquitous nanomaterials [45,46]. The oxidation of graphene yields graphene oxide (GO), which has various physicochemical characteristics. It is a two-dimensional honeycomb structure with a thickness of just one atom and is a hydrophilic variant of graphene [47]. GO's adaptability and biocompatibility make it a good fit for use in the life sciences. It can be used in bioimaging and biosensing because of fluorescence in the visible and infrared sections of the electromagnetic spectrum and Raman signals in the D, G, and 2D regions [48]. As shown in **Figure 8.1** [43], the functional oxygenated entities are located on the GO nanosheets' leading and trailing edge planes. In addition to its valuable properties, GO may be used to make composites when combined with polymers and other additives. The incorporation of chitosan, polyacrylic acid (PAA), polyethylene glycol (PEG), folic acid, and others can improve GO's biocompatibility, loading capacity, targetability, and structural properties [43].

rGO and GO have the same basic structure as graphene but also have oxygen-enriched functional regions of various strengths [47]. Before GO or rGO may be used in the biological sciences, their surfaces must be functionalized. As a result of the presence of these oxygenated functional groups, GO may be grafted or doped with a wide variety of additional functional components to improve its surface properties without compromising its fundamental characteristics [47,49].

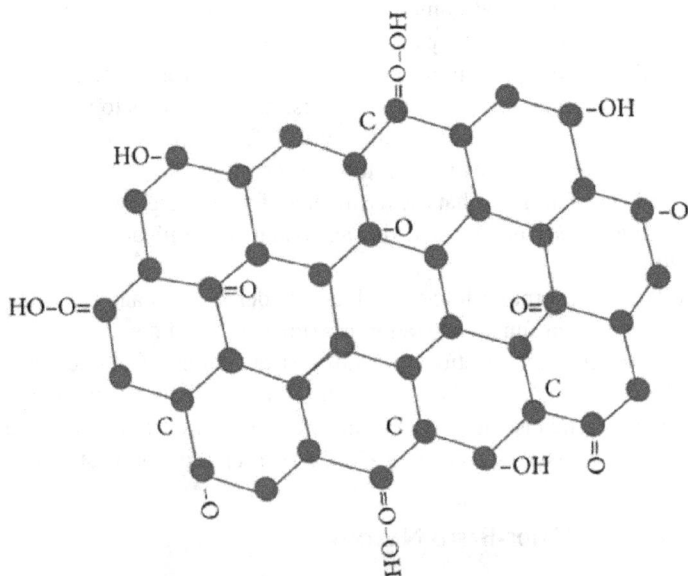

FIGURE 8.1 Schematic Representation of Graphene Oxide's Molecular Structure. [Reprinted with permission from *Sontakke et al. (2023)*] [43].

Another major hurdle for GO in the pharmaceutical industry is its instability in water. As GO tends to collect in physiological fluids like proteins and salt due to nonspecific binding and electrostatic interactions, it is difficult to use it as a building block for biological probes [43]. By adding certain functional groups, GO can be made more physiologically soluble and hence more useful in biological settings. Moreover, GO is one of the most popular and extensively investigated nanomaterials for uses involving drug delivery due to its better features, including a higher surface area. A distinct graphene derivative, reduced graphene oxide (rGO), is readily available by thermal or chemical reduction of GO and has been used in various practical settings, including drug delivery [44].

Cancer, neurological disease, gene delivery, and tissue engineering are just a few of the medical fields that have explored GO and rGO extensively [43]. In 2021, Liu et al. reviewed the most recent GO-based nanocarriers for cancer therapy advances. Nevertheless, the specifics of GO synthesis, functionalization, stimulus-responsive behavior, and the prospective uses of these nanocarriers in other biological disciplines have not been discussed [44]. Recent advances in the usage of GO/rGO-based nanocomposites for biological purposes were illustrated by Bellier et al. (2022) [50]. Nevertheless, the authors did not examine these nanocomposites' toxicological features, stimulus responsiveness, or future prospects. Wound healing, cancer treatments, and drug delivery are just some of the many uses listed for GO-based stimuli-responsive nanoplatforms by Patil et al. (2021) [51]. Similar to this, in 2022, Jafari et al. reported a stimuli-responsive drug delivery method utilizing graphene-based nanocomposites [52]. Jain et al. (2021) developed ways for functionalizing nanographene oxide and its applications in cancer therapy, gene transfer, and bioimaging [53].

While many studies have shown the value of GO in the medical profession, there have been few in-depth analyses pointing out the current gaps in the research and suggesting ways to remedy them. Previous reviews on GO and GO-based nanomaterials mainly focus on their synthesis and application in the biomedical field, particularly for anticancer DDS. However, they lack a thorough discussion of the toxicity, biodistribution, bioavailability, and the factors affecting the adaptability of GO-based nanocarriers for these applications. Nevertheless, there is a dearth of knowledge on functionalizing GO-based nanocarriers with a wide variety of biomolecules and how to modify their morphology into one- or zero-dimensional nano-morphologies to improve their versatility in the state-of-the-art literature. There are a few methodologies for functionalizing GO with metal-organic frameworks (MOFs) [54] for biomedical applications and chemotherapeutic agents in cancer therapy. In a study by Sontakke et al., it was reported to incorporate GO with MIL-100(Fe) for the controlled anticancer drug release [55]. Notably, the synthesis and functionalization of GO-based nanocarriers are subject to a variety of process- and property-related criticalities that directly impact the nanocarriers' physicochemical properties. Highlighting these problems and looking for answers are paramount [43].

8.2.4 Hydrogels

Three-dimensional networks of hydrogel polymers have special surface properties, including porosity, swelling, hydrophilicity, mechanical flexibility, and softness.

Hydrogels are capable of absorbing over 90% of water molecules without breaking down. Also, the interior holes of the hydrogels enable the release of tiny molecules into the environment. Because of their unique properties, hydrogels are excellent for various biological applications, such as medication delivery for a number of illnesses, tissue engineering scaffolds, and tissue enhancement. The creation of hydrogels involves the extensive use of both synthetic and natural polymers. Moreover, adding nanoparticles like GO and changing the kind of monomer utilized might change the surface properties. Notwithstanding their adaptability, flexibility, and usefulness, hydrogels in biological applications have advantages and disadvantages [43].

For some drug compounds, notably hydrophobic ones, hydrogels frequently have a poor loading capacity and release behavior when it comes to drug delivery. The uneven dosing behavior of the drug-loaded composite may be caused by this variance in release behavior. After that, several techniques were created to enhance hydrogels' mechanical strength and drug-release properties [56,57]. These techniques included using double networks, polyampholytes, and nanocomposites. The oxygenated functional groups in GO considerably improve drug loading and release behavior. Strong cross-links can be produced by these GO functional groups' interactions with the hydrophilic polymeric chains. For usage in drug delivery applications, hybrid hydrogel nanocarriers' loading capacity, biocompatibility, and release behavior are all enhanced by cross-linking. It has previously been possible to create composite hydrogels with enhanced surface properties by combining different nanomaterials, such as metal and organic nanoparticles. GO exhibits superior molecular interactions with therapeutic compounds compared to conventional nanomaterials and greater flexibility, surface-to-volume ratio, biological activity, biocompatibility, loading capacity, and loading capacity [57,58].

Fong et al. (2017) have created a folic acid (FA) conjugated GO nanocarrier (GO-FA) for the targeted delivery of DOX [59]. The drug-loaded nanocomposite (GO-FA-DOX) was included in the injectable and thermosensitive hyaluronic acid-chitosan-g-poly(N-isopropyl acrylamide) (HACPN) hydrogel for intratumoral drug administration. The HACPN hydrogel's configurable breakdown time enables fine control of the DOX release when used with a GO-FA nanocarrier. Due to its high drug loading efficiency and time-dependent toxicity impact *in-vitro*, GOFA-DOX/HACPN has shown promise as a potential *in-vivo* treatment. Blood tests and major organ biopsies both revealed no signs of side effects, supporting the treatment's safety [59]. In another work, Zhu et al. (2015) developed an injectable hydrogel composed of chitosan and glycerophosphate salt that increased the therapeutic efficiency of DOX [60]. The chemotherapeutic drug DOX was preloaded into a super-paramagnetic graphene oxide (GO/IONP/PEI) gel via polyethyleneimine (PEI) modification. It has been demonstrated that DOX-GO/IONP/PEI has more cytotoxicity and anticancer activity than free DOX [60]. Its improved capacity to infiltrate cell membranes was the cause of this.

8.2.5 POLYMERIC NANOHYBRIDS

For biodistribution and precise cell targeting, polymeric nanohybrid materials contain a biological surface modification, a therapeutic "payload," and a core substance

[61]. Nanovector drug delivery systems, such as the anticancer drug paclitaxel, are used in biomedical applications to encapsulate and transport medications with low water solubility [62,63]. Abraxane, a drug marketed as paclitaxel coupled to albumin nanoparticles, is an FDA-approved therapy for metastatic breast cancer [63]. Tumors can be noninvasively targeted with polymeric nanovectors. Nanohybrid materials facilitate drug delivery, imaging, and targeting. Polylactide-polyglycolide copolymers entrapping luteinizing hormone-releasing hormone (LHRH), marketed as goserelin (Zoladex) and leuprolide (Lupron Depot) and liposomes encapsulating daunorubicin and doxorubicin, marketed as DaunoXome and Doxil/Caelyx, have also received attention in cancer drug delivery [43,64]. Other polymers include poly-caprolactones, N-(2-hydroxyl propyl)methacrylamide (HPMA) copolymers, polygly-colic acid (PGA) containing paclitaxel (XyotaxTM), and natural polymers such as albumin, gelatin, alginate, collagen, and chitosan. Many studies have been conducted on polymer-drug conjugates [65].

Drug polymer conjugates increase a drug's plasma half-life and tumor site accumulation because polymers have a greater hydrodynamic volume. Doxorubicin and PHPMA copolymer had drug stability in plasma of five minutes when given separately but one hour when combined, increasing drug accumulation in solid tumors [66]. Antibodies, peptides, and saccharides are connected in the PHPMA copolymer [61]. HPMA-doxorubicin uses Galactosamine to target the hepatocyte asialoglycoprotein receptors [67]. Styrene maleic anhydride, in combination with neocarzinostatin (SMANCS), is used to treat hepatocellular cancer [68]. Targeting the treatment of tumor cells by receptor-mediated endocytosis is made possible by the conjugation of transferrin, folate, epidermal growth factor, and arginine-glycine-aspartic acid (RGD) tripeptide to the polymer backbone [61]. It is advisable to use non-cationic or surface-modified polymers when administering nanoparticles systemically to prevent plasma protein adsorption to the nanoparticle surface and RES absorption.

To increase the nanovector systemic retention and circulation time, hydrophilic polymers with neutral charges like polyethylene glycol (PEG) or polyethylene oxide (PEO) are frequently used for surface modification [69]. PEG disguises polymers, reducing hydrophobic interactions with RES. The ether oxygen of PEG forms a hydrogen bond with water molecules, creating a hydrating shell around the nanovector [70]. The nanovector is steric due to the molecular weight and molar ratio of PEG. Recently, PEG conjugates with anticancer drugs were evaluated [71]. To transport paclitaxel, PEO altered a Poly(3-caprolactone) (PCL) nanovector. Also used for surface modification include polyvinyl alcohol, polyacryl amide, polyvinyl pyrrolidone, polysorbate-80, and block copolymers such as poloxamer (Pluronic) and poloxamine (Tectronic) [61].

Synthetic polymers are produced via dispersion and emulsion (EP) polymerization. In DP, a polymeric stabilizer stabilizes the precipitated monomer chains after they precipitate in an insoluble phase and are formed by an initiator in a continuous aqueous phase. As the initiator produces ions, ionic polymerization takes place, which can result in either cationic or anionic polymers. When a radical nucleates the monomer, radical polymerization takes place. By emulsifying the monomer in a surfactant that does not include a solvent, EP synthesis produces monomer-swollen micelles and stable monomer droplets. Similar to DP, an initiator produces radicals or ions to initiate the polymerization of monomeric molecules. This method may be used as the continuous phase with organic or aqueous solutions.

EP creates poly(alkyl cyanoacrylate) (PACA) nanoparticles in the continuous organic phase and takes the shape of nanocapsules, shell-like structures with liquid chambers [72]. To create a microemulsion with drug-carrying water-swollen micelles, the medicine is dissolved in an aqueous phase such as iso-octane, cyclohexane-chloroform, isopropyl myristate-butanol, and hexane with surfactants. EP polymerizes monomers such as alkylcyanoacrylates in a continuous aqueous phase with the least amount of surfactants. It only works to stabilize brand-new polymer particles. Emulsifiers and stabilizers control the polymer's particle size. Poly(isobutyl cyanoacrylate) (PIBCA) nanoparticles were reduced in size by high concentrations of poloxamer 188 (> 2%) from 200 nm to 31–56 nm [73]. Zeta potential and drug release were both higher in DP nanovectors than in EP ones. The stabilizing effect of dextran channels the release of medicines.

Mostly during polymerization or absorption into prepared particles, drugs are loaded onto PACA nanoparticles. Drug-polymer covalent bonding may result from this. The kind of drug loading affects the carrier capacity, which is the amount of drug attached to a certain number of nanoparticles in comparison to the original drug concentration [74,75]. Actinomycin D was covalently bonded during manufacture, while betaxololchlorhydrate, hematoporphyrin, primaquine, and doxorubicin were all adsorbed on PACA nanoparticles. Poly(alkyl cyanoacrylate) (PACA) nanovectors loaded with doxorubicin can avoid tumor cell multidrug-resistance-1-type efflux pumps [61].

Drug binding and polymer breakdown significantly impact how quickly drugs are released. Lipophilic, oligomeric PACAs encapsulate amphiphilic doxorubicin to interact with it during polymerization—conjugation results from hydrogen linkages between the cyano groups of alkylcyanoacrylate and doxorubicin's N and H functions. Hydrophobic forces, H-bonds, and dipole-charge interaction hold together the drug-polymer conjugate. Furthermore, 5-fluorouracil (5-FU) polymerizes [76]. 5-FU amino groups produce zwitterions at an acidic pH of 1–2, which may prevent polymerization from starting. The amino terminal groups on PEG were used to attach folic acid to a nano-precipitated copolymer poly[aminopoly(ethylene glycol) cyanoacrylate-co-hexadecyl cyanoacrylate] [poly(H2NPEGCA-co-HDCA)] to target tumor cells [77].

Due to their biodegradability via hydrolytic cleavage of the ester linkage, biocompatibility, and existing FDA approval for use in humans as resorbable sutures, bone implants and screws, contraceptive implants, as scaffolds in tissue engineering, and as graft materials polylactides (PLA) and poly (D,L-lactide-coglycolide) (PLGA) have all been extensively investigated for drug delivery applications [78]. Delivering anticancer and other therapeutic chemicals are PLGA/PLA hybrid nanovectors. Prostate cancer models received intratumoral injections of transferrin-PLGA nanovectors loaded with paclitaxel. These specifically targeted nanoparticles improved cellular uptake, reducing the whole tumor's size and improving animal survival [61,79]. The IC50 for paclitaxel was five times lower when transferrin-coupled nanovector particles were used. Cationic di-block copolymer poly(l-lysine)-poly(ethylene glycol)-folate (PLL-PEG-FOL) surface-coated PLGA nanovectors increased intracellular delivery in KB cells overexpressing folate receptors [80]. By targeted receptor-mediated endocytosis, paclitaxel-loaded PLGA nanoparticles conjugated to wheat germ agglutinin (WGA) demonstrated enhanced anti-proliferation effect in A549 and H1299 cells in another study [81]. Cystatin inhibits the cysteine proteases cathepsins B and L linked to tumors when enclosed in PLGA nanovectors. MCF-10A neoT cells were destroyed by cytostatin-loaded PLGA nanovectors 160 times faster than by the free drug [61]. Doxorubicin was delivered via PLGA nanovectors by chemical conjugation via an ester link to PLGA polymer, and it showed sustained drug release over a month, improved drug uptake in the HepG2 cell line, and a marginally lower IC50 than free doxorubicin [82].

When internalized, the pH-sensitive PBAE nanovectors release their contents in the acidic tumor microenvironment and the endosomes and lysosomes of cells, making them ideal for the delivery of anticancer drugs. Paclitaxel-loaded PEO-PBAE nanovectors were studied in MDAMB231 human breast cancer cells [83,84]. The surface of a triblock copolymer (PEO/PPO/PEO) was modified to extend the half-life of nanovectors from 10 to 21 hours. Within five hours, it boosted the drug concentration in solid tumors by 5.2 to 23 times. Pluronics, which are polymeric micelles made of ethylene and propylene oxide, can defeat MDR but may also activate complement [85].

The requirement of entirely biodegradable material drives the creation and ongoing study of biodegradable fillers. Biodegradable fillers have been made by combining several natural polymers, such as cellulose, to achieve this goal. The advantages of cellulose nanostructures include the biopolymer's widespread availability. Moreover, cellulose nanostructures may be generated from trash collected from agricultural leftovers, a move toward circular economy principles. Bacterial nanocellulose (BNC), cellulose nanofibrils (CNFs) or microfibrils (CMFs), and cellulose nanocrystals (CNCs) are the three types of cellulose nanostructures found according to their origin and structure [86,87]. To produce bacterial nanocellulose, bacteria, namely, Acetobacters, are used. Fibrillar structures called CNFs or CMFs have a diameter of 10–100 nm and a length on the micrometer scale. The diameter of CNF is on the nanometer scale, whereas that of CMF is in the micron range [15]. However, the literature commonly confuses the two concepts. Mechanical delamination of fibers at high pressures was the first source for these materials. Nevertheless, due to the process's high energy requirements, various options have been developed, such as the use of homogenizers and microfluidizers, as well as pretreatments prior to the delamination, such as oxidizing or enzymatic treatments [87]. Very crystalline cellulose nanostructures (CNCs) have a single-dimensional size of less than 100 nm and take the form of rods, needles, or whiskers [88]. Acid hydrolysis, in which the cellulose starting material is processed by strong acid conditions, is the most often used way to generate CNC. After that, centrifugation and filtration methods are often used to separate the material into a final nano product [88].

More than two decades of study have gone into the incorporation of cellulose nanostructures (CNFs) into biodegradable polymers like PLA, with the seminal work coming from Iwatake et al., who used CNF as a reinforcement of PLA [89]. PLA was added gradually to a CNF suspension in water/acetone to make these nanocomposites. The CNF suspension was crucial in ensuring the nanofiller was uniformly distributed throughout the polymeric matrix. Once the solvents were removed, the residual material was treated using a twin rotary roller mixer. The addition of the scattered nanoparticles led to a significant increase in Young's modulus and tensile strength. In addition to the mechanical strengthening, CNC has been shown to increase miscibility between two biodegradable polymer blends, such as PLA and PBS [90].

To enhance the interaction between the polymer and the filler, certain alternate approaches might be used. The usage of silanes in the synthesis of CNF and PLA is one example. Surface modification is another strategy for enhancing fiber and PLA dispersion [91]. CNF was esterified first, and then the modified CNF was put to a PLA dissolution using an Ultra Turrax homogenizer.

Chitosan nanoparticles are yet another remarkable biodegradable nanofillers (CHT NPs) family. Ionotropic gelation and polyelectrolyte complex are the two most common techniques used in laboratories to generate nanoparticles. The ionotropic gelation approach is based on the interaction between the amine group in an acidic chitosan solution and a polyanion added to the mixture, forming nanoparticles. Nevertheless, when DNA is introduced to chitosan dissolved in acetic acid, charge neutralization between the macromolecules occurs, forming CHT NPs [92]. Chitosan fibers may also be manufactured; electrospinning is the most common technique for producing these nanostructures [93]. CHT NPs have several uses, including tissue engineering, drug delivery, water purification, and food packaging [92,94]. Nanocomposites composed of CHT NPs show potential as a food packaging material. In addition to the antibacterial properties of the final nanocomposite, the drawbacks of CHT NPs can be minimized by mixing them with other carbonaceous, metal, and inorganic nanofillers, as demonstrated in earlier cases [94].

8.2.6 Metal Impregnated Nanohybrids

Due to their special characteristics, metallic or metal nanoparticles have grown in significance. These noble metal nanoparticles, which are often made from silver, gold, platinum, or metal oxides, have a variety of applications but are particularly useful in the domains of optics, catalysis, electronics, and biomedicine [36].

The top-down and bottom-up techniques are the two basic strategies for producing metallic nanoparticles [36]. Typically, in top-down techniques, the bulk macroscopic material is put through a physical or chemical process that transforms it into nanoparticles. These techniques include mechanical milling, laser ablation, and sputtering. On the other hand, in bottom-up procedures, nanoparticles are created by connecting smaller particles, such as ions, atoms, or tiny molecules. Several techniques have been developed, including physical or chemical vapor deposition, chemical reduction of metallic salts in liquid or gas phase, and electrochemical techniques.

Green synthetic techniques that prevent the use of harmful solvents and reagents are strongly advised for the production of nanoparticles in line with the current research trend [12,37,95]. In this line, research into the manufacture of metallic particles utilizing plants and extracts is fresh and expanding. In a nutshell, this biogenic technique involves using plant extracts as a reducing agent to help metal ions create nanoparticles later on [38]. This technology has been widely used for biomedical applications because it creates these nanoparticles safely, eliminating the need for additional synthetic chemicals. It is essential to highlight that metal nanoparticle form, size distribution, and antibacterial capabilities are directly influenced by the plant extract employed during manufacture [39].

A colloidal dispersion of the nanoparticles is typically obtained by synthesizing gold nanoparticles (Au NPs) in liquid aqueous solutions. Typically, a chemical reagent reduces AuCl3 salts to create chemical ions. The production of the Au NPs then follows a process known as nucleation. A surfactant is often added to create a stable colloidal solution for this reaction [40]. Labeling, drug delivery systems, hyperthermia therapy, and optical sensors are all used for Au NPs [36,40].

Au NPs have been effectively employed in biodegradable polymer-based nanocomposites to enhance the electrical conductivity, dielectric properties, and ion mobility of the polymer due to the electrical characteristics of noble metal particles [96]. For instance, environmentally friendly nanocomposite materials have been created by employing a variety of plant extracts and green Au NP synthesis. These nanocomposites contain them. To create a film with a thickness varying from 55 to 100 m, different quantities of nanoparticles were added to carboxy methyl cellulose (CMC) solutions. At a temperature of 353 K, a 3-magnitude order increase in electrical conductivity was seen compared to pure CMC. Similar to the previous work, another one supports the effectiveness of Au NPs utilized as active fillers in PVA-based green nanocomposites [41]. More recently, Au NPs-reinforced biodegradable polymer-based nanocomposites have been developed. *Mentha Spicata L.* leaf extract was used to create Au NPs. The produced Au NPs were incorporated into a solution with a 70:30 weight ratio of PVA and CMC. A drop in the dielectric permittivity and increased direct electrical conductivity of 4 magnitude orders were noted [42].

Using biodegradable polymers like chitosan as a reducing and stabilizing agent is another intriguing method for the environmentally friendly production of Au NPs. In this regard, a solid film made of the nanocomposite material was made and employed for surface-enhanced Raman scattering (SERS) to detect tryptophan, a model analyte molecule. Begines et al. reported the creation of an Au NP nanocomposite stabilized by polyurethanes derived from sugars [97]. Because of its antibacterial qualities, the chosen material was subsequently treated and employed via an inkjet printing approach for controlled medication release applications or in cellulose/keratin nanocomposite packaging [98]. Another study focused on a nanocomposite formed of xanthan gum grafted with polyacrylic acid by an in-situ microwave-assisted polymerization with greenly produced Au NPs [99]. Au NPs were created from the plant extract *Nepeta leucophylla* and were included in a biodegradable hydrogel for amoxicillin-controlled release. A maximum medication loading efficiency of 85% was attained in addition to the nanoparticles' ability to modulate the diffusion rate. Several biodegradable polymers have been employed to stabilize Au NPs, including alginates, polysaccharides, poly(-caprolactone) copolymers, and PVA copolymers [100].

Due to their antibacterial, optical, electrical, and catalytic capabilities, silver nanoparticles (Ag NPs) are widely recognized [101]. Ag NPs production is frequently carried out via chemical reduction techniques, perhaps due to their simplicity. Reducing substances such as sodium citrate, sodium borohydride, thio-glycerol, hydrazine, and 2-mercaptoethanol are frequently used to produce Ag NPs [102,103]. However, green synthesis techniques are now preferred because of their toxicity, particularly for biomedical and packaging applications.

An *M. frondose* leaf extract was used as a reducing agent to create Ag NPs. By using solution casting, a nanocomposite material made of Ag NPs, chitosan, and gelatin was created for use in food packaging as an environmentally friendly material that increased the shelf life of carrots [104]. In a different environmentally friendly synthesis procedure, Ag NPs were created using lemon juice as a reducing agent, and they were then mixed with starch to form a polymer film before being used as a nanofiller [105]. These films showed an efficient ability to inhibit microbial growth and a reduction in water vapor permeability, making them an appropriate material for use in food packaging. Silver-coated Au NPs were created by combining the biocompatibility of Au NPs with the antibacterial capabilities of Ag NPs. These core-shell nanoparticles were placed on cellulose paper to create a biodegradable, antibacterial layer. The following references thoroughly analyze green nanocomposites based on Au and Ag NPs utilized in food packaging applications [106,107]. *Ocimum sanctum* was used as the reducing agent in a composite of cellulose and Ag NPs described in another study [108]. In this instance, the cellulose sheets that had been previously impregnated with the plant extracts were processed by dipping them in AgNO3 solutions. The material demonstrated good effectiveness against *E. coli* germs and has intriguing potential for use in medical dressing.

It is widely known that chitosan has the ability to function as a stabilizer and reducing agent during the creation of metal nanoparticles. Ag NPs, PVA, and chitosan were used to create the hydrogel that Popescu et al. created [109]. Oxalic acid produced an ionic cross-linking that was used with the freeze-thawing process to cross-link the material. The cross-linked gel demonstrated significant antibacterial action against *S. aureus*, *P. gingivalis*, and *K. pneumoniae*, three types of harmful bacteria. This substance was suggested as a potential therapeutic option for periodontitis because of its exceptional antibacterial characteristics. On the other hand, an electrospun PVA/chitosan/Ag NPs nanocomposite was created. A chitosan/Ag NPs composite was first created. The previously created nanocomposite was then combined with PVA, which was processed by electrospinning to create a fiber mat. Compared to the control materials, the hybrid materials demonstrated that adding Ag NPs increased mechanical parameters, including elastic modulus and hardness, making them suitable materials for biomedical applications [110].

It has been investigated if combining metallic nanoparticles with other nanofillers has a synergistic impact. Using PCL as the host polymer matrix, Ag NPs and SWCNTs have been combined [111]. According to reports, the combination of SWCNTs with Ag NPs has a synergistic impact that improves mechanical and electrical characteristics. The nucleation effects of both nanoparticles and the manner that Ag NPs act as a conductor between the SWCNTs were used to explain this phenomenon. Ag NPs and graphene oxide were shown to have a similar synergistic effect [112].

8.2.7 DENDRIMERS

Weakly water-soluble medications are dispersed and dissolved using dendrimers, which are artificial, highly branching, globular, monodispersed, nanometric macromolecules.

Iterative reaction procedures create dendrimers with unique branching structures. Due to their monodispersity, regulated molecular weight, a large number of surface functional groups, and ability to enclose guest molecules in the inner hydrophobic environment, dendrimers are potential scaffolds for drug delivery [113]. Controlled bioactive delivery made possible by nanotechnology has shown promise and may pave the way for successful tailored therapies and therapeutic drug monitoring. Genetic material, vaccines, diagnostic tools, and drug administration are all being studied using nanotechnology [114].

Dendrimers offer a variety of biological and pharmaceutical applications; however, due to reticuloendothelial system (RES) absorption, drug outflow, resistance, stability, hemolytic toxicity, and hydrophobicity, their cationic surface charge limits clinical use. These limitations can be circumvented by PEGylation, surface engineering, and dual drug delivery systems [114]. Recently, some researchers have shown interest in dual drug delivery systems that use dendrimers coupled to a variety of carriers, including microspheres, liposomes, nanoparticles, carbon nanotubes (CNTs), microspheres, and microspheres. Dendrimers may easily be encapsulated to form a nanohybrid, absorbed on surfaces, or chemically connected to CNTs since they are smaller than liposomes, NPs, and microspheres. QDs easily fit within dendrimer cavities. The desired role of nanocarriers is to protect bioactives from cellular endosomal degradation and first-pass metabolism. The ideal solution for biological issues like drug delivery may be nanohybrids. There is a wealth of research on dendrimer-based nanohybrid systems with conventional nanocarriers and several medical and nonmedical applications. All dendrimer-based nanohybrids are discussed.

Liposomes are nonimmunogenic, biodegradable, and biocompatible nanocarriers with an aqueous phase and phospholipid bilayer. The lipids used to make them determine their size and charge. Targeted nanocarriers include liposomes [115]. Few commercial products use dendrimers as carriers because of the cytotoxicity caused by the cationic charge on the surface, which limits their clinical application [114]. Several research organizations have released articles on dendrimer manufacturing. The toxicity brought on by the dendrimer's cationic charge can be lessened by new dendrimers like biodegradable, polyester, melamine, triazine, and poly-l-lysine as surface modifications like PEGylation, carbohydrate coating, acetylation, and amino acid and peptide conjugation [114,116,117]. To increase biocompatibility, our group combined dendrimers with lipoproteins. Hybrid dendrimers reduce toxicity and enhance drug loading when combined with liposomes, CNTs, microspheres, QDs, and NPs. Dendrimers have opposing charges and a size that is similar to the aqueous gap between the two bilayers, which allows them to be encapsulated or adsorbed on liposomes. All liposomes absorbed dendrimers; however, 8- and 16-amino-group dendrimers were less well absorbed. Amphipathic partial dendrimers dissolve liposomes. Positively charged liposomes were expanded using 32-amino-group dendrimers. It may have been brought on by hydrophobic contact, quantum size, and the dendrimers' larger surface area containing 32 amino groups. When head size increased, the amount of adsorbed partial dendrimers decreased [118]. The charge of a liposome has no impact on adsorption.

Cationic poly(amido amine) (PAMAM) in liposomes with opposing charges. The loading of an acidic methotrexate (MTX) drug increased significantly in the nanohybrid due to the pH and solubility gradient influx generated by dendrimer charge interaction, which may also obstruct drug release. Pharmaceuticals can be trapped at higher quantities in dendrimer-liposome hybrids because dendrimer synthesis increases drug loading [119]. Drug loading effectiveness is impacted by the drug dendrimer-to-lipid molar ratio in the liposome. A molar ratio of 10:10:0.1 was found in two liposomes containing hexadecylphosphocholine (HePC), egg yolk phosphatidylcholine (EPC), and stearylamine (SA) (molar ratio). Efficiency was 91% and 95%, respectively, when Doxorubicin (Dox)-PAMAM dendrimer (3:1 and 6:1 molar ratio) was coupled with both kinds of liposomes. At pH 7.4 (TES buffer) compared to pH 4.5 (acetate buffer), drug encapsulation was greater, and Dox release from the liposome was very sluggish (17% at pH 7.4 and 25 °C even after 24 h). Dox entrapment was enhanced at pH 7.4. Due to the interaction between the drug and the dendrimer, Dox-dendrimer incorporation into liposomes was higher at 3:1 than 6:1 in both buffers. The study claimed cytotoxic experiments against lungs (DMS114, NCI-H460), colon (HT29, HCT116), breast (MB435k, MCF7), prostate (DU145), and central nervous system (CNS) (SF268) cancer cell lines and discovered that MDA-MB435, DMS114, and NCI-H460 were the most sensitive [120]. As drug carriers, dendrimer-liposome hybrids are commonly utilized because of their enhanced permeability and retention (EPR) effect and better drug encapsulation efficiency. Due to their ability to overcome hurdles, it is vital to research dendrimer-liposome hybrids as feasible nanocarriers in nanotherapeutics.

NPs range in size from 1 to 100 nm and can be amorphous or crystalline. NPs are the most common nanocarrier for the delivery of medications due to their increased surface area and quantum size effects. In 2002, PEG-grafted PAMAM-NH$_2$ dendrimers were used to create gold and cadmium sulfide nanoparticles (NPs). As a template, star polymer can strengthen polydispersed NPs and improve miscibility in organic solvents. Dendrimer-grafted NPs is depicted in **Figure 8.2** [114]. On magnetite-modified aminosilane NPs, PAMAM dendrimer was generated. Due to the enormous size of BSA and the small surface area of NPs, BSA immobilization increased linearly with dendrimer production. Immobilization outperformed amino silane-modified NPs by 3.9–7.7 times [121].

Dendrimers are typically mononuclear micelles. In the aqueous phase, SiO$_2$ NPs are stabilized by dendrimers by preventing photocatalysis [122]. Unexpectedly, dendrimers also significantly influenced the size, shape, size distribution, and stability of silver NPs produced using co-mediators such as polyvinyl pyrrolidone (PVP) and PAMAM G1.5 dendrimers. The diameter of spherical NPs was around 5 nm. During at least two months at room temperature, these NPs did not aggregate. NP size and distribution are similarly impacted by oligosaccharide (maltose)-modified poly(propylene imine) glycodendrimers as templates. G4 (1–2 nm) (1–2 nm) Due to their autoreductive property, maltose-modified dendrimers produced the smallest NPs; unmodified dendrimers did not. Due to the interfacial absorption of larger NPs, lower-generation dendrimers (G2-G3) were more stable. In well-defined cavities, dendrimers can serve to stabilize smaller NPs [123]. Platinum (Pt) NPs stabilized by carbosilane dendrimers via the Pt-C link and showed excellent dispersibility in situ with a range of sizes [124].

Terminal functionality allows NPs to self-assemble into the G2-G5 thiol-terminated PAMAM dendrimer. Bridging aggregation regulated NP-dendrimer aggregation. Dendrimer production increased steric hindrance, shrinking the cluster. Dendrimer production and NP diameter influence interparticle spacing.

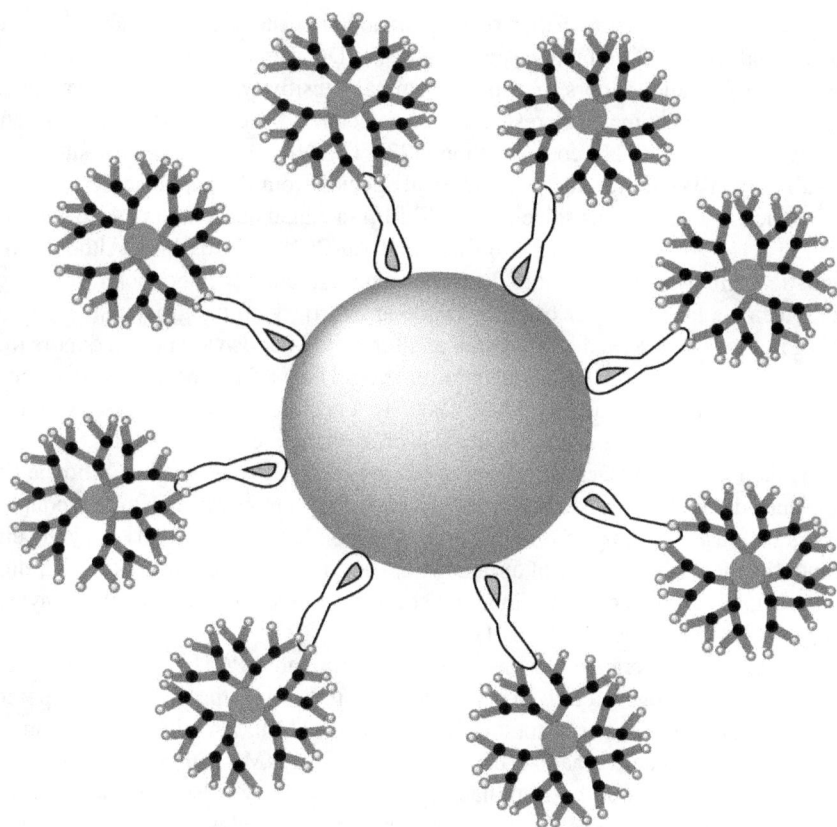

Drug Discovery Today

FIGURE 8.2 Dendrimer-Grafted Nanohybrid. Reprinted with permission from *Kesharwani et al. (2018)*] [114].

Higher-generation PAMAM stabilized silver (Ag)/AuNPs (G5). Dendrimer-entrapped and dendrimer-stabilized NPs (DENPs and DSNPs) for computed tomography (CT) imaging and other biological applications were promisingly cytocompatible [125]. Dendrimers dictate NP sizes and morphology. The polypropylene imine (PPI) G3 dendrimer molar ratio affects the size of the AuNP nanocomposite. Dendrimer-AuNP interaction and particle growth at higher molar ratios yield smaller NPs [126]. PAMAM- dendrimer-modified ternary magnetic iron oxide NPs/DNA/PEI magnetoplexes improve NP transfection. Magnetofection swiftly accumulated magnetoplexes and absorbed them in a magnetic field in COS-7 cells [127].

The dendrimer-NP hybrid has been used in a number of different fields, both biological and nonbiological, such as electrochemistry, catalysis, and immunological sensors. Palladium (Pd)NP forms the 2.7 nm carbon-Pd stabilized Frechet type G1 dendrimer (Pd-G1). It catalyzes double-bonded compounds. The complex is reusable, responds fast, and produces a lot of products at room temperature. Halogens and endocyclic double bonds were unaffected [33]. PPI-dendrimers were used to make a chemoresistor, vapor-sensing nanocomposite film, and layer-by-layer (LbL) dendrimer self-assembly AuNPs (G1–5). Dendrimer synthesis solvated toluene and 1-propanol vapors, boosting chemical sensitivity. Water vapor was unaffected, and nanocomposites' resistivity was dictated by dendrimer synthesis and size, which controlled NP concentration [128]. The NP-dendrimer composite was a stimuli-responsive sensor because chemical species from the vapor phase impacted its conductance. In various solvents, AuNP film included dendrimers PAMAM (G3) and PPI (G4). Au-PPI was 27.8 nm thick and Au-PAMAM 36.6 nm. Although the aliphatic chain was insufficient to form a strong interaction with nonpolar molecules like toluene, a large number of polar amide and tertiary amine groups of PAMAM and PPI of the films served as receptors and formed H-bonds with proton donors like water, suggesting that the NP-dendrimer film could be used as a chemiresistive vapor sensor [129]. Electrochemically, PAMAM (G4) dendrimer-encapsulated AuNP nanocomposites recognized α-synuclein. Parkinson's, Alzheimer's, and Huntington's have α-synuclein pathology. Dendrimer encapsulated in AuNP was covalently bonded to the electrode, and horseradish-peroxidase-secondary-antibody (HRP-Ab2) coupled to NPs increased signals (15.6 nm). Systems responded at 14.6 pg mL^{-1}α-synuclein. Due to the increased number of amino groups in the dendrimer and HRP-Ab2, dual signal amplification occurred. Thus, the study recommended expanding the hybrid to approaches for protein analysis [114].

Bimetallic NPs were synthesized from OH-terminated PAMAM G4 dendrimers that partially hydrogenated 1,3-cyclooctadiene, indicating the dendrimer's potential application as a nanoreactor in NP production [130]. An LbL film was made utilizing an electroactive nanostructure membrane (ENM) with alternating layers of AuNP-dendrimer (amine-terminated, G4) and poly (vinylsulfonic acid). PVS/PAMAM-AuNP electrodes reduced oxygen for three bilayers better than ITO electrodes [131]. A dendrimer-NP cisplatin delivery method was reported wherein Herceptin-conjugated PAMAM dendrimers and diglycolamic acid were utilized. HER-2-positive and HER-2-negative ovarian cancer cell line tests showed that the nanoconstruct lowered IC50 values for cisplatin. Targeted conjugate administration boosted anticancer activity in SKOV-3 tumor xenografts [132]. EPR stabilized a multistage nanocarrier in systemic circulation and accumulated in the tumor by encapsulating PAMAM dendrimer (5 nm). Loading MTX enhanced tumor penetration and effectiveness [133]. Dendrimers increased magnetic nanoparticle tumor cell capture, water solubility, and antibody conjugation (MNPs). Nanosubstrate accelerates tumor cell identification and collects 86 ± 5% [134].

Dendrimer-quantum-dot hybrid QDs are semiconducting, spherical, bright nanocrystals with a radius of 10–100. Size influences their attributes. QDs are employed for *in-vivo* applications, *in-vitro* bioimaging, fluorescence, greater chemical stability, readily changeable spectrum characteristics, narrow emission, broad UV excitation, and superior photo-stability. Dendrimer-QD hybrids improved QD quantum yield, water solubility, and toxicity [114].

PAMAM dendrimers encapsulate Cadmium Sulfide (CdS) QDs in a nanocomposite with all the previously mentioned properties [135]. PAMAM G4 dendrimers tagged with 525 ITKTM(PEG) QDs target the vimentin shRNA plasmid for imaging. The EGF-conjugated dendrimer targeted NIH3T3 and HN12 cells via EGFR, which is overexpressed in the cell lines. EGFR on the cell membrane, nuclear membrane, and cytoplasm allowed the conjugate system into endosomes. EGF's positive charge attracts receptors. Drugs or nucleic acids feed growth factors. The QD-PAMAM G4-aptamer GBI-10 combination improves targeted administration, water solubility, and Apt-QD nanoprobe binding affinity against U251 glioblastoma cells. GBI-10 recognizes tenacin-C, an extracellular protein on human U251 cells; nanoprobes strongly bind to the cells [136]. RGD peptide enhances dendrimer-QD hybrid imaging and targeting. Melanoma, sprouting tumor vasculature, glioblastoma, breast, prostate, and ovarian cancer overexpress integrin V3, which interacts with the RGD peptide—conjugated nanoprobes image A375 melanoma cells and HUVECs *in-vitro* and *in-vivo*. RGD-conjugated QDs were biocompatible and non-cytotoxic [137].

Dendrimer-CdTe QDs reduce Cd release and cytotoxicity. PAMAM G3.0 dendrimer-CdTe QD nanoconjugate may be transfected into PK15 cells for cell-imaging. CdTe-PAMAM cell survival was 75.28% after 48 hours and 25.23% after 12 hours using CdSe QDs. Dendrimer-modified QDs have significantly low cytotoxicity [114]. Graded band gap construction and QD LbL deposition enabled FRET to detect DNA hydrolysis. QDs modified with PAMAM dendrimer improve cellular uptake, cytosolic distribution, and intracellular fluorescence in primary MSCs.

Nonbiological applications used diaminobutane-based CdS, ZnS, and CdS/ZnS-QDS nanocomposites. pH, ionic strength, and Hg(II) nanosensors use nanocomposites [138]. Glass carbon electrodes can electrochemically monitor waterborne bisphenol A [2,2-bis(4-hydroxyphenyl)propane] using CoTe QDs with PAMAM dendrimer. The method has a lower oxidation potential, improved sensitivity, lower detection limits, and shorter reaction time than previous electrochemical methods [139]. The nanocomposite detected BPA in milk after extensive testing. Nanocomposites have reduced oxidation potential, higher sensitivity, lower detection limits, and faster reactions [83,84].

Carbon sp^2 hybridized 3D hexagonal dendrimer-carbon-nanotube hybrid CNTs. CNTs are intriguing nanomaterials with pharmacological and biological applications, but their dispersibility, hydrophobicity, degradability, and toxicity limit clinical usage. Functionalization and hybrid nanocarriers are being studied to overcome CNT limitations [140]. CNTs are suitable biosensors and biocatalysts, but their low dispersibility in solvents, especially water, is an issue. Partial oxidation, hydrophilic groups, and polymers improve CNT water dispersibility. CNTs were conjugated with dendrimers to improve water dispersibility [114].

Multiwall nanotube mats were synthesized by dendrimer-aided catalytic annealing in air. Dendrimers affect nanofiber size. Dendrimer-based Co32 nanoclusters were employed as uniform-size catalytic probes for diameter-controlled SWCNT production. Topographical studies showed that the nanotubes had a restricted diameter range and were no thicker than 1.3 nm [141]. Dendrimer-CNT hybrids also used innovative methods. Enzyme immobilization generated unknown dendrimer-CNT hybrids. Bienzymatic CNT-PAMAM dendrimer conjugate immobilized GOx and HRP primed—glucose-sensitive conjugate. The bienzymatic conjugate's 0.34 V negative potential allows glucose monitoring without ascorbic acid. Fluoroalkyls have better thermal and chemical stability than water dispersibility, surface energy, and dielectric constant. Fluorinated-dendrimer copolymer self-aggregates, making water dispersibility high. Copolymers spread SWCNTs and fullerenes in water at 21.5–67.3 and 4.2–13.3 μg/mL. In fluorinated-dendrimer copolymer, SWCNTs, fullerene, and MNPs improve aqueous dispersibility [142]. Electropolymerized poly-pyrrole film served as a hybrid self-aggregation probe by self-assembling glutamate dehydrogenase (GLDH) and poly(amidoamine) dendrimer-encapsulated platinum NPs (Pt-DENs) onto multiwall CNTs. A nano bioconjugated biosensor evaluated glutamate-oxidized NADH with high sensitivity, low detection limit, quick response, and no interference. CNTs had equally spaced 3 nm-wide NPs. Biosensor response depends on polypyrrole layer thickness, which increased with electro-polymerization but lost biostability after six cycles [143]. The self-assembly of dendrimer-encapsulated PtNP (Pt-PAMAM) and glutamate dehydrogenase (GLDH) on multi-wall CNTs developed the first amperometric glutamate biosensor (MWCNTs). CNTs' GLDH-Pt-PAMAM multilayer enhanced electron transport surface area. GLDH polyanionic material was used to make LbL film at pH 7.4.10 nm thick CNT layer. Repeatable, stable, and sensitive modified enzymatic biosensors prevent enzyme leakage and maintain enzyme activity [65]. MWCNTs and pure dendrimers lost 38% cytotoxicity. Grafting silver nanoparticles (AgNPs) boosts CNT-dendrimer hybrid stability, water dispersibility, and antibacterial activity [144]. CNT-dendrimer hybrids can be used in electrochemistry, while PAMAM G4 dendrimer templates PdNPs on MWNTs. The nanocomposite converted hydrazine, a direct fuel cell fuel, electrocat-alytically [145]. Most of the published research describes the synthesis of dendrimer-CNT hybrids to achieve the greater dispersibility of CNTs in the aqueous phase.

Microspheres are protein or synthetic polymer powders with biodegradable nano-carriers and diameters < 200 m. Controlled and prolonged medicine distribution requires microsphere delivery. Microspheres are nanocarriers too. Drug accumu-lation rather than other organs or tissue protects unstable drugs in the circulatory system with microspheres. Hybrid dendrimer-microsphere carriers can bioengineer, biocatalyze, and detect biomolecules [146]. Hybrid dendrimer-microsphere systems are understudied. Microsphere-dendrimer glucose biosensors are noninvasive. Con-canavaline A-glycodendrimer in biocompatible PEG microspheres is a minimally invasive glucose sensor. PEG hydrogel matrix microporation generated micro-spheres. Throughout 14 days, the fluorescent tag Con A measures physiological glu-cose levels via competitive binding. Leaching prevented pores from functioning and reversing [147].

Bioengineering and catalysis employ dendrimer-microsphere hybrids. Since PLLA hydrolyzes fast, dendrimer-like copolymers of poly(l-lactide) and polystyrene make biocatalysis and bioengineering microspheres. Once hydrolyzed micromolecules and solvents evaporated, 295 nm microspheres had one or two tiny surface holes [148]. Polystyrene microspheres stabilize PAMAM dendrimer, NPs coated in SiO_2 for immobilization and the nanocomposite. PAMAM (G5) dendrimer was grafted onto polystyrene microspheres and dispersed in $AgNO_3$ to form AgNPs. PS@PAMAM@ SiO_2-Ag nanocomposite reduced 4-nitrophenol better in the catalytic column [149]. Dendrimers and microspheres may absorb hazardous chemicals from aqueous solu-tions. Stepwise reaction with methylate acrylate and ethylene diamine produced magnetic poly-(methyl acrylate-divinyl benzene) microspheres on NH2-terminated dendrimers. Nanohybrids absorbed aqueous hexavalent chromium. Due to several surface functions, a suitable pH of 3, and rising temperature, G3 adsorption was 231.8 mg/g [150]. Dendrimer-microsphere hybrids were largely employed for bioengineering and catalysis, not medication delivery.

Gelation creates pharmaceutical and biological hydrogels. Hydrogels with amphiphilic Janus dendrimers increased payload and drug release [151]. Wróblewska and Winnicka found that PAMAM dendrimer-based erythromycin hydrogels released erythromycin faster in a concentration- and generation-dependent way. Erythromycin release increased, and non-Newtonian thixotropic systems shear-thinned in rheograms. Later dendrimers' bactericidal activity increased somewhat with stability at 40 ± 2 °C and $75 \pm 5\%$ RH [152]. Dendrimers were changed with integrin-binding sequences, pN-modified hyaluronan, and propargylamine-derived azido-hyaluronic acid to generate hydrogels. Dendrimers were thermoresponsive biological carriers and did not affect hyaluronan hydrogel rheology [153].

With their 3D hyperbranched macromolecular architecture, precise molecular weight, size, and shape, and excellent host-guest interactions conferred by a large number of cavities in the internal structure and the presence of multifunctional surface groups, dendrimers are emerging as promising nanomaterials in the delivery of drug and genetic material. These tiny macromolecules are getting a lot of attention as potential nanocarriers with a wide variety of applications because of their unique physical and chemical characteristics. Dendrimers have several potential benefits as drug carriers, but their toxicity due to their surface cationic charge and plush price have limited their clinical usage. Thus, hybrid carrier systems constructed with dendrimers and other nanomaterials are being studied as a means to lessen these issues and guarantee clinical applicability. One promising approach being investigated in the realm of nanomedicine is the creation of hybrid nanomaterials for the transportation of bioactives. Dendrimers have recently been described in the literature as being used in hybrids with other nanocarriers to increase medication delivery.

8.3 PROPERTIES OF NANOHYBRIDS

Composites combine two or more elements to create a material with superior properties than those of its constituent parts. This type of material typically consists of a reinforcement to add stiffness and strength and a matrix to add geometry and cohesion. According to the intended use, we provide a wide variety of organic, metallic, polymeric, and ceramic matrices. Popular reinforcements include carbon fibers, glass, natural fibers, and others. As these materials are sourced from the natural world, they represent a sizable subset of the composite materials that we have available. Examples of these kinds of natural composites are bone and wood. Wood comprises a lignin matrix and cellulose fibers, whereas bone comprises collagen, which serves as the matrix, and fibers formed of a mineral called apatite [7].

According to this definition, a nanocomposite is a multiphase material in which all the phases have sizes less than 10 nm. The idea behind this type of material is to use building blocks on the nanoscale scale to create and produce materials with improved properties [29].

Research into nanocomposites has increased dramatically after discovering that graphene has desirable properties. Graphene's two-dimensional structure endows it with a wide range of desirable properties, including mechanical strength, thermal conductivity, and electrical conductivity. The advantageous features of graphene have led to several attempts to integrate it into polymeric matrices. Graphene's measured mechanical properties are Young's modulus of 1.0 TPa, a tensile strength of 42 N/m, and fracture toughness of 4.0 0.6 MPa. These values are evidence of the extraordinary durability of graphene. Graphene and its derivatives have the potential to enhance the performance of polymer nanocomposites when utilized as fibers. One example is offered by Cheng-An et al., who studied the effect of adding 20% graphene to PVA films to increase their strength [154]. The resultant material had a tensile strength of 59.6 MPa, which is almost five times that of pure PVA.

This dramatic improvement in mechanical properties can be attributed to the strength of the matrix, the hydroxyl groups in the PVA, the hydroxyl groups in the graphene, and the functionalities of the oxygen in the graphene, which resulted in the formation of hydrogen bridges. Compared to traditional ways of producing carbon-based nanomaterials, hydrothermal carbonization stands out as a more eco-friendly option for producing nanocomposites. Hydrothermal carbonization is not a recent synthesis process, but it has become an essential technique for making hybrid materials from carbon [7]. Hydrothermal carbonization is attractive because it allows for producing a wide variety of hybrid and carbon nanostructures while being environmentally friendly, controllable, and scalable. CO_2 sequestration, water purification, and catalysts are just a few of the many chemical industry applications for the products of this process. Plant-based, animal-based, and mineral-based natural fibers are each classified separately. Plant fibers generally comprise cellulose, whereas animal fibers comprise proteins (hair, silk, wool). Throughout the past decade, scientists have investigated using fibers of natural origin as the primary building blocks for nanomaterials because of their wide availability, low cost, recyclable nature, and superior mechanical and chemical properties.

Nanocomposites used or aimed at the biological and food industries nowadays often have antibacterial properties. This is because biomedical practitioners are having trouble treating infected wounds and foods that have been preserved for extended periods of time. While developing multicomponent nanocomposites, scientists focus on a wide range of active agents to provide antibacterial activity; some metals, such as silver nanoparticles or zinc oxide nanoparticles, stand out in this respect, as do specific transition metals like Cu [155]. Although the inhibitory efficacy of antimicrobial medicines varies depending on the bacteria they are intended to combat, different natural extracts have been used to offer these qualities to nanocomposites [156].

To produce chitosan-based nanocomposite films with various clay loadings of 0, 5, 10, and 15% cross-linked with glycerol at concentrations of 10, 20, and 30%, respectively, Kusmono et al. 2019 reported using a casting procedure [157]. The study proved that incorporating clay into nanocomposites significantly increased their tensile strength and tensile modulus, from 5% to 20%, respectively. Nevertheless, no nanocomposite produced inhibitory zones against E. coli just by touch, ruling it out as a practical possibility for use in packaging material [157].

Cell viability and biocompatibility studies showed no cytotoxicity in NIH3T3 or MG-63 cells. A study on the development of porous 3D scaffolds utilizing the freeze-drying approach based on gallium-apatite/chitin/pectin was reported by Cui et al. [158]. The cells also grew in number and stuck to the scaffolds. Implantation of the scaffolds showed the creation of mature bone via the generation of new bone layers and the differentiation of osteoblasts; therefore, it is regarded as a material that fits the conditions to be considered for orthopedic applications.

Nazir et al. produced a hydrogel nanocomposite composed of arabinoxylan (ARA) and loaded with graphene oxide functionalized with the chemotherapeutic medication fluorouracil (5FU) [159]. According to the study, many types of bacteria, including *S. aureus* and *P. aeruginosa*, and the skin cancer cell line U-87 were killed by it. This has led to their classification as a promising nanomaterial for treating and preventing skin cancer [159].

In 2022, Li et al. developed polyurethane foams that were both flexible and infused with Cu nanoparticles with a size distribution of 100 to 130 nm [160]. Researchers found that the addition of nanoparticles to polyurethane foam did not alter the foam's chemical makeup and that the foam exhibited potent antimicrobial activity against a range of pathogens, including *E. coli*, *P. aeruginosa*, and *S. aureus* [160]. This finding suggests the foam could find application in water purification and medicine.

Environmental pollution has emerged as a major problem worldwide due to the devastating consequences of various pollutants on ecosystems and human health. Thus, it is crucial for the world's population that these poisons be treated and eventually eradicated. Contaminant removal by biodegradation is an adaptable process. Nanocomposites with unique chemical and physical stability, large surface area, and adsorption capacity can boost the efficiency of biodegradation processes [161]. Biodegradation is believed to be a green process since it does not need additional energy, thereby conserving both renewable and nonrenewable resources. Enzymatic, cellular, and bacterial breakdown are the principal areas of study [162].

In 2021, Candotto Carniel et al. studied the ambient biodegradation of graphene using axenic cultures of basidiomycetes such *Bjerkandera adusta*, *Phanerochaete chrysosporium*, and *Morchella esculenta* [163]. They report that the selected fungus can oxidize graphene to a compound comparable to graphene oxide, and they recommend continuing the experiment for longer than four months to test if the product can entirely degrade to CO_2 [163].

The chemical composition of the components determines the properties of natural nanocomposites. Although natural polymers are notoriously abrasive and chemically inert, they are flexible and biodegradable. They frequently have antimicrobial and bacteriostatic biological properties. However, several additives or fillers are utilized to improve their poor mechanical qualities, the most notable of which are metallic nanoparticles, polymer nanoparticles, and carbon-based nanostructures, including multiwall or single-wall carbon nanotubes, nanofibers, graphene, fullerenes, etc. Natural composites are fascinating because they improve the natural polymer's impressive characteristics. Natural inorganic nanocomposites containing zeolites, different sands, feldspars, and clays combined with metallic nanoparticles or carbon-based nanostructures are more challenging regarding breakdown or biodegradation. Nonetheless, positive characteristics like mechanical strength, corrosion resistance, hardness, etc. are present [7].

8.4 APPLICATION OF NANOHYBRIDS IN DRUG DELIVERY

8.4.1 CANCER THERAPY

Problems with solubility and cell penetration are common when using chemotherapeutic drugs. The lack of specific therapeutic targeting for cancer cells further restricts clinical uses by causing systemic toxicity [61]. The search for safe and efficient medication administration has become the forefront of scientific inquiry. The potential of CNTs as a novel and developing nanomaterial for use in drug delivery carriers has garnered considerable interest in recent years. Functionalized carbon nanotubes delivered several tiny molecules of anticancer medication to tumor cells. Several types of human cancer have been successfully treated with the chemotherapeutic drug doxorubicin (DOX). Branched PL-PEG functionalized SWCNTs have had DOX loaded onto their sidewalls by π-π stacking [164]. The DOX loading ratio tested in this research was 2.5 g/g of SWCNTs. Unlike free DOX and DOXIL, SWCNT-formulated DOX demonstrated significantly higher therapeutic effectiveness in a mouse breast cancer model while exhibiting significantly reduced toxicity. The same research team also used SWCNTs with paclitaxel loaded onto them; they did this by attaching the medication to the amino group of the branching phospholipid-PEG chains via cleavable ester linkages, which are hydrolyzed in the cellular milieu [165]. The resulting substance, SWCNT-PEG-paclitaxel, is soluble in water. In a 4T1 murine breast cancer model, the generated SWCNT-PTX conjugate showed more efficiency than clinical Taxol in reducing tumor development [166]. The SWCNT-PTX was also more blood-stable and less toxic than the control. The anticancer prodrug cisplatin was conjugated to PL-PEG-SWCNT using a similar method [167].

Peptide linkages were used to attach the amino end group of PL-PEG to the carbon nanotubes, where the platinum (IV) complex c,c,t-$[Pt(NH_3)_2Cl_2(OEt)(O_2CCH_2CH_2CO_2H)]$ was deposited. Endocytosis was used by testicular cancer cells to absorb the SWCNTs, and a subsequent decrease in compartmental pH allowed for drug release. In addition, toxicity was significantly reduced in the SWCNT-formulated platinum (IV) complex compared to the free drug therapy. SWCNTs conjugated with quantum dots (QDs) or the targeting ligand epidermal growth factor (EGF) have been used to provide targeted delivery of anticancer medicines like cisplatin to squamous carcinoma cells. As squamous carcinoma cells have EGF receptors, the QD luminescence makes it easy to follow the SWCNT formulation, and the conjugation of EGF shows that the formulation was quickly taken up [168]. SWCNTs have also been investigated for their potential to transport small interfering RNAs (siRNAs) through non-covalent interactions [169]. To suppress the expression of telomerase reverse transcriptase (TERT) and to decrease cell proliferation in-vitro and in-vivo in tumor models, a recent study investigated the capacity of cationic SWCNTs to form stable complexes with siRNAs [170].

Using a 1,3-dipolar cycloaddition strategy, CNTs could be covalently functionalized with methotrexate (MTX). Two connecting sites, one for FITC and one for MTX, were introduced onto the sidewalls of carbon nanotubes in this study's protocol [171]. Increased cellular uptake of MTX was achieved by conjugation to carbon nanotubes. Nevertheless, neither the in-vitro nor the in-vivo effectiveness of the drugs nor their release patterns were examined. The anticancer drug 10-hydroxycamptothecin (HCPT) was given using an MWNT that had been covalently modified [172]. By amidation, the carboxylic groups on the oxidized nanotube were linked to drug molecules using diaminotriethylene glycol as a spacer. The MWNT-HCPT conjugates had a longer blood circulation and a larger drug accumulation at the tumor site, and the MWNT-HCPT formed HCPT demonstrated better anticancer efficacy *in-vitro* and *in-vivo* compared to the current HCPT formulation [61].

Using biocompatible polymeric membranes like alginate-poly-l-lysine-alginate (APA), we microencapsulate carbon nanotubes for site-specific delivery [173]. Microencapsulation serves to shield payloads from hostile surroundings while letting targeted solutes through a polymeric membrane. The regulated, continuous, and extended release of the therapeutics at the intended location allows for the optimal delivery of bioactive compounds. To encapsulate the CNTs, a microencapsulator was used to create beads out of a solution of calcium chloride and sodium alginate, which had been mixed with a suspension of functionalized SWCNTs. During our early research, we analyzed how the SWCNTs were dispersed throughout the polymeric core. Using the results of optimization and characterization of the microencapsulated SWCNT formulation, we are now concentrating on delivering the therapy to specific areas in the gastrointestinal tracts of animals to treat colon cancer. Our lab coupled SWCNTs to pEGFP in an *in-vitro* investigation of a colon cancer cell line to improve transfection efficiency while minimizing cellular damage [174].

8.4.2 Neurodegenerative Diseases

Neurodegenerative disease refers to a collection of disorders that affect the brain and spinal cord and result in the malfunction or death of neurons. Alzheimer's, Parkinson's, and Huntington's illnesses are the three most prevalent kinds of neurodegeneration, according to experts [175]. Alzheimer's disease, the most frequent form of dementia, is characterized by the neuroinflammatory development of amyloid plaques and neurofibrillary tangles. A deficit in acetylcholine is another indication of the condition [175]. Subcellular and molecular characteristics of NDs include faulty synapses, neuronal loss, and the creation of cerebral deposits, all of which are produced by the accumulation of improperly folded proteins [176]. These mechanisms, which contribute to cellular homeostasis, make it possible to prevent neurological illnesses. Hence, monitoring ion levels and dynamics in the brain is a valuable tool for analyzing and interpreting cerebral activity, giving a fresh way of considering and tracking neurological illnesses such as Alzheimer's [177]. For the treatment of neurodegenerative illnesses, medication delivery based on solid lipid nanoparticles should be prioritized. Specifically, SLNs can deliver the active component to the appropriate location with minimal off-target effects, overcome physiological barriers to boost bioavailability without the need for enormous dosages, and protect pharmaceuticals against chemical and enzymatic degradation [178].

Alzheimer's disease (AD) is a progressive, deadly neurological condition that mostly affects the elderly and is the major cause of dementia in this group. AD is characterized by diminished cholinergic transmission, which is notably evident in the cerebral cortex and hippocampus, two brain areas associated with improved cognitive and memorizing capacities [179]. It is defined by the gradual shrinkage of the brain's cortex and the loss of cortical neurons [180]. AD has a 10% prevalence among those 65 and older and a 50% prevalence among those 85 and older. The likelihood of developing AD in women is 1.5 times that of men. AD is now afflicting 15 million individuals worldwide [180]. Typically, neurodegenerative disorders are associated with cell death in the brain and spinal cord. In Alzheimer's disease and Parkinson's disease, for example, neuronal damage is linked to aberrant protein processing and accumulation, resulting in a steady decline in cognitive and motor functions [181]. It is now employed as a therapy option for the condition's advanced stages. Memantine combined with a cholinesterase inhibitor appears to be the most effective therapy for moderate to severe AD [178].

Due to breakthroughs in nanotechnology, we can now combine therapy and diagnostics more firmly [176]. The construction of this nanosensor, which was demonstrated to be more sensitive than regular carbon nanotubes, led to the enhanced sensitivity of the sensors [179]. Due to the brain's fragility, nature has equipped it with incredibly effective defenses. Yet the same mechanisms may hinder treatment attempts [180]. Ion sensors are in great demand because monitoring ion changes in the brain is crucial. To address the challenges provided by the brain's complex microenvironment and the ion dynamics spanning healthy and pathological processes, sensors must be sensitive, selective, and biocompatible [177]. When metal ion levels grow over time, the effects on the brain become catastrophic [182]. Medication distribution to the brain remains a formidable obstacle in the treatment of AD [182]. In addition to the tau kinase cyclin-dependent kinase 5, which is downregulated in Alzheimer's disease, sensors target ADAM10, which is necessary for APP processing [183]. The disorder is distinguished by an increase in the frequency of neuronal severances. By activating the brain regions near to the damaged connections, it is possible to rebuild or replace the missing route [184]. Directly disrupting the amyloid plaque might be a viable new treatment for AD. Several lines of evidence indicate that the transformation of the peptide from its soluble to insoluble form plays a significant role in the onset of AD [185]. Atomic force microscopy (AFM) has been utilized to examine the molecular mechanisms behind the creation of the insoluble plaques associated with Alzheimer's disease [185]. Much fewer peptide plaques were seen in mice exposed to radiofrequency radiation [184]. In recent years, several possible Alzheimer's disease therapies have been researched. These include 1. inhibiting or modulating secretase activity, 2. using antibodies or nano particulate systems to increase A clearance from the brain, 3. reducing cholesterol levels (since elevated cholesterol is associated with an increased risk of developing AD), 4. chelating metallic ions required for A aggregation, and 5. protecting neurons from synaptic dysfunction [186].

Various drug delivery systems have been investigated to administer regulated and targeted doses of medicine to the brain in order to more effectively treat neurodegenerative diseases [187]. In the last decade, nanotechnology has had a significant influence on the development of delivery systems for DNA, proteins, and other tiny molecules [188]. Proteomics is crucial to the target selection and validation phases of drug development [185]. There are two fundamental features of nanoparticles that make them advantageous for medication delivery. First, nanoparticles are less likely to be absorbed by immune cells and to spread beyond the initial site of infection due to their tiny size and limited surface area. Microparticles and nanoparticles can be used to improve vaccination [188]. Active or passive targeting can be used to accomplish targeted distribution [188]. Alzheimer's disease is closely associated with human plasma concentrations of beta-amyloid40, beta-amyloid42, and phosphorylated tau protein Thioflavin-T (ThT) has been reported as a probe for detecting amyloid in Alzheimer's disease senile plaques [179,182]. Many studies show that miRNAs may serve as significant biomarkers in a wide range of disorders, including cancer, diabetes, cardiovascular disease, aging, asthma, autoimmune disease, renal diseases, and neurodegenerative diseases [183]. This demonstrates the significance of microRNAs in the distribution of pharmaceuticals. The nanoparticles were first produced by emulsion polymerization. Analyses were conducted on the particle size, drug loading capacity, and process yield of poly (n-butyl cyanoacrylate) nanoparticles. Usually, the size of drug-loaded nanoparticles was 40.5 6.9 nm [180]. Mechanisms for drug delivery must be capable of penetrating the arterial wall and entering the interstitium [189]. Only receptor systems capable of transcytosis (the migration of a complex ligand-receptor from the luminal to the abluminal membranes of the endothelial cells) are of interest for drug delivery across the blood-brain barrier (BBB) [189]. Within nanotechnology, the subject of employing gold nanoparticles (AuNPs) to deliver medications is increasing quickly. Nontoxic and biocompatible, AuNPs have attracted considerable interest as a possible pharmaceutical delivery technique [187]. One benefit of genetically encoded nanosensors is that they may drive proteins to particular sites within cells, as proven in an animal model of Alzheimer's disease [187]. Its genetic programming enables the sensors to be utilized in living cells and targeted to certain subcellular compartments, where concentration variations may be monitored [190]. Hence, applications such as ND assessment may benefit from the library of genetically encoded glutamate nanosensors [190]. To effectively treat Alzheimer's disease, it is necessary to create a non-oral, long-term delivery strategy for donepezil. It has been demonstrated that nanoparticles may transport medications across the BBB to malignancies of the central nervous system (CNS), and key characteristics of such tools have been found [189,191]. The detection of high quantities of donepezil in the brain might be a game-changer for Alzheimer's disease treatment. NPs are tiny enough to be absorbed by cells and pass through capillaries, enabling efficient medication accumulation at the body's chosen target sites [191]. No *in-vivo* examples of an antibody-coated nanoparticle-based therapy for Alzheimer's disease that led to complete memory recovery have ever been recorded, which is a significant challenge for the science [186].

8.4.3 INFLAMMATORY DISEASES

Wound healing is an example of a regeneration process, including inflammation, which contributes to maintaining homeostasis. In addition, it alters both acute-phase and immunological responses to infections [192]. Immunometabolism, a term used to explain the links between inflammatory response and metabolic problems and obesity in light of current discoveries, is a frequent term for describing these links [193]. During the complex process of inflammation, B lymphocytes, T lymphocytes, and myeloid cells interact with one another via chemicals present on their membranes [192]. Inflammatory disorders span a broad spectrum of inflammatory signs and conditions, including autoimmune diseases, glomerulonephritis, inflammatory bowel disease, etc.

The majority of research examining the etiology of inflammatory bowel disease (IBD) has pointed to the interplay between the mucosal immune system and the bacterial ecology of the gut [194]. According to one interpretation of this idea, the mucosal immune system is the source of the problem, as microfloras are responsible for the mucosal inflammation that defines human illness. Colitis ulcerative and Crohn's disease are the two most prevalent inflammatory bowel diseases. Twin concordance studies likely provide the greatest evidence that genetic variables contribute to susceptibility to inflammatory bowel disease [195]. IBD is defined as chronic, recurrent inflammation of the gastrointestinal system that has a detrimental effect on the quality of life of those affected [196]. *E. coli* can cause inflammatory bowel disease in certain individuals. Several tried-and-true methods for recognizing *E. coli* include multi-tube fermentation, membrane, dilution plate counting, and Raman spectroscopic testing [197]. Early research on IBD concentrated on finding a single pathogenic microbe or illness-causing pathway; however, more recent research has revealed the limits of this strategy. The dynamic, complex system generated by interactions between gut microbes and hosts is always developing [198].

Polyethylene glycol (PEG) is the most prevalent surface modification used in nano-based IBD therapy. Being hydrophilic, PEG coatings prevent nanoparticles from interacting sterically with other nanoparticles and blood components. In addition to avoiding surface aggregation, opsonization, and phagocytosis, PEG also boosts the surface's resistance to these processes so that the molecule remains in circulation for a longer period of time [199]. Manganese Prussian blue nanozymes (MPBZs) with multienzyme activity were manufactured using a simple hydrothermal technique under easy and moderate reaction conditions by mixing the Mn^{2+} ion source solution with polyvinylpyrrolidone (PVP) and a $[Fe(CN)_6]^{4-}$ ion source with PVP while magnetically stirring [200]. After that, we investigated the potential mechanism of MPBZ-mediated nano therapy for IBD. Many possible stimuli have been associated with the activation of the cellular immune response in inflammatory diseases. Specifically, the inflamed region often has an increased number of immune-related cells, such as macrophages. Since macrophages are responsible for clearing particles from the circulation, they may be the cells targeted by nanoparticle-based rheumatoid arthritis treatment [194].

8.5 SUMMARY

Nanomaterials have the potential for early detection and diagnosis of diseases, drug targeting, and delivery of genes and proteins. Natural nanocomposites are multiphase compounds generated from natural sources such as plants, vegetables, trees, seeds, microorganisms, and animals. Graphene-based nanohybrids (GNs) are composed of carbon atoms organized in a honeycomb configuration in two dimensions. To produce GNs, they must be functionalized to enhance their dispersion and overcome restrictions in technical applications. Nanohybrid materials are used in biomedical applications to encapsulate and transport medications with low water solubility.

Synthetic polymers are produced via the polymerization of dispersion and emulsion (EP). Drug delivery involves the use of lipophilic, oligomeric PACAs encapsulating amphiphilic doxorubicin to interact with it during polymerization. Cationic di-block copolymer poly(l-lysine)-poly(ethylene glycol)-folate (PLL-PEG-FOL) surface-co biodegradable fillers are made by combining several natural polymers, such as cellulose, and have advantages such as biopolymer availability and the ability to be generated from trash collected from agricultural leftovers. Bacterial nanocellulose (BNC) is one of the three types of cellulose nanostructures, while CNCs have a single-dimensional size of less than 100 nm and take the form of rods, needles, or whiskers. Chitosan nanoparticles are a family of biodegradable nanofillers that have several uses, such as tissue engineering, drug delivery, water purification, and food packaging.

Metal impregnated nanohybrids have grown significantly in significance due to their special characteristics. Drug delivery is a biogenic technique that uses plant extracts as a reducing agent to create nanoparticles. Au NPs are synthesized gold nanoparticles in liquid aqueous solutions, and biodegradable polymer-based nanocomposites have been used to enhance electrical conductivity, dielectric properties, and ion mobility. Dendrimers offer a variety of NPs, ranging in size from 1 to 100 nm and can be amorphous or crystalline. PAMAM-dendrimer-modified ternary magnetic iron oxide NPs/DNA/PEI magnetoplexes increase NP transfection efficiency.

CNTs are a promising nanomaterial for drug delivery carriers, with DOX, paclitaxel, cisplatin, and QDs being used to provide targeted delivery of anticancer medicines. SWCNTs also have the potential to transport siRNAs through non-covalent interactions. Microencapsulated CNTs were used to deliver therapies to specific areas in the gastrointestinal tracts of animals. Alzheimer's disease is characterized by neuroinflammatory development of amyloid plaques and neurofibrillary tangles, deficit in acetylcholine, faulty synapses, neuronal loss, and cerebral deposits. Ion sensors are essential for monitoring ion changes in the brain, while drug delivery systems have been investigated to administer targeted doses of medicine to the brain. Nanotechnology has been advantageous for medication delivery due to its tiny size.

REFERENCES

[1] G.A. Hughes, Nanostructure-mediated drug delivery, Nanomed. Nanotechnol. Biol. Med. 1 (2005) 22–30. doi:10.1016/j.nano.2004.11.009.

[2] G. Cirillo, S. Hampel, U.G. Spizzirri, O.I. Parisi, N. Picci, F. Iemma, Carbon nanotubes hybrid hydrogels in drug delivery: A perspective review, BioMed Res. Int. 2014 (2014) e825017. doi:10.1155/2014/825017.

[3] N.S. Satarkar, D. Biswal, J. Zach Hilt, Hydrogel nanocomposites: A review of applications as remote controlled biomaterials, Soft Matter. 6 (2010) 2364–2371. doi:10.1039/B925218P.

[4] K.J. Morrow, R. Bawa, C. Wei, Recent advances in basic and clinical nanomedicine, Med. Clin. N. Am. 91 (2007) 805–843. doi:10.1016/j.mcna.2007.05.009.

[5] L. Yang, X. Zhang, M. Ye, J. Jiang, R. Yang, T. Fu, Y. Chen, K. Wang, C. Liu, W. Tan, Aptamer-conjugated nanomaterials and their applications, Adv. Drug Deliv. Rev. 63 (2011) 1361–1370. doi:10.1016/j.addr.2011.10.002.

[6] N. Daum, C. Tscheka, A. Neumeyer, M. Schneider, Novel approaches for drug delivery systems in nanomedicine: Effects of particle design and shape, WIREs Nanomed. Nanobiotechnol. 4 (2012) 52–65. doi:10.1002/wnan.165.

[7] Y.D. Franco-Aguirre, J.J. Cedillo-Portillo, O.A. Martínez-Anguiano, A.O. Castañeda-Facio, M.E. Castañeda-Flores, J.G. Fuentes-Avilés, S.C. Esparza-Gonzalez, A. Sáenz-Galindo, Overview of natural nanocomposites and applications, in: F. Avalos

Belmontes, F.J. González, M.Á. López-Manchado (Eds.), Green-Based Nanocomposite Materials and Applications, Springer International Publishing, Cham (2023): pp. 63–79. doi:10.1007/978-3-031-18428-4_4.

[8] P. Anastas, N. Eghbali, Green chemistry: Principles and practice, Chem. Soc. Rev. 39 (2010) 301–312. doi:10.1039/B918763B.

[9] K. Maldonado-Lara, G. Luna-Bárcenas, E. Luna-Hernández, F. Padilla-Vaca, E. Hernández-Sánchez, R. Betancourt-Galindo, J.L. Menchaca-Arredondo, B.L. España-Sánchez, Preparación y caracterización de nanocompositos quitosano-cobre con actividad antibacteriana para aplicaciones en ingeniería de tejidos, Rev. Mex. de Ing. Biomed. 38 (2017) 306–313. doi:10.17488/RMIB.38.1.26.

[10] M.C. Urrejola, L.V. Soto, C.C. Zumarán, J.P. Peñaloza, B. Álvarez, I. Fuentevilla, Z.S. Haidar, Polymeric nanoparticle systems: Structure, elaboration methods, characteristics, properties, biofunctionalization and self-assembly layer by layer technologies, Int. J. Morphol. 36 (2018) 1463–1471. doi:10.4067/S0717-95022018000401463.

[11] R.A. Ilyas, H.A. Aisyah, A.H. Nordin, N. Ngadi, M.Y.M. Zuhri, M.R.M. Asyraf, S.M. Sapuan, E.S. Zainudin, S. Sharma, H. Abral, M. Asrofi, E. Syafri, N.H. Sari, M. Rafidah, S.Z.S. Zakaria, M.R. Razman, N.A. Majid, Z. Ramli, A. Azmi, S.P. Bangar, R. Ibrahim, Natural-fiber-reinforced chitosan, chitosan blends and their nanocomposites for various advanced applications, Polymers. 14 (2022). doi:10.3390/POLYM14050874.

[12] P. Mondal, A. Anweshan, M.K. Purkait, Green synthesis and environmental application of iron-based nanomaterials and nanocomposite: A review, Chemosphere. 259 (2020) 127509. doi:10.1016/j.chemosphere.2020.127509.

[13] S.A. Bhawani, A.H. Bhat, F.B. Ahmad, M.N.M. Ibrahim, Green polymer nanocomposites and their environmental applications, in: Polymer-Based Nanocomposites for Energy and Environmental Applications: A Volume in Woodhead Publishing Series in Composites Science and Engineering, Woodhead Publishing, Cambridge (2018): pp. 617–633. doi:10.1016/B978-0-08-102262-7.00023-4.

[14] S. Hema, A. Krishnan, A. Akther, A. Suresh, S. Sambhudevan, B. Shankar, Green nanocomposites based on natural rubber latex containing xylan from sugarcane bagasse—synthesis, characterization and dye absorption studies, Mater. Today. Proceed. 46 (2021) 2950–2954. doi:10.1016/j.matpr.2020.12.414.

[15] F.J. González, E.I. González-Castillo, A. Peña, F. Avalos Belmontes, Nanofillers and nanomaterials for green based nanocomposites, Eng. Mater. (2023) 13–30. doi:10.1007/978-3-031-18428-4_2/COVER.

[16] C. Lee, X. Wei, J.W. Kysar, J. Hone, Measurement of the elastic properties and intrinsic strength of monolayer graphene, Sci. 321 (2008) 385–388. doi:10.1126/SCIENCE. 1157996.

[17] O.C. Compton, S.T. Nguyen, Graphene oxide, highly reduced graphene oxide, and graphene: Versatile building blocks for carbon-based materials, Small. 6 (2010) 711–723. doi:10.1002/SMLL.200901934.

[18] K.S. Kim, Y. Zhao, H. Jang, S.Y. Lee, J.M. Kim, K.S. Kim, J.H. Ahn, P. Kim, J.Y. Choi, B.H. Hong, Large-scale pattern growth of graphene films for stretchable transparent electrodes, Nature. 457 (2009) 706–710. doi:10.1038/NATURE07719.

[19] C. Soldano, A. Mahmood, E. Dujardin, Production, properties and potential of graphene, Carbon. 48 (2010) 2127–2150. doi:10.1016/J.CARBON.2010.01.058.

[20] J. Liu, J. Tang, J.J. Gooding, Strategies for chemical modification of graphene and applications of chemically modified graphene, J. Mat. Chemistry. 22 (2012) 12435–12452. doi:10.1039/C2JM31218B.

[21] V. Georgakilas, M. Otyepka, A.B. Bourlinos, V. Chandra, N. Kim, K.C. Kemp, P. Hobza, R. Zboril, K.S. Kim, Functionalization of graphene: Covalent and non-covalent approaches, derivatives and applications, Chem. Rev. 112 (2012) 6156–6214. doi:10.1021/CR3000412.

[22] I. Choi, Y. Choi, Plasmonic nanosensors: Review and prospect, IEEE J. Select. Topic. Q. Electr. 18 (2012) 1110–1121. doi:10.1109/JSTQE.2011.2163386.

[23] P.K.S. Mural, M. Sharma, G. Madras, S. Bose, A critical review on in situ reduction of graphene oxide during preparation of conducting polymeric nanocomposites, RSC Adv. 5 (2015) 32078–32087. doi:10.1039/C5RA02877A.

[24] A.J. Glover, M. Cai, K.R. Overdeep, D.E. Kranbuehl, H.C. Schniepp, In situ reduction of graphene oxide in polymers, Macromol. 44 (2011) 9821–9829. doi:10.1021/MA2008783.

[25] S. Ye, J. Feng, A new insight into the in situ thermal reduction of graphene oxide dispersed in a polymer matrix, Polymer Chemistry. 4 (2013) 1765–1768. doi:10.1039/C3PY00019B.

[26] N.G. Sahoo, S. Rana, J.W. Cho, L. Li, S.H. Chan, Polymer nanocomposites based on functionalized carbon nanotubes, Prog. Polymer Sci. (Oxford). 35 (2010) 837–867. doi:10.1016/j.progpolymsci.2010.03.002.

[27] I. Armentano, M. Dottori, E. Fortunati, S. Mattioli, J.M. Kenny, Biodegradable polymer matrix nanocomposites for tissue engineering: A review, Polymer Degrad. Stab. 95 (2010) 2126–2146. doi:10.1016/J.POLYMDEGRADSTAB.2010.06.007.

[28] A. Chen, S. Chatterjee, Nanomaterials based electrochemical sensors for biomedical applications, Chem. Soc. Rev. 42 (2013) 5425–5438. doi:10.1039/C3CS35518G.

[29] Z. Alves, N.M. Ferreira, P. Ferreira, C. Nunes, Design of heat sealable starch-chitosan bioplastics reinforced with reduced graphene oxide for active food packaging, Carbhydr. Polym. 291 (2022). doi:10.1016/J.CARBPOL.2022.119517.

[30] S. Sinha Ray, M. Okamoto, Polymer/layered silicate nanocomposites: A review from preparation to processing, Prog. Polymer Sci. (Oxford). 28 (2003) 1539–1641. doi:10.1016/J.PROGPOLYMSCI.2003.08.002.

[31] F.N. Molinari, E. Barragán, E. Bilbao, L. Patrone, G. Giménez, A.V. Medrano, A. Tolley, L.N. Monsalve, An electrospun polymer composite with fullerene-multiwalled carbon nanotube exohedral complexes can act as memory device, Polymer. 194 (2020). doi:10.1016/J.POLYMER.2020.122380.

[32] H.B.M.Z. Islam, M.A.B.H. Susan, A.B. Imran, High-strength potato starch/hectorite clay-based nanocomposite film: Synthesis and characterization, Iranian Polymer J. (English Edition). 30 (2021) 513–521. doi:10.1007/S13726-021-00907-Y.

[33] N. Moazeni, Z. Mohamad, N. Dehbari, Study of silane treatment on poly-lactic acid(PLA)/sepiolite nanocomposite thin films, J. Appl. Polym. Sci. 132 (2015). doi:10.1002/APP.41428.

[34] F. Masood, H. Haider, T. Yasin, Sepiolite/poly-3-hydroxyoctanoate nanocomposites: Effect of clay content on physical and biodegradation properties, Appl. Clay Sci. 175 (2019) 130–138. doi:10.1016/J.CLAY.2019.04.012.

[35] L. García-Quiles, Á.F. Cuello, P. Castell, Sustainable materials with enhanced mechanical properties based on industrial polyhydroxyalkanoates reinforced with organomodified sepiolite and montmorillonite, Polym. 11 (2019). doi:10.3390/POLYM11040696.

[36] P.G. Jamkhande, N.W. Ghule, A.H. Bamer, M.G. Kalaskar, Metal nanoparticles synthesis: An overview on methods of preparation, advantages and disadvantages, and applications, J Drug Deliv Sci Technol. 53 (2019). doi:10.1016/J.JDDST.2019.101174.

[37] Y. Khane, K. Benouis, S. Albukhaty, G.M. Sulaiman, M.M. Abomughaid, A. Al Ali, D. Aouf, F. Fenniche, S. Khane, W. Chaibi, A. Henni, H.D. Bouras, N. Dizge, Green synthesis of silver nanoparticles using aqueous citrus limon zest extract: Characterization and evaluation of their antioxidant and antimicrobial properties, Nanomater. 12 (2022). doi:10.3390/NANO12122013.

[38] A.K. Mittal, Y. Chisti, U.C. Banerjee, Synthesis of metallic nanoparticles using plant extracts, Biotech. Adv. 31 (2013) 346–356. doi:10.1016/J.BIOTECHADV.2013.01.003.

[39] G.M. Asnag, A.H. Oraby, A.M. Abdelghany, Green synthesis of gold nanoparticles and its effect on the optical, thermal and electrical properties of carboxymethyl cellulose, Compos. B. Eng. 172 (2019) 436–446. doi:10.1016/J.COMPOSITESB.2019.05.044.

[40] R.A. Sperling, P.R. Gil, F. Zhang, M. Zanella, W.J. Parak, Biological applications of gold nanoparticles, Chem. Soc. Rev. 37 (2008) 1896–1908. doi:10.1039/B712170A.

[41] S. Chowdhury, Y.L. Teoh, K.M. Ong, N.S. Rafflisman Zaidi, S.K. Mah, Poly(vinyl) alcohol crosslinked composite packaging film containing gold nanoparticles on shelf life extension of banana, Food Packag. Shelf Life. 24 (2020). doi:10.1016/J.FPSL.2020.100463.

[42] M.A. Morsi, A.H. Oraby, A.G. Elshahawy, R.M. Abd El-Hady, Preparation, structural analysis, morphological investigation and electrical properties of gold nanoparticles filled polyvinyl alcohol/carboxymethyl cellulose blend, J. Mater. Res. Technol. 8 (2019) 5996–6010. doi:10.1016/J.JMRT.2019.09.074.

[43] A.D. Sontakke, S. Tiwari, M.K. Purkait, A comprehensive review on graphene oxide-based nanocarriers: Synthesis, functionalization and biomedical applications, FlatChem. 38 (2023) 100484. doi:10.1016/j.flatc.2023.100484.

[44] L. Liu, Q. Ma, J. Cao, Y. Gao, S. Han, Y. Liang, T. Zhang, Y. Song, Y. Sun, Recent progress of graphene oxide-based multifunctional nanomaterials for cancer treatment, Cancer Nano. 12 (2021) 18. doi:10.1186/s12645-021-00087-7.

[45] H.M. Hegab, L. Zou, Graphene oxide-assisted membranes: Fabrication and potential applications in desalination and water purification, J. Membr. Sci. 484 (2015) 95–106. doi:10.1016/J.MEMSCI.2015.03.011.

[46] S.I. Siddiqui, S.A. Chaudhry, A review on graphene oxide and its composites preparation and their use for the removal of As3+and As5+ from water under the effect of various parameters: Application of isotherm, kinetic and thermodynamics, Process Saf. Environ. Prot. 119 (2018) 138–163. doi:10.1016/J.PSEP.2018.07.020.

[47] A.D. Sontakke, M.K. Purkait, Fabrication of ultrasound-mediated tunable graphene oxide nanoscrolls, Ultrason. Sonochem. 63 (2020) 104976. doi:10.1016/j.ultsonch.2020.104976.

[48] F. Alemi, R. Zarezadeh, A.R. Sadigh, H. Hamishehkar, M. Rahimi, M. Majidinia, Z. Asemi, A. Ebrahimi-Kalan, B. Yousefi, N. Rashtchizadeh, Graphene oxide and reduced graphene oxide: Efficient cargo platforms for cancer theranostics, J. Drug Deliv. Sci. Technol. 60 (2020). doi:10.1016/J.JDDST.2020.101974.

[49] S.-F. Pan, Y. Dong, Y.-Ming. Zheng, L.-B. Zhong, Z.-H. Yuan, Self-sustained hydrophilic nanofiber thin film composite forward osmosis membranes: Preparation, characterization and application for simulated antibiotic wastewater treatment, J. Membr. Sci. 523 (2017) 205–215. doi:10.1016/j.memsci.2016.09.045.

[50] N. Bellier, P. Baipaywad, N. Ryu, J.Y. Lee, H. Park, Recent biomedical advancements in graphene oxide- and reduced graphene oxide-based nanocomposite nanocarriers, Biomater. Res. 26 (2022). doi:10.1186/S40824-022-00313-2.

[51] T.V. Patil, D.K. Patel, S.D. Dutta, K. Ganguly, K.T. Lim, Graphene oxide-based stimuli-responsive platforms for biomedical applications, Mol. 26 (2021). doi:10.3390/MOLECULES26092797.

[52] A. Jafari, K. Khanmohammadi Chenab, H. Malektaj, F. Farshchi, S. Ghorbani, A. Ghasemiamineh, M. Khoshakhlagh, B. Ashtari, M.R. Zamani-Meymian, An attempt of stimuli-responsive drug delivery of graphene-based nanomaterial through biological obstacles of tumor, FlatChem. 34 (2022). doi:10.1016/J.FLATC.2022.100381.

[53] R.K. Jain, Delivery of molecular medicine to solid tumors: Lessons from in vivo imaging of gene expression and function, J. Con. Rel. 74 (2001) 7–25. doi:10.1016/S0168-3659(01)00306-6.

[54] A. Bhattacharjee, S. Gumma, M.K. Purkait, Fe3O4 promoted metal organic framework MIL-100(Fe) for the controlled release of doxorubicin hydrochloride, Microporous and Mesoporous Mater. 259 (2018) 203–210. doi:10.1016/j.micromeso.2017.10.020.

[55] A.D. Sontakke, A. Bhattacharjee, R. Fopase, L.M. Pandey, M.K. Purkait, One-pot, sustainable and room temperature synthesis of graphene oxide-impregnated iron-based metal-organic framework (GO/MIL-100(Fe)) nanocarriers for anti-cancer drug delivery systems, J. Mater. Sci. 57 (2022) 19019–19049. doi:10.1007/S10853-022-07773-W.

[56] F. Song, X. Li, Q. Wang, L. Liao, C. Zhang, Nanocomposite hydrogels and their applications in drug delivery and tissue engineering, J. Biomed. Nanotechnol. 11 (2015) 40–52. doi:10.1166/JBN.2015.1962.

[57] J. Yi, G. Choe, J. Park, J.Y. Lee, Graphene oxide-incorporated hydrogels for biomedical applications, Polym. J. 52 (2020) 823–837. doi:10.1038/S41428-020-0350-9.

[58] S. Zhang, Y. Chen, H. Liu, Z. Wang, H. Ling, C. Wang, J. Ni, B. Çelebi-Saltik, X. Wang, X. Meng, H.J. Kim, A. Baidya, S. Ahadian, N. Ashammakhi, M.R. Dokmeci, J. Travas-Sejdic, A. Khademhosseini, Room-temperature-formed PEDOT:PSS hydrogels enable injectable, soft, and healable organic bioelectronics, Adv. Mater. 32 (2020). doi:10.1002/ADMA.201904752.

[59] Y.T. Fong, C.H. Chen, J.P. Chen, Intratumoral delivery of doxorubicin on folate-conjugated graphene oxide by in-situ forming thermo-sensitive hydrogel for breast cancer therapy, Nanomater. 7 (2017). doi:10.3390/NANO7110388.

[60] X. Zhu, H. Zhang, H. Huang, Y. Zhang, L. Hou, Z. Zhang, Functionalized graphene oxide-based thermosensitive hydrogel for magnetic hyperthermia therapy on tumors, Nanotechnol. 26 (2015). doi:10.1088/0957-4484/26/36/365103.

[61] S. Prakash, M. Malhotra, W. Shao, C. Tomaro-Duchesneau, S. Abbasi, Polymeric nano-hybrids and functionalized carbon nanotubes as drug delivery carriers for cancer therapy, Adv. Drug Del. Rev. 63 (2011) 1340–1351. doi:10.1016/J.ADDR.2011.06.013.

[62] V. Torchilin, Lipid-core micelles for targeted drug delivery, Curr. Drug Del. 2 (2005) 319–327. doi:10.2174/156720105774370221.

[63] A. Roby, S. Erdogan, V.P. Torchilin, Solubilization of poorly soluble PDT agent, meso-tetraphenylporphin, in plain or immunotargeted PEG-PE micelles results in dramatically improved cancer cell killing in vitro, Eur. J. Pharm. Biopharm. 62 (2006) 235–240. doi:10.1016/j.ejpb.2005.09.010.

[64] I. Brigger, C. Dubernet, P. Couvreur, Nanoparticles in cancer therapy and diagnosis, Adv. Drug Del. Rev. 54 (2002) 631–651. doi:10.1016/S0169-409X(02)00044-3.

[65] R. Duncan, Polymer conjugates as anticancer nanomedicines, Nat. Rev. Cancer. 6 (2006) 688–701. doi:10.1038/NRC1958.

[66] P. Rejmanová, J. Kopeček, R. Duncan, J.B. Lloyd, Stability in rat plasma and serum of lysosomally degradable oligopeptide sequences in N-(2-hydroxypropyl) methacrylamide copolymers, Biomater. 6 (1985) 45–48. doi:10.1016/0142-9612(85)90037-7.

[67] L.W. Seymour, K. Ulbrich, P.S. Steyger, M. Brereton, V. Subr, J. Strohalm, R. Duncan, Tumour tropism and anti-cancer efficacy of polymer-based doxorubicin prodrugs in the treatment of subcutaneous murine B16F10 melanoma, Br. J. Cancer. 70 (1994) 636–641. doi:10.1038/BJC.1994.363.

[68] H. Maeda, SMANCS and polymer-conjugated macromolecular drugs: Advantages in cancer chemotherapy, Adv. Drug Del. Rev. 46 (2001) 169–185. doi:10.1016/S0169-409X(00)00134-4.

[69] V.P. Torchilin, Drug targeting, Eur. J. Pharm. Sci. 11 (2000). doi:10.1016/S0928-0987(00)00166-4.

[70] R. Gref, A. Domb, P. Quellec, T. Blunk, R.H. Müller, J.M. Verbavatz, R. Langer, The controlled intravenous delivery of drugs using PEG-coated sterically stabilized nanospheres, Adv. Drug Del. Rev. 16 (1995) 215–233. doi:10.1016/0169-409X(95)00026-4.

[71] R.B. Greenwald, C.D. Conover, Y.H. Choe, Poly(ethylene glycol) conjugated drugs and prodrugs: A comprehensive review, Crit. Rev. Ther. Drug Carrier Syst. 17 (2000). doi:10.1615/CritRevTherDrugCarrierSyst.v17.i2.20.

[72] A.N. Murthy, I. Etsion, F.E. Talke, Analysis of surface textured air bearing sliders with rarefaction effects, Tribol. Lett. 28 (2007) 251–261. doi:10.1007/S11249-007-9269-Y.

[73] B. Seijo, E. Fattal, L. Roblot-Treupel, P. Couvreur, Design of nanoparticles of less than 50 nm diameter: Preparation, characterization and drug loading, Int. J. Pharm. 62 (1990) 1–7. doi:10.1016/0378-5173(90)90024-X.

[74] P. Couvreur, B. Kante, M. Roland, P. Speiser, Adsorption of antineoplastic drugs to polyalkylcyanoacrylate nanoparticles and their release in calf serum, J. Pharm. Sci. 68 (1979) 1521–1524. doi:10.1002/jps.2600681215.

[75] J. Kreuter, H.R. Hartmann, Comparative study on the cytostatic effects and the tissue distribution of 5-fluorouracil in a free form and bound to polybutylcyanoacrylate nanoparticles in sarcoma 180-bearing mice, Oncol. (Switzerland). 40 (1983) 363–366. doi:10.1159/000225763.

[76] A. Erdely, T. Hulderman, R. Salmen, A. Liston, P.C. Zeidler-Erdely, D. Schwegler-Berry, V. Castranova, S. Koyama, Y.-A. Kim, M. Endo, P.P. Simeonova, Cross-talk between lung and systemic circulation during carbon nanotube respiratory exposure. potential biomarkers, Nano Lett. 9 (2009) 36–43. doi:10.1021/nl801828z.

[77] B. Stella, S. Arpicco, M.T. Peracchia, D. Desmaële, J. Hoebeke, M. Renoir, J. D'Angelo, L. Cattel, P. Couvreur, Design of folic acid-conjugated nanoparticles for drug targeting, J. Pharm. Sci. 89 (2000) 1452–1464. doi:10.1002/1520-6017 (200011)89:11<1452::AID-JPS8>3.0.CO;2-P.

[78] J. Panyam, V. Labhasetwar, Biodegradable nanoparticles for drug and gene delivery to cells and tissue, Adv. Drug Del. Rev. 55 (2003) 329–347. doi:10.1016/ S0169-409X(02)00228-4.

[79] S.H. Kim, J.H. Jeong, K.W. Chun, T.G. Park, Target-specific cellular uptake of PLGA nanoparticles coated with poly(L-lysine)-poly(ethylene glycol)-folate conjugate, Langmuir. 21 (2005) 8852–8857. doi:10.1021/LA0502084.

[80] Y. Mo, L.-Y. Lim, Paclitaxel-loaded PLGA nanoparticles: Potentiation of anticancer activity by surface conjugation with wheat germ agglutinin, J. Con. Rel. 108 (2005) 244–262. doi:10.1016/j.jconrel.2005.08.013.

[81] M. Cegnar, A. Premzl, V. Zavašnik-Bergant, J. Kristl, J. Kos, Poly(lactide-co-glycolide) nanoparticles as a carrier system for delivering cysteine protease inhibitor cystatin into tumor cells, Exp. Cell Res. 301 (2004) 223–231. doi:10.1016/j.yexcr.2004.07.021.

[82] L. Zhang, J.M. Chan, F.X. Gu, J.W. Rhee, A.Z. Wang, A.F. Radovic-Moreno, F. Alexis, R. Langer, O.C. Farokhzad, Self-assembled lipid-polymer hybrid nanoparticles: A robust drug delivery platform, ACS Nano. 2 (2008) 1696–1702. doi:10.1021/NN800275R.

[83] H. Yin, L. Cui, Q. Chen, W. Shi, S. Ai, L. Zhu, L. Lu, Amperometric determination of bisphenol A in milk using PAMAM–Fe3O4 modified glassy carbon electrode, Food Chem. 125 (2011) 1097–1103. doi:10.1016/j.foodchem.2010.09.098.

[84] A. Anweshan, P.P. Das, S. Dhara, M.K. Purkait, Chapter 12 - Nanosensors in food science and technology, in: A. Husen, K.S. Siddiqi (Eds.), Advances in Smart Nanomaterials and Their Applications, Elsevier (2023): pp. 247–272. doi:10.1016/ B978-0-323-99546-7.00015-X.

[85] P.D. Scholes, A.G.A. Coombes, L. Illum, S.S. Davis, J.F. Watts, C. Ustariz, M. Vert, M.C. Davies, Detection and determination of surface levels of poloxamer and PVA surfactant on biodegradable nanospheres using SSIMS and XPS, J. Con. Rel. 59 (1999) 261–278. doi:10.1016/S0168-3659(98)00138-2.

[86] C.R. Bauli, D.B. Rocha, S.A. de Oliveira, D.S. Rosa, Cellulose nanostructures from wood waste with low input consumption, J. Clean. Prod. 211 (2019) 408–416. doi:10.1016/J.JCLEPRO.2018.11.099.

[87] D. Klemm, E.D. Cranston, D. Fischer, M. Gama, S.A. Kedzior, D. Kralisch, F. Kramer, T. Kondo, T. Lindström, S. Nietzsche, K. Petzold-Welcke, F. Rauchfuß, Nanocellulose as a natural source for groundbreaking applications in materials science: Today's state, Mater. Today. 21 (2018) 720–748. doi:10.1016/J.MATTOD.2018.02.001.

[88] D. Trache, M.H. Hussin, M.K.M. Haafiz, V.K. Thakur, Recent progress in cellulose nanocrystals: Sources and production, Nanoscale. 9 (2017) 1763–1786. doi:10.1039/C6NR09494E.

[89] A. Iwatake, M. Nogi, H. Yano, Cellulose nanofiber-reinforced polylactic acid, Compos. Sci. Technol. 68 (2008) 2103–2106. doi:10.1016/J.COMPSCITECH.2008.03.006.

[90] Y. Wang, Z. Ying, W. Xie, D. Wu, Cellulose nanofibers reinforced biodegradable polyester blends: Ternary biocomposites with balanced mechanical properties, Carbhydr. Polym. 233 (2020). doi:10.1016/J.CARBPOL.2020.115845.

[91] A.N. Frone, S. Berlioz, J.F. Chailan, D.M. Panaitescu, Morphology and thermal properties of PLA-cellulose nanofibers composites, Carbhydr. Polym. 91 (2013) 377–384. doi:10.1016/J.CARBPOL.2012.08.054.

[92] K. Divya, M.S. Jisha, Chitosan nanoparticles preparation and applications, Environ. Chem. Lett. 16 (2018) 101–112. doi:10.1007/s10311-017-0670-y.

[93] R. Jayakumar, M. Prabaharan, S.V. Nair, H. Tamura, Novel chitin and chitosan nanofibers in biomedical applications, Biotechnol. Adv. 28 (2010) 142–150. doi:10.1016/j.biotechadv.2009.11.001.

[94] F. Garavand, I. Cacciotti, N. Vahedikia, A. Rehman, Ö. Tarhan, S. Akbari-Alavijeh, R. Shaddel, A. Rashidinejad, M. Nejatian, S. Jafarzadeh, M. Azizi-Lalabadi, S. Khoshnoudi-Nia, S.M. Jafari, A comprehensive review on the nanocomposites loaded with chitosan nanoparticles for food packaging, Crit. Rev. Food Sci. Nutr. 62 (2022) 1383–1416. doi:10.1080/10408398.2020.1843133.

[95] P. Duarah, A. Bhattacharjee, P. Mondal, M.K. Purkait, Green synthesized carbon and metallic nanomaterials for biofuel production: Effect of operating parameters, in: M. Srivastava, M.A. Malik, P.K. Mishra (Eds.), Green Nano Solution for Bioenergy Production Enhancement, Springer Nature, Singapore (2022): pp. 105–126. doi:10.1007/978-981-16-9356-4_5.

[96] M.R. Atta, Q.A. Alsulami, G.M. Asnag, A. Rajeh, Enhanced optical, morphological, dielectric, and conductivity properties of gold nanoparticles doped with PVA/CMC blend as an application in organoelectronic devices, J. Mater. Sci. Mater. Electron. 32 (2021) 10443–10457. doi:10.1007/S10854-021-05701-3.

[97] B. Begines, A. Alcudia, R. Aguilera-Velazquez, G. Martinez, Y. He, R. Wildman, M.J. Sayagues, A. Jimenez-Ruiz, R. Prado-Gotor, Design of highly stabilized nanocomposite inks based on biodegradable polymer-matrix and gold nanoparticles for inkjet printing, Sci. Rep. 9 (2019). doi:10.1038/S41598-019-52314-2.

[98] C.D. Tran, F. Prosenc, M. Franko, Facile synthesis, structure, biocompatibility and antimicrobial property of gold nanoparticle composites from cellulose and keratin, J. Colloid Interface Sci. 510 (2018) 237–245. doi:10.1016/J.JCIS.2017.09.006.

[99] J. Singh, S. Kumar, A.S. Dhaliwal, Controlled release of amoxicillin and antioxidant potential of gold nanoparticles-xanthan gum/poly (Acrylic acid) biodegradable nanocomposite, J. Drug Deliv. Sci. Technol. 55 (2020). doi:10.1016/J.JDDST.2019.101384.

[100] A. Buonerba, A. Grassi, Trends in sustainable synthesis of organics by gold nanoparticles embedded in polymer matrices, Catalysts. 11 (2021). doi:10.3390/CATAL11060714.

[101] A.A. Yaqoob, K. Umar, M.N.M. Ibrahim, Silver nanoparticles: Various methods of synthesis, size affecting factors and their potential applications–a review, Appl. Nanosci. (Switzerland). 10 (2020) 1369–1378. doi:10.1007/S13204-020-01318-W.

[102] X.F. Zhang, Z.G. Liu, W. Shen, S. Gurunathan, Silver nanoparticles: Synthesis, characterization, properties, applications, and therapeutic approaches, Int. J. Mol. Sci. 17 (2016). doi:10.3390/IJMS17091534.

[103] K. Ranoszek-Soliwoda, E. Tomaszewska, E. Socha, P. Krzyczmonik, A. Ignaczak, P. Orlowski, M. Krzyzowska, G. Celichowski, J. Grobelny, The role of tannic acid and sodium citrate in the synthesis of silver nanoparticles, J. Nanopart. Res. 19 (2017). doi:10.1007/S11051-017-3973-9.

[104] S. Ediyilyam, B. George, S.S. Shankar, T.T. Dennise, S. Wacławek, M. Cerník, V.V.T. Padil, Chitosan/gelatin/silver nanoparticles composites films for biodegradable food packaging applications, Polym. 13 (2021). doi:10.3390/POLYM13111680.

[105] F. Ortega, V.B. Arce, M.A. Garcia, Nanocomposite starch-based films containing silver nanoparticles synthesized with lemon juice as reducing and stabilizing agent, Carbhydr. Polym. 252 (2021). doi:10.1016/J.CARBPOL.2020.117208.

[106] T.T. Tsai, T.H. Huang, C.J. Chang, N. Yi-Ju Ho, Y.T. Tseng, C.F. Chen, Antibacterial cellulose paper made with silver-coated gold nanoparticles, Sci. Rep. 7 (2017). doi:10.1038/S41598-017-03357-W.

[107] K. Kraśniewska, S. Galus, M. Gniewosz, Biopolymers-based materials containing silver nanoparticles as active packaging for food applications–a review, Int. J. Mol. Sci. 21 (2020). doi:10.3390/IJMS21030698.

[108] V. Sadanand, N. Rajini, B. Satyanarayana, A.V. Rajulu, Preparation and properties of cellulose/silver nanoparticle composites with in situ-generated silver nanoparticles using Ocimum sanctum leaf extract, Int. J. Polym. Anal. Charact. 21 (2016) 408–416. doi:10.1080/1023666X.2016.1161100.

[109] I. Popescu, M. Constantin, I.M. Pelin, D.M. Suflet, D.L. Ichim, O.M. Daraba, G. Fundueanu, Eco-friendly synthesized pva/chitosan/oxalic acid nanocomposite hydrogels embedding silver nanoparticles as antibacterial materials, Gels. 8 (2022). doi:10.3390/GELS8050268.

[110] K. Santiago-Castillo, A.M. Torres-Huerta, D. Del Ángel-López, M.A. Domínguez-Crespo, H. Dorantes-Rosales, D. Palma-Ramírez, H. Willcock, In situ growth of silver nanoparticles on chitosan matrix for the synthesis of hybrid electrospun fibers: Analysis of microstructural and mechanical properties, Polym. 14 (2022). doi:10.3390/POLYM14040674.

[111] E. Fortunati, F. D'Angelo, S. Martino, A. Orlacchio, J.M. Kenny, I. Armentano, Carbon nanotubes and silver nanoparticles for multifunctional conductive biopolymer composites, Carbon. 49 (2011) 2370–2379. doi:10.1016/J.CARBON.2011.02.004.

[112] S. Kumar, S. Raj, S. Jain, K. Chatterjee, Multifunctional biodegradable polymer nanocomposite incorporating graphene-silver hybrid for biomedical applications, Mater. Design. 108 (2016) 319–332. doi:10.1016/J.MATDES.2016.06.107.

[113] P. Kesharwani, V. Gajbhiye, N.K. Jain, A review of nanocarriers for the delivery of small interfering RNA, Biomater. 33 (2012) 7138–7150. doi:10.1016/j.biomaterials.2012.06.068.

[114] P. Kesharwani, A. Gothwal, A.K. Iyer, K. Jain, M.K. Chourasia, U. Gupta, Dendrimer nanohybrid carrier systems: An expanding horizon for targeted drug and gene delivery, Drug Dis. Today. 23 (2018) 300–314. doi:10.1016/j.drudis.2017.06.009.

[115] S. Chandrasekaran, M.R. King, Microenvironment of tumor-draining lymph nodes: opportunities for liposome-based targeted therapy, Int. J. Mol. Sci. 15 (2014) 20209–20239. doi:10.3390/ijms151120209.

[116] D. Bhadra, S. Bhadra, S. Jain, N.K. Jain, A PEGylated dendritic nanoparticulate carrier of fluorouracil, Int. J. Pharm. 257 (2003) 111–124. doi:10.1016/S0378-5173(03)00132-7.

[117] P. Agrawal, U. Gupta, N.K. Jain, Glycoconjugated peptide dendrimers-based nanoparticulate system for the delivery of chloroquine phosphate, Biomater. 28 (2007) 3349–3359. doi:10.1016/j.biomaterials.2007.04.004.

[118] G. Purohit, T. Sakthivel, A.T. Florence, Interaction of cationic partial dendrimers with charged and neutral liposomes, Int. J. Pharm. 214 (2001) 71–76. doi:10.1016/S0378-5173(00)00635-9.

[119] A.J. Khopade, F. Caruso, P. Tripathi, S. Nagaich, N.K. Jain, Effect of dendrimer on entrapment and release of bioactive from liposomes, Int. J. Pharm. 232 (2002) 157–162. doi:10.1016/S0378-5173(01)00901-2.

[120] A. Papagiannaros, K. Dimas, G.T. Papaioannou, C. Demetzos, Doxorubicin–PAMAM dendrimer complex attached to liposomes: Cytotoxic studies against human cancer cell lines, Int. J. Pharm. 302 (2005) 29–38. doi:10.1016/j.ijpharm.2005.05.039.

[121] B. Pan, F. Gao, L. Ao, H. Tian, R. He, D. Cui, Controlled self-assembly of thiol-terminated poly(amidoamine) dendrimer and gold nanoparticles, Colloids Surf. A Physicochem. Eng. Asp. 259 (2005) 89–94. doi:10.1016/j.colsurfa.2005.02.009.

[122] Y. Nakanishi, T. Imae, Synthesis of dendrimer-protected TiO2 nanoparticles and photodegradation of organic molecules in an aqueous nanoparticle suspension, J. Colloid Interface Sci. 285 (2005) 158–162. doi:10.1016/j.jcis.2004.11.055.

[123] T. Pietsch, D. Appelhans, N. Gindy, B. Voit, A. Fahmi, Oligosaccharide-modified dendrimers for templating gold nanoparticles: Tailoring the particle size as a function of dendrimer generation and -molecular structure, Colloids Surf. A Physicochem. Eng. Asp. 341 (2009) 93–102. doi:10.1016/j.colsurfa.2009.03.044.

[124] C. Li, D. Li, Z.-S. Zhao, X.-M. Duan, W. Hou, Platinum nanoparticles from hydrosilylation reaction: Carbosilane dendrimer as capping agent, Colloids Surf. A Physicochem. Eng. Asp. 366 (2010) 45–49. doi:10.1016/j.colsurfa.2010.05.013.

[125] H. Liu, M. Shen, J. Zhao, R. Guo, X. Cao, G. Zhang, X. Shi, Tunable synthesis and acetylation of dendrimer-entrapped or dendrimer-stabilized gold–silver alloy nanoparticles, Colloids Surf. B Biointerfaces. 94 (2012) 58–67. doi:10.1016/j.colsurfb.2012.01.019.

[126] X. Sun, Y. Luo, Size-controlled synthesis of dendrimer-protected gold nanoparticles by microwave radiation, Mater. Lett. 59 (2005) 4048–4050. doi:10.1016/j.matlet.2005.07.060.

[127] W.-M. Liu, Y.-N. Xue, W.-T. He, R.-X. Zhuo, S.-W. Huang, Dendrimer modified magnetic iron oxide nanoparticle/dna/pei ternary complexes: A novel strategy for magnetofection, J. Con. Rel. 152 (2011) e159–e160. doi:10.1016/j.jconrel.2011.08.061.

[128] N. Krasteva, B. Guse, I. Besnard, A. Yasuda, T. Vossmeyer, Gold nanoparticle/PPI-dendrimer based chemiresistors: Vapor-sensing properties as a function of the dendrimer size, Sens. Actuators B Chem. 92 (2003) 137–143. doi:10.1016/S0925-4005(03)00250-8.

[129] N. Krasteva, H. Möhwald, R. Krastev, Structural changes in stimuli-responsive nanoparticle/dendrimer composite films upon vapor sorption, Comptes Rendus Chimie. 12 (2009) 129–137. doi:10.1016/j.crci.2008.09.001.

[130] Y.-M. Chung, H.-K. Rhee, Partial hydrogenation of 1,3-cyclooctadiene using dendrimer-encapsulated Pd–Rh bimetallic nanoparticles, J. Mol. Catal. A Chem. 206 (2003) 291–298. doi:10.1016/S1381-1169(03)00418-7.

[131] F.N. Crespilho, F.C. Nart, O.N. Oliveira, C.M.A. Brett, Oxygen reduction and diffusion in electroactive nanostructured membranes (ENM) using a layer-by-layer dendrimer-gold nanoparticle approach, Electrochim. Acta. 52 (2007) 4649–4653. doi:10.1016/j.electacta.2007.01.048.

[132] A. Kesavan, P. Ilaiyaraja, W. Sofi Beaula, V. Veena Kumari, J. Sugin Lal, C. Arunkumar, G. Anjana, S. Srinivas, A. Ramesh, S.K. Rayala, D. Ponraju, G. Venkatraman, Tumor targeting using polyamidoamine dendrimer–cisplatin nanoparticles functionalized with diglycolamic acid and herceptin, Eur. J. Pharm. Biopharm. 96 (2015) 255–263. doi:10.1016/j.ejpb.2015.08.001.

[133] Y. Fan, S. Yuan, M. Huo, A.S. Chaudhuri, M. Zhao, Z. Wu, X. Qi, Spatial controlled multistage nanocarriers through hybridization of dendrimers and gelatin nanoparticles for deep penetration and therapy into tumor tissue, Nanomed. Nanotechnol. Biol. Med. 13 (2017) 1399–1410. doi:10.1016/j.nano.2017.01.008.

[134] P. Zhang, Y. Zhang, M. Gao, X. Zhang, Dendrimer-assisted hydrophilic magnetic nanoparticles as sensitive substrates for rapid recognition and enhanced isolation of target tumor cells, Talanta. 161 (2016) 925–931. doi:10.1016/j.talanta.2016.08.064.

[135] B.I. Lemon, R.M. Crooks, Preparation and characterization of dendrimer-encapsulated CdS semiconductor quantum dots, J. Am. Chem. Soc. 122 (2000) 12886–12887. doi:10.1021/ja0031321.

[136] Z. Li, P. Huang, R. He, J. Lin, S. Yang, X. Zhang, Q. Ren, D. Cui, Aptamer-conjugated dendrimer-modified quantum dots for cancer cell targeting and imaging, Mater. Lett. 64 (2010) 375–378. doi:10.1016/j.matlet.2009.11.022.

[137] Z. Li, P. Huang, J. Lin, R. He, B. Liu, X. Zhang, S. Yang, P. Xi, X. Zhang, Q. Ren, D. Cui, Arginine-glycine-aspartic acid-conjugated dendrimer-modified quantum dots for targeting and imaging melanoma, J. Nanosci. Nanotechnol. 10 (2010) 4859–4867. doi:10.1166/jnn.2010.2217.

[138] B. Reddy, Advances in Nanocomposites: Synthesis, Characterization and Industrial Applications, BoD—Books on Demand, Rijeka (2011).

[139] H. Yin, Y. Zhou, S. Ai, Q. Chen, X. Zhu, X. Liu, L. Zhu, Sensitivity and selectivity determination of BPA in real water samples using PAMAM dendrimer and CoTe quantum dots modified glassy carbon electrode, J. Hazard. Mater. 174 (2010) 236–243. doi:10.1016/j.jhazmat.2009.09.041.

[140] P. Kesharwani, R. Ghanghoria, N.K. Jain, Carbon nanotube exploration in cancer cell lines, Drug Dis. Today. 17 (2012) 1023–1030. doi:10.1016/j.drudis.2012.05.003.

[141] J. Geng, H. Li, D. Zhou, W.T.S. Huck, B.F.G. Johnson, A dendrimer-based Co32 nanocluster: Synthesis and application in diameter-controlled growth of single-walled carbon nanotubes, Polyhedron. 25 (2006) 585–590. doi:10.1016/j.poly.2005.08.036.

[142] H. Yoshioka, M. Suzuki, M. Mugisawa, N. Naitoh, H. Sawada, Synthesis and applications of novel fluorinated dendrimer-type copolymers by the use of fluoroalkanoyl peroxide as a key intermediate, J. Colloid Interface Sci. 308 (2007) 4–10. doi:10.1016/j.jcis.2006.12.046.

[143] L. Tang, Y. Zhu, X. Yang, C. Li, An enhanced biosensor for glutamate based on self-assembled carbon nanotubes and dendrimer-encapsulated platinum nanobiocomposites-doped polypyrrole film, Anal. Chim. Acta. 597 (2007) 145–150. doi:10.1016/j.aca.2007.06.024.

[144] E. Murugan, G. Vimala, Effective functionalization of multiwalled carbon nanotube with amphiphilic poly(propyleneimine) dendrimer carrying silver nanoparticles for better dispersability and antimicrobial activity, J. Colloid Interface Sci. 357 (2011) 354–365. doi:10.1016/j.jcis.2011.02.009.

[145] Y. Shen, Q. Xu, H. Gao, N. Zhu, Dendrimer-encapsulated Pd nanoparticles anchored on carbon nanotubes for electro-catalytic hydrazine oxidation, Electrochem. Comm. 11 (2009) 1329–1332. doi:10.1016/j.elecom.2009.05.005.

[146] S. Choudhary, A. Jain, M.C.I.M. Amin, V. Mishra, G.P. Agrawal, P. Kesharwani, Stomach specific polymeric low density microballoons as a vector for extended delivery of rabeprazole and amoxicillin for treatment of peptic ulcer, Colloids Surf. B Biointerfaces. 141 (2016) 268–277. doi:10.1016/j.colsurfb.2016.01.048.

[147] B.M. Cummins, J. Lim, E.E. Simanek, M.V. Pishko, G.L. Coté, Encapsulation of a Concanavalin A/dendrimer glucose sensing assay within microporated poly (ethylene glycol) microspheres, Biomed. Opt. Express. 2 (2011) 1243–1257. doi:10.1364/BOE.2.001243.

[148] L.-Z. Kong, C.-Y. Pan, Preparation of dendrimer-like copolymers based on polystyrene and poly(l-lactide) and formation of hollow microspheres, Polymer. 49 (2008) 200–210. doi:10.1016/j.polymer.2007.11.042.

[149] G. Dang, Y. Shi, Z. Fu, W. Yang, Polymer particles with dendrimer@SiO2–Ag hierarchical shell and their application in catalytic column, J. Colloid Interface Sci. 369 (2012) 170–178. doi:10.1016/j.jcis.2011.11.054.

[150] A.Z. Wilczewska, K. Niemirowicz, K.H. Markiewicz, H. Car, Nanoparticles as drug delivery systems, Pharm. Rep. 64 (2012) 1020–1037. doi:10.1016/S1734-1140(12)70901-5.

[151] S. Nummelin, V. Liljeström, E. Saarikoski, J. Ropponen, A. Nykänen, V. Linko, J. Sep-
     pälä, J. Hirvonen, O. Ikkala, L.M. Bimbo, M.A. Kostiainen, Self-assembly of amphi-
     philic janus dendrimers into mechanically robust supramolecular hydrogels for sustained
     drug release, Chem. Eur. J. 21 (2015) 14433–14439. doi:10.1002/chem.201501812.
[152] M. Wróblewska, K. Winnicka, The effect of cationic polyamidoamine dendrimers
     on physicochemical characteristics of hydrogels with erythromycin, Int. J. Mol. Sci.
     16 (2015) 20277–20289. doi:10.3390/ijms160920277.
[153] R.J. Seelbach, P. Fransen, M. Peroglio, D. Pulido, P. Lopez-Chicon, F. Duttenhoefer,
     S. Sauerbier, T. Freiman, P. Niemeyer, C. Semino, F. Albericio, M. Alini, M. Royo,
     A. Mata, D. Eglin, Multivalent dendrimers presenting spatially controlled clusters
     of binding epitopes in thermoresponsive hyaluronan hydrogels, Acta Biomaterialia.
     10 (2014) 4340–4350. doi:10.1016/j.actbio.2014.06.028.
[154] T. Cheng-An, Z. Hao, W. Fang, Z. Hui, Z. Xiaorong, W. Jianfang, Mechanical properties
     of graphene oxide/polyvinyl alcohol composite film, Polym. Polym. Compos. 25 (2017)
     11–16. doi:10.1177/096739111702500102.
[155] A. Mohandas, S. Deepthi, R. Biswas, R. Jayakumar, Chitosan based metallic nanocom-
     posite scaffolds as antimicrobial wound dressings, Bioact. Mater. 3 (2018) 267–277.
     doi:10.1016/J.BIOACTMAT.2017.11.003.
[156] R. Chawla, S. Sivakumar, H. Kaur, Antimicrobial edible films in food packaging: Cur-
     rent scenario and recent nanotechnological advancements- a review, Car. Polym. Tech-
     nol. Appl. 2 (2021). doi:10.1016/J.CARPTA.2020.100024.
[157] Kusmono, I. Abdurrahim, Water sorption, antimicrobial activity, and thermal and
     mechanical properties of chitosan/clay/glycerol nanocomposite films, Heliyon.
     5 (2019). doi:10.1016/J.HELIYON.2019.E02342.
[158] Y. Cui, Q. Wu, J. He, M. Li, Z. Zhang, Y. Qiu, Porous nano-minerals substituted apa-
     tite/chitin/pectin nanocomposites scaffolds for bone tissue engineering, Arab. J. Chem.
     13 (2020) 7418–7429. doi:10.1016/J.ARABJC.2020.08.018.
[159] S. Nazir, M. Umar Aslam Khan, W. Shamsan Al-Arjan, S. Izwan Abd Razak, A. Javed,
     M. Rafiq Abdul Kadir, Nanocomposite hydrogels for melanoma skin cancer care and
     treatment: In-vitro drug delivery, drug release kinetics and anti-cancer activities, Arab.
     J. Chem. 14 (2021). doi:10.1016/J.ARABJC.2021.103120.
[160] C. Li, H. Ye, S. Ge, Y. Yao, B. Ashok, N. Hariram, H. Liu, H. Tian, Y. He, G. Guo,
     A.V. Rajulu, Fabrication and properties of antimicrobial flexible nanocomposite pol-
     yurethane foams with in situ generated copper nanoparticles, J. Mater. Res. Technol.
     19 (2022) 3603–3615. doi:10.1016/J.JMRT.2022.06.115.
[161] H. Munir, K. Tahira, A.R. Bagheri, M. Bilal, Biodegradation of materials in pres-
     ence of nanoparticles, Biodegr. Biodet. Nanoscale. (2021) 9–30. doi:10.1016/
     B978-0-12-823970-4.00002-6.
[162] Z. Peng, X. Liu, W. Zhang, Z. Zeng, Z. Liu, C. Zhang, Y. Liu, B. Shao, Q. Liang,
     W. Tang, X. Yuan, Advances in the application, toxicity and degradation of carbon
     nanomaterials in environment: A review, Environ. Int. 134 (2020). doi:10.1016/J.
     ENVINT.2019.105298.
[163] F. Candotto Carniel, L. Fortuna, D. Zanelli, M. Garrido, E. Vázquez, V.J. González,
     M. Prato, M. Tretiach, Graphene environmental biodegradation: Wood degrading
     and saprotrophic fungi oxidize few-layer graphene, J. Hazard. Mater. 414 (2021).
     doi:10.1016/J.JHAZMAT.2021.125553.
[164] R.P. Feazell, N. Nakayama-Ratchford, H. Dai, S.J. Lippard, Soluble single-walled car-
     bon nanotubes as longboat delivery systems for platinum(IV) anticancer drug design,
     J. Am. Chem. Soc. 129 (2007) 8438–8439. doi:10.1021/JA073231F.
[165] W. Wu, R. Li, X. Bian, Z. Zhu, D. Ding, X. Li, Z. Jia, X. Jiang, Y. Hu, Covalently
     combining carbon nanotubes with anticancer agent: Preparation and antitumor activity,
     ACS Nano. 3 (2009) 2740–2750. doi:10.1021/NN9005686.

[166] A. Kulamarva, P.M.V. Raja, J. Bhathena, H. Chen, S. Talapatra, P.M. Ajayan, O. Nalamasu, S. Prakash, Microcapsule carbon nanotube devices for therapeutic applications, Nanotechnol. 20 (2009). doi:10.1088/0957-4484/20/2/025612.

[167] A. Kulamarva, J. Bhathena, M. Malhotra, S. Sebak, O. Nalamasu, P. Ajayan, S. Prakash, In vitro cytotoxicity of functionalized single walled carbon nanotubes for targeted gene delivery applications, Nanotoxicol. 2 (2008) 184–188. doi:10.1080/17435390802464994.

[168] A.A. Bhirde, V. Patel, J. Gavard, G. Zhang, A.A. Sousa, A. Masedunskas, R.D. Leapman, R. Weigert, J.S. Gutkind, J.F. Rusling, Targeted killing of cancer cells in vivo and in vitro with EGF-directed carbon nanotube-based drug delivery, ACS Nano. 3 (2009) 307–316. doi:10.1021/nn800551s.

[169] R. Krajcik, A. Jung, A. Hirsch, W. Neuhuber, O. Zolk, Functionalization of carbon nanotubes enables non-covalent binding and intracellular delivery of small interfering RNA for efficient knock-down of genes, Biochem. Biophys. Res. Comm. 369 (2008) 595–602. doi:10.1016/j.bbrc.2008.02.072.

[170] Z. Zhang, X. Yang, Y. Zhang, B. Zeng, S. Wang, T. Zhu, R.B.S. Roden, Y. Chen, R. Yang, Delivery of telomerase reverse transcriptase small interfering RNA in complex with positively charged single-walled carbon nanotubes suppresses tumor growth, Clin. Cancer Res. 12 (2006) 4933–4939. doi:10.1158/1078-0432.CCR-05-2831.

[171] G. Pastorin, W. Wu, S. Wieckowski, J.P. Briand, K. Kostarelos, M. Prato, A. Bianco, Double functionalisation of carbon nanotubes for multimodal drug delivery, Chem. Comm. (2006) 1182–1184. doi:10.1039/B516309A.

[172] M.J. O'Connell, S.M. Bachilo, C.B. Huffman, V.C. Moore, M.S. Strano, E.H. Haroz, K.L. Rialon, P.J. Boul, W.H. Noon, C. Kittrell, J. Ma, R.H. Hauge, R.B. Weisman, R.E. Smalley, Band gap fluorescence from individual single-walled carbon nanotubes, Sci. 297 (2002) 593–596. doi:10.1126/science.1072631.

[173] N.W.S. Kam, M. O'Connell, J.A. Wisdom, H. Dai, Carbon nanotubes as multifunctional biological transporters and near-infrared agents for selective cancer cell destruction, Proc. Natl. Acad. Sci. U.S.A. 102 (2005) 11600–11605. doi:10.1073/PNAS.0502680102.

[174] N. Shao, S. Lu, E. Wickstrom, B. Panchapakesan, Integrated molecular targeting of IGF1R and HER2 surface receptors and destruction of breast cancer cells using single wall carbon nanotubes, Nanotechnol. 18 (2007). doi:10.1088/0957-4484/18/31/315101.

[175] N. Poovaiah, Z. Davoudi, H. Peng, B. Schlichtmann, S. Mallapragada, B. Narasimhan, Q. Wang, Treatment of neurodegenerative disorders through the blood–brain barrier using nanocarriers, Nanoscale. 10 (2018) 16962–16983. doi:10.1039/C8NR04073G.

[176] S. Ramanathan, G. Archunan, M. Sivakumar, S. Tamil Selvan, A.L. Fred, S. Kumar, B. Gulyás, P. Padmanabhan, Theranostic applications of nanoparticles in neurodegenerative disorders, Int. J. Nanomed. 13 (2018) 5561–5576. doi:10.2147/IJN.S149022.

[177] M. Wei, P. Lin, Y. Chen, J.Y. Lee, L. Zhang, F. Li, D. Ling, Applications of ion level nanosensors for neuroscience research, Nanomed. 15 (2020) 2871–2881. doi:10.2217/nnm-2020-0320.

[178] I. Cacciatore, M. Ciulla, E. Fornasari, L. Marinelli, A. Di Stefano, Solid lipid nanoparticles as a drug delivery system for the treatment of neurodegenerative diseases, Expert Opin. Drug Deliv. 13 (2016) 1121–1131. doi:10.1080/17425247.2016.1178237.

[179] M. Bilal, M. Barani, F. Sabir, A. Rahdar, G.Z. Kyzas, Nanomaterials for the treatment and diagnosis of Alzheimer's disease: An overview, NanoImpact. 20 (2020) 100251. doi:10.1016/j.impact.2020.100251.

[180] B. Wilson, M.K. Samanta, K. Santhi, K.P.S. Kumar, N. Paramakrishnan, B. Suresh, Poly(n-butylcyanoacrylate) nanoparticles coated with polysorbate 80 for the targeted delivery of rivastigmine into the brain to treat Alzheimer's disease, Brain Res. 1200 (2008) 159–168. doi:10.1016/j.brainres.2008.01.039.

[181] J.L. Gilmore, X. Yi, L. Quan, A.V. Kabanov, Novel nanomaterials for clinical neuroscience, J. Neuroimmune Pharmacol. 3 (2008) 83–94. doi:10.1007/s11481-007-9099-6.

[182] G. Modi, V. Pillay, Y.E. Choonara, V.M.K. Ndesendo, L.C. du Toit, D. Naidoo, Nanotechnological applications for the treatment of neurodegenerative disorders, Prog. Neurobiol. 88 (2009) 272–285. doi:10.1016/j.pneurobio.2009.05.002.

[183] P. Shah, S.K. Cho, P.W. Thulstrup, M.J. Bjerrum, P.H. Lee, J.-H. Kang, Y.-J. Bhang, S.W. Yang, MicroRNA biomarkers in neurodegenerative diseases and emerging nanosensors technology, J. Movement Dis. 10 (2017) 18. doi:10.14802/jmd.16037.

[184] F. Mesiti, P.A. Floor, A.N. Kim, I. Balasingham, On the modeling and analysis of the RF exposure on biological systems: A potential treatment strategy for neurodegenerative diseases, Nano Comm. Net. 3 (2012) 103–115. doi:10.1016/j.nancom.2012.02.001.

[185] K.K. Jain, The role of nanobiotechnology in drug discovery, Drug Dis. Today. 10 (2005) 1435–1442. doi:10.1016/S1359-6446(05)03573-7.

[186] D. Carradori, C. Balducci, F. Re, D. Brambilla, B. Le Droumaguet, O. Flores, A. Gaudin, S. Mura, G. Forloni, L. Ordoñez-Gutierrez, F. Wandosell, M. Masserini, P. Couvreur, J. Nicolas, K. Andrieux, Antibody-functionalized polymer nanoparticle leading to memory recovery in Alzheimer's disease-like transgenic mouse model, Nanomed. Nanotechnol. Biol. Med. 14 (2018) 609–618. doi:10.1016/j.nano.2017.12.006.

[187] T. Ali, M.J. Kim, S.U. Rehman, A. Ahmad, M.O. Kim, Anthocyanin-loaded PEG-gold nanoparticles enhanced the neuroprotection of anthocyanins in an Aβ1–42 mouse model of Alzheimer's disease, Mol. Neurobiol. 54 (2017) 6490–6506. doi:10.1007/s12035-016-0136-4.

[188] S.K. Sahoo, V. Labhasetwar, Nanotech approaches to drug delivery and imaging, Drug Dis. Today. 8 (2003) 1112–1120. doi:10.1016/S1359-6446(03)02903-9.

[189] L. Juillerat-Jeanneret, The targeted delivery of cancer drugs across the blood–brain barrier: Chemical modifications of drugs or drug-nanoparticles? Drug Dis. Today. 13 (2008) 1099–1106. doi:10.1016/j.drudis.2008.09.005.

[190] S. Okumoto, L.L. Looger, K.D. Micheva, R.J. Reimer, S.J. Smith, W.B. Frommer, Detection of glutamate release from neurons by genetically encoded surface-displayed FRET nanosensors, Proc. Natl. Acad. Sci. U.S.A. 102 (2005) 8740–8745. doi:10.1073/pnas.0503274102.

[191] Bhavna, S. Md, M. Ali, S. Baboota, J.K. Sahni, A. Bhatnagar, J. Ali, Preparation, characterization, in vivo biodistribution and pharmacokinetic studies of donepezil-loaded PLGA nanoparticles for brain targeting, Drug Dev. Indus. Pharm. 40 (2014) 278–287. doi:10.3109/03639045.2012.758130.

[192] T. Hirano, IL-6 in inflammation, autoimmunity and cancer, Int. Immunol. 33 (2021) 127–148. doi:10.1093/intimm/dxaa078.

[193] Y.S. Lee, J. Olefsky, Chronic tissue inflammation and metabolic disease, Genes Dev. 35 (2021) 307–328. doi:10.1101/gad.346312.120.

[194] T. Palaniyandi, K. B, P. Prabhakaran, S. Viswanathan, M. Rahaman Abdul Wahab, S. Natarajan, S. Kumar Kaliya Moorthy, S. Kumarasamy, Nanosensors for the diagnosis and therapy of neurodegenerative disorders and inflammatory bowel disease, Acta Histochemica. 125 (2023) 151997. doi:10.1016/j.acthis.2023.151997.

[195] D.C. Baumgart, S.R. Carding, Inflammatory bowel disease: Cause and immunobiology, Lancet. 369 (2007) 1627–1640. doi:10.1016/S0140-6736(07)60750-8.

[196] J. Lu, T. Van Stappen, D. Spasic, F. Delport, S. Vermeire, A. Gils, J. Lammertyn, Fiber optic-SPR platform for fast and sensitive infliximab detection in serum of inflammatory bowel disease patients, Biosens. Bioelectron. 79 (2016) 173–179. doi:10.1016/j.bios.2015.11.087.

[197] R. Akrofi, P.-L. Zhang, Q.-Y. Chen, Functional BOD-Ad-Cmyc@BSA complex nano-sensor for Cu(II) and the detection of live E. coli, Spectrochim. Acta A Mol. Biomol. Spectrosc. 239 (2020) 118483. doi:10.1016/j.saa.2020.118483.

[198] M. Wlodarska, A.D. Kostic, R.J. Xavier, An integrative view of microbiome-host interactions in inflammatory bowel diseases, Cell Host Microbe. 17 (2015) 577–591. doi:10.1016/j.chom.2015.04.008.

[199] M. Yang, Y. Zhang, Y. Ma, X. Yan, L. Gong, M. Zhang, B. Zhang, Nanoparticle-based therapeutics of inflammatory bowel diseases: A narrative review of the current state and prospects, J. Bio-X Res. 03 (2020) 157–173. doi:10.1097/JBR.0000000000000078.

[200] J. Zhao, W. Gao, X. Cai, J. Xu, D. Zou, Z. Li, B. Hu, Y. Zheng, Nanozyme-mediated catalytic nanotherapy for inflammatory bowel disease, Theranostics. 9 (2019) 2843. doi:10.7150/thno.33727.

9 Smart Carbon-Based Nanocarriers for Drug Delivery

9.1 INTRODUCTION TO INTELLIGENT NANOMATERIALS FOR DRUG DELIVERY

Humans have been trying to imitate nature by modeling the behavior of other species since prehistoric times. It is well established that natural biological systems can dynamically alter their attributes to adapt to their surroundings intelligently. "Intelligent materials," or those that can "react to changes in the surroundings at the most optimum scenario and exhibit their particular activities according to these changes," were initially reported in detail for the first time by Toshinori Takagi in the 1990s [1]. Though the scope and feasibility of this idea were incomprehensible at the time, it was believed that it would pave the way for novel discoveries and innovations in the scientific and technological arenas. With the advent of cutting-edge technology and the subsequent demand for novel materials to fulfill these needs, the concept of "intelligent material" (also known as "stimuli-responsive material" or "smart material") has attracted increasing attention from researchers [2].

Researchers were inspired to develop "stimuli-responsive" substances with biomimetic functionality having excellent potential for use in sophisticated or intelligent technologies by the remarkable ability of biological systems to transform energy and perform numerous functions. In the first decade of the 21st century, nanomaterials were intensely investigated and eventually implemented in practice. The need for highly functionalized biomaterials is growing due to advancements in biomedical engineering. A common ability throughout all biological systems is the ability to respond to shifts in their environment, which is vital for maintaining the optimal functioning of any organism. Due to this need for adaptability, "smart nanomaterials" that can change their physical properties in response to external stimuli have been developed. These properties include morphology, permeability, solubility, and mechanical attributes. The ability of the nanomaterial to recover from the altered state determines whether or not the reaction may be reversed.

In recent years, the space between biology and the materials sciences has shrunk significantly, allowing significant advancements in interdisciplinary techniques, notably those that utilize nanostructures for applications in medicine and biology. The pharmaceutical industry has been at the forefront of the rapid growth of nanotechnology. Many medications are now being produced in nanostructured delivery systems to treat and diagnose a wide range of disorders; these systems offer several benefits, including fewer adverse effects, more precise drug dosing, and enhanced

DOI: 10.1201/9781003358114-9

pharmacokinetics. Many of the drawbacks associated with free therapeutic entities, including poor solubility, low stability, nonspecific toxicity, rapid inactivation or degradation *in-vivo*, poor biodistribution, and unfavorable pharmacokinetics, can be overcome by the use of drug-loaded nanoparticles as pharmaceutical carriers, which can appropriately be called a drug delivery system (DDS) [3]. It is possible to create nanocarriers that can encapsulate both hydrophilic and hydrophobic molecules as drugs, increase their stability, enable drug targeting to pathological organs and tissues, provide controlled release, and modify the pharmacokinetics as desirable, that is, supersede the drug's pharmacokinetics with the explicitly designed pharmacokinetics of the DDS. **Figure 9.1** illustrates the plethora of nanomaterials that can be employed to deliver therapeutics at targeted locations. Unwanted side effects of the therapy can thereby be significantly reduced. In response to certain inherent stimuli features of diseased tissues or external stimuli provided from outside the body, nano-sized DDSs can be precisely tailored to modify some parameters or functions (for example, improve medication release or intracellular absorption) [4,5]. Pathological areas, including atherosclerotic lesions, infarcts, tumors, infection sites, and transplant rejection zones, differ from normal tissues due to the presence of internal stimuli, such as local changes in pH, temperature, and chemical concentrations, that is, the presence of specific hormones, enzymes, protein factors, antigens, and other bioactive molecules. External stimuli include magnetic field, electric field, heat, electromagnetic waves, and ultrasound [3], as shown in **Figure 9.2**.

Several new materials and engineering methodologies have been created to produce DDSs that can specifically respond to the peculiar circumstances of afflicted tissues, owing to a more profound knowledge of the microenvironmental changes at diseased sites. The stimuli-sensitive DDSs are able to activate specific mechanisms that regulate drug release or the effectiveness of cellular ingestion with exposure to an extrinsic or endogenous stimulus. Drug release is regulated through morphological changes, such as degradation or permeability enhancement, and the breakdown of chemical bonds intended to bind the medication to the nano-sized carriers. The stimuli-responsive DDSs are designed to exploit the unique biochemistry of each

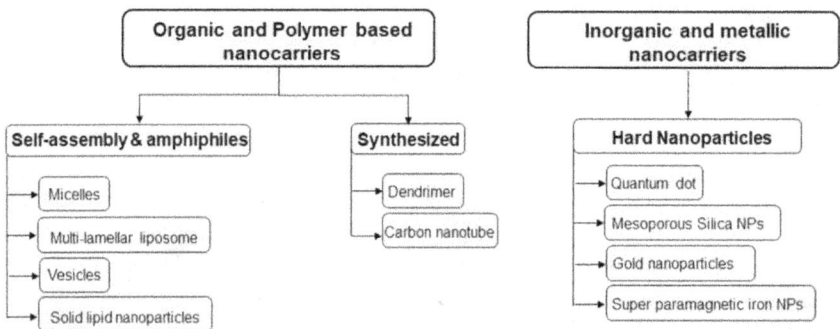

FIGURE 9.1 Various Nanomaterials as Carriers for Drug Delivery.

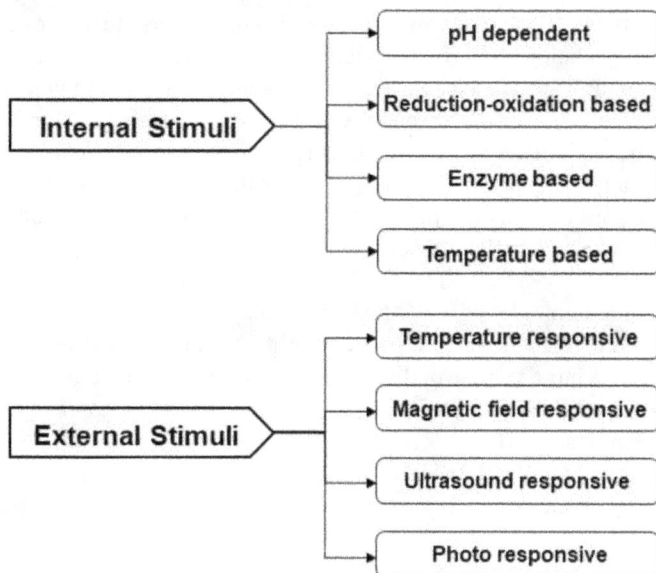

FIGURE 9.2 Classification of Stimuli.

afflicted region, enabling them to acclimatize to the local environment, ensuing in targeted drug delivery at precisely the correct time and location to enhance efficacy while minimizing adverse effects [6,7].

This chapter focuses on targeted drug delivery strategies via smart or intelligent nanomaterials that are aware of their surroundings and respond to either internal or external stimuli. Primary emphasis has been given to pH-responsive nanocarriers and their application in different therapies. The oral administration of medicine and its release in the gastrointestinal tract (GIT) is also discussed in detail.

9.2 STRATEGIES FOR THERAPEUTIC TARGETING AND CONTROLLED DELIVERY OF DRUGS

Modern DDSs consider a variety of factors, including the ideal time to administer medication, the drug's bioavailability, the body's drug absorption capacity, and its pharmacokinetics. Following are the four conditions that any effective drug delivery system must accomplish:

1. Retention.
2. Evasion.
3. Targeting.
4 Releasing.

The DDS must have a long residence time in circulation so that it can travel to the site of interest and be released there at the precise time required for the drug to function effectively. The carrier must survive different environments inside the body and prevent degradation by the body's secretions, such as enzymes, antigens, reactive oxygen species (ROS), etc., to achieve a long residence time in circulation. A precise targeting mechanism avoids accidental release at unintended sites. The smart nanocarriers can be engineered for either a burst release [8], where the entire drug load is discharged at a go, or sustained release [9], where the medication is slowly disbursed at the target over a certain period. If a DDS satisfies all four of these conditions, it is optimal and will not harm healthy cells or organs, and it can be reasonably termed a targeted drug delivery system (TDDS) [10]. A TDDS is therefore recommended over more typical medicine delivery methods. Conventional drugs have various limitations compared to TDDSs, such as poor solubility, instability, half-lives, absorption, and the need for a large volume of distribution. Traditional medications are notorious for their poor specificity and low therapeutic index. The TDD approach is intended to resolve these issues [11].

Targeting a medicine to a specific organ or part of the body can improve its therapeutic efficacy and lessen its side effects. Six prominent strategies (**Figure 9.3**) are

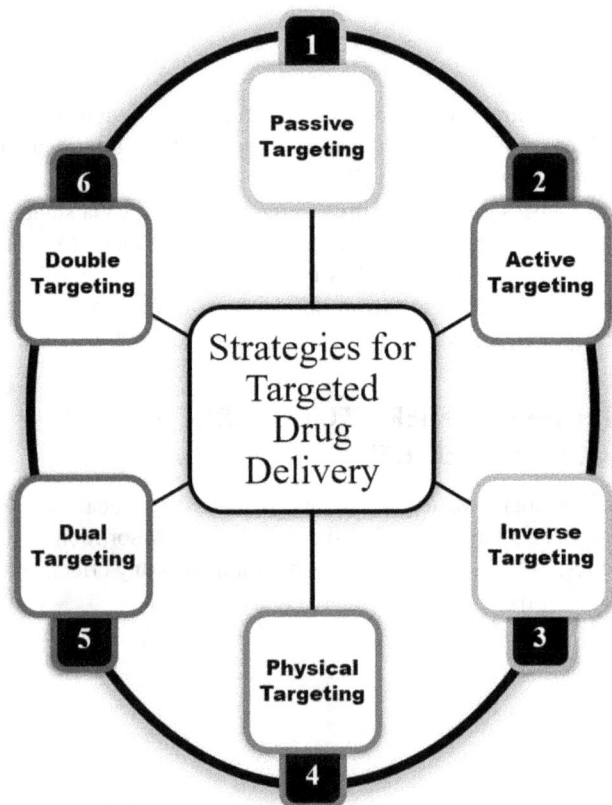

FIGURE 9.3 Strategies Employed by DDS for Precise Targeting.

employed to target a specific organ or tissue for administering medicine, and they are as follows:

1. Passive targeting.
2. Active targeting.
3. Inverse targeting.
4. Physical targeting.
5. Dual targeting.
6. Double targeting.

Passive targeting DDS relies on the circulatory system, specifically the systemic circulation, to reach the desired site. In this method, the body's intrinsic reaction to the physicochemical attributes of the therapeutic compound or therapeutic system results in drug targeting. Passive targeting DDS exploits the medication's tendency to collect more in the tissues around the target, such as tumors, than in the healthy surrounding tissue [10]. NPs carriers are directed into the blood arteries, specifically at the disease location, allowing for a high concentration of medications. The enhanced permeability retention (EPR) effect or the slow lymphatic drainage facilitates this process [12]. Tumor vasculature is aberrant in solid tumors. Traditional anticancer treatments exploit passive targeting because a greater concentration of the medication accumulates in malignant cells due to better blood flow to these cells. The malignant tissue secretes angiogenic factors and stimulates new blood vessel development. Tumor abnormalities can be used to target cancer medications, especially nanoparticulate anticancer therapeutics, passively. The capacity of antimalarial medications to cure microbial illnesses such as brucellosis, candidiasis, and leishmaniasis is another instance of passive targeting [13].

Active targeting DDS relies on a biochemical interface to lock on target cells. A specific ligand-receptor interaction occurs with the NP carrier-associated ligand and the receptors on the target cell after extravasation and blood circulation. Proteins, polysaccharides, nucleic acids, peptides, and other small molecules have all been used as ligands [10]. Ligands with high affinity to receptors may be purposefully added directly into therapeutics or co-encapsulated with it, and the essential ligands can be coated on nanoparticles to generate ligand-receptor interactions. However, for ligand-receptor interactions to occur, the distance between the two molecules must be shorter than 0.5 nanometers. Therefore, active receptor targeting does not commence until after the drug has circulated throughout the body and is extravasated into the malignant cells. The folic acid-folate receptor is a well-studied example of this type of interaction.

Based on the location of administration of the drug-laden nano-sized carriers, active targeting can be further classified into three subcategories, namely, 1. first order, 2. second order, and 3. third order. The first-order active targeting DDS is distributed to capillary beds of broad target areas such as organs or tissues. Such lymphatic tissue targeting areas include the cerebral ventricles, eyes, joints, peritoneal cavity, and pleural cavity. Second-order drug targeting targets the treatment of disease-causing microenvironments, such as cancer cells. The Kupffer cells of the liver are an ideal pharmaceutical target. Third-order drug targeting necessitates intracellular localization to the target site via endocytosis or receptor-based ligand-mediated interactions.

Inverse targeting of DDS refers to the mechanism by which reticuloendothelial systems (RESs) actively work to prevent the absorption of the colloidal carrier. A significant volume of blank colloidal carriers or macromolecules, such as dextran sulfate, are injected before testing to prevent the RES from functioning normally. RES can be overloaded in this method, and defensive mechanisms may be suppressed with ease. This method is often considered efficient for delivering drugs to non-RES tissues and organs [12].

Physical targeting can direct the drug carrier to a particular area by modifying environmental parameters such as pH, temperature, light intensity, magnetic field, electric field, or ionic strength, as well as smaller, more specific stimuli such as glucose concentration or gaseous concentration. Nanoparticle drug targeting tumors and cytosolic injection of encapsulated medicine or genetic elements favor this strategy. It is a result of these physical characteristics that can control drug delivery to the tumor [14,15].

Dual targeting is when temporal and spatial techniques are used to target a carrier system. Here, spatial placement focuses medications on precisely designated organs, tissues, cells, or even subcellular compartments, while temporal delivery permits the regulation of the pace of drug administration to the target location [16].

Double targeting strategy focuses on the therapeutic activity of the carrier molecule, which improves medicine efficacy, which is unique to this method of pharmaceutical administration. For example, an antibacterial or antifungal medicine can be conjugated to a carrier molecule that also has antibacterial or antifungal activity, and the combined impact of the drug conjugation or composite can be studied. Antibacterial drugs coupled with porous ZnO nanoparticles are both efficient against bacteria, resulting in a TDD with dual targeting [10].

The selection of a strategy should only be finalized after a careful analysis of factors such as the drug's and nanocarrier's characteristics, the disease's location, and the environment surrounding the ailing tissue or organ.

9.3 pH-RESPONSIVE NANOCARRIERS FOR CONTROLLED DRUG DELIVERY

Targeted, stimulus-responsive delivery of active pharmacological compounds has made extensive use of the vast pH range of the human body. Polymers with ionizable groups, which change conformation and solubility in response to changes in environmental pH, and polymeric systems with acid-sensitive bonds, whose cleavage results in the release of the bioactive molecule from the polymer backbone, modification of the polymer's charge, or exposure of the targeting ligands, are two common approaches to achieving this objective. Products using pH-sensitive coatings for the digestive tract are among the most prominent uses of pH-responsive technology [17].

Due to the prevalence of pH variations in various specific and pathological systems, smart nanomaterials that demonstrate unique functional capabilities in response to pH are enticing in the biomedical sector. Since the pH of various human bodily fluids varies (chronic wounds have a pH between 7.4 and 5.4, while saliva ranges from 6.5 to 7.5, and the pH of the digestive tract varies from 4 to 6.5 in the stomach to 7.5 in the intestines), using such materials might be beneficial (5 to 8). It is also worth noting that the pH levels are abnormal in the diseased state as opposed to the healthy state. For instance, the pH of the tumor's surroundings is lower, between 6.5 and 6.9, whereas the pus of a bacterial infection is acidic, with a range of 6.0 to 6.6, and the pH of irritated tissues is between 6 and 7.

Tumors, inflammation, and hypoxic regions are all characterized by low pH. It was hypothesized that lactic acid (pK 3.7) was the primary source of tumor acidity after research conducted by Warburg and colleagues in the 1930s demonstrated that tumor cells preferentially convert glucose and other substrates to lactic acid. New evidence suggests that elevated CO_2 and the increased expression and activity of vascular-type proton pumps also contribute to the acidification of the body. Tumors have a low pH because of unregulated cell growth and proliferation (tumorigenesis), which causes hypoxia, poor blood flow, and metabolic abnormalities. **Table 9.1** [2] lists a few pH-responsive nanomaterials and their applications as DDSs.

Different pH-responsive materials have been developed up to this point, considering the exceptional range of pH values found. The majority of pH-sensitive materials may be split into two categories: those that include ionizable moieties and those that have acid-labile links. The first type essentially requires the existence of ionizable, fragile, basic, or acidic moieties (amines and carboxylic acids) that adhere to a hydrophobic backbone, such as polyelectrolytes [18]. Such pH-sensitive material demonstrates protonation/deprotonation processes by distributing charge among the molecule's ionizable regions. The second category is composed of materials with acid-labile covalent backbone linkages, which are primarily polymers. Breaking these bonds determines if the substance aggregates dissociate or polymer chains break following a fall in pH. The second kind, which undergoes less internal change as a result of covalent bonding, is more appropriate for usage as a DDS. In

---

TABLE 9.1

List of pH-Responsive Nanocarriers and Their Therapeutic Applications. Reproduced with permission from *M. Aflori (2021)*[2].

Sl. No.	Nanocarriers	Application
1	Ppoly (ethylene glycol)-Ag nanoparticle PEG-Ag NPs	Antibacterial, wound healing
2	Hybrid ultra-pH-sensitive (HyUPS) nanotransistor HyUPS nanotransistors	Receptor-mediated endocytosis in tumor cells
3	Layered double hydroxides-zinc (II) phthalocyanine containing octasulfonate nanohybrid LDH-ZnPcS$_8$ nanohybrid	Theranostics
4	Melanin-like nanoparticles	Photoacoustic imaging of tumors
5	polylactic acid-resveratrol PLA-RSV	Drug delivery
6	Poly(carboxybetaine methacrylate)-nanodiamonds PCBSA-@-NDs	Theranostics

pH-sensitive polymers, a pH shift results in a phase transition. A phase transition may occur within a pH variation typically between 0.2 and 0.3. Among the most well-known pH-sensitive polymers are poly(L-lysine), poly(N,N -dimethylaminoethyl methacrylate), poly(methacrylic acid), poly(acrylic acid), poly(N,N -dialkyl amino-ethyl methacrylates), poly(ethylenimine), chitosan, aginate, and hyaluronic acid [19].

Due to the interaction between the negatively charged octasulfonate-modified zinc (II) phthalocyanine ($ZnPcS_8$) and the positively charged hydroxide layers of layered double hydroxide (LDH), a novel pH-responsive supramolecular nanomaterial has been developed. LDH-$ZnPcS_8$ is inert in basic environments and photoactive in acid media (pH 6.5) [20]. **Figure 9.4** illustrates the co-precipitation process used to create the LDH-$ZnPcS_8$ nanohybrid. The nanohybrid had 20.87 wt% magnesium, 7.13 wt% aluminum, and 0.27 wt% zinc. LDH -$ZnPcS_8$ has a $ZnPcS_8$ loading percentage of 7.35% by weight. The likely mechanism as an aPS for PDT is depicted, in which $ZnPcS_8$ is released from LDH-$ZnPcS_8$ in response to low acidity, hence reactivating its photoactivities.

A melanin-like nanoparticle (MelNP) was created to harness its particular property to build a highly pH-sensitive device for *in-vivo* imaging cancer targets [21]. Polysaccharides (e.g., chitosan) that undergo conformational changes and/or pH-responsive solubility and polymers with weak acid bonds (vinyl ester, ketal, acetal, orthoester, etc.) whose breaking initiates surface charge changes or the release of molecules are examples of pH-responsive nanomaterials. Chitosan, for instance, is a polysaccharide whose activity varies based on the surrounding environment. In a healthy environment, its surface charge is either negative or neutral. However, in a pathological environment, its surface charge is positive (due to the protonation of the amino group), allowing it to interact quickly with the negative charge of the cells. Based on this feature, chitosan can target therapeutic effects in specific

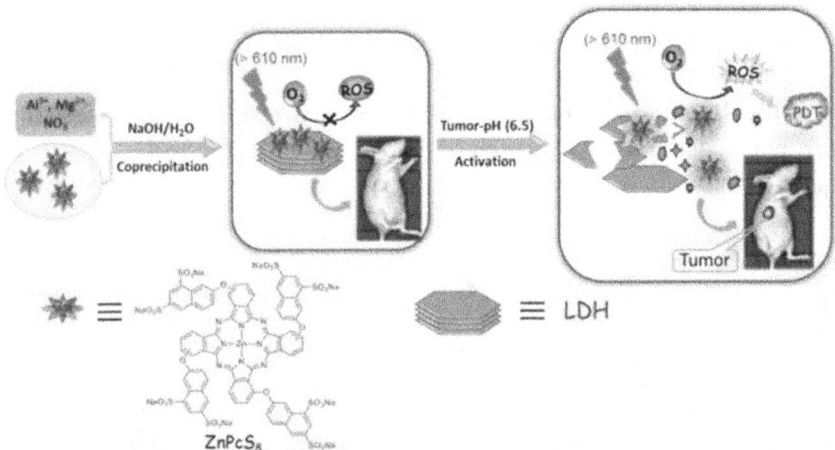

FIGURE 9.4 Schematic Depiction of Formation and Subsequent Activation of Photoactivity in LDH-$ZnPcS_8$ as a Response to Low pH Environment Surrounding a Tumor. [Reproduced with permission from *Li et al. (2017)*] [20].

areas [22]. The polylactic acid PLA system developed by Bonadies et al. (2020) is pH-responsive and may be utilized as an implant covering for lengthy periods. They described an electrospun membrane that rapidly produced resveratrol (RSV) when the pH was changed from neutral to slightly acidic (around 5.5). They demonstrated that the use of a PLA-RSV membrane could prevent implant-associated infections [23].

9.4 NANOCARRIERS FOR SMART DRUG RELEASE IN THE GASTROINTESTINAL TRACT

The vast majority of FDA-approved drugs need parenteral administration, which is associated with several drawbacks, including high cost, limited patient compliance, and significant systemic toxicity. Therefore, significant efforts have been directed at the creation of carriers for the oral administration of therapeutics. Oral administration is preferred because it is noninvasive and has a high percentage of patient compliance. Traditional excipient-based approaches have garnered much attention to facilitate the transit of oral biologics via the GIT, which is a challenging pathway for them to traverse. The extreme stomach pH, digesting enzymes, gut bacteria, gut mucosa, and epithelium disrupt biologics' tertiary/quaternary structure, and absorption into the systemic circulation is inhibited [24].

Many physiological impediments in the gastrointestinal system dramatically decrease drug absorption when medications are taken orally. First, the immensely acidic environment and proteolytic enzymes of the stomach function as a first barrier, disrupting the formulation. Second, the mucus layer also functions as a barrier, preventing positive and hydrophobic molecules from flowing through the epithelium of the stomach. Third, the tight junctions, goblet cells, M cells, and enterocytes that comprise the intestinal epithelium cooperate to keep medicines out. After the gastrointestinal tract, the submucosal lamina propria is a second barrier to medicine absorption into the blood [25].

The gastric residency duration is extended for systems meant to target the stomach to enhance absorption or localize the effects of medications. Localization of the drug's effects on the stomach must first be retained there, which may help inhibit the degradation of the medication in the intestines. Similarly, medications that are soluble at low pH may dissolve more readily in such environments. However, their stomach solubility is enhanced. Consequently, they undergo stomach solubilization during retention and are subsequently made available in a soluble condition to the colon for increased absorption. Regarding giving drugs with a narrow window for absorption, such as site-specific absorption, gastro-retentive devices may be generally advantageous. Some study indicates that the gastro-retentive processes assist set up the stomach as a drug reservoir, making the treatment more slowly and precisely available to the absorption site (the intestine) [26].

The formulation of a targeted oral DDS must consider the medication, the transport mode, and the intended receiver. With the use of reformulation research, the physicochemical properties of drugs, such as pK_a, pH, solubility, incompatibility, and stability, may be better understood. The partition coefficient of a drug determines how effectively it may traverse these membrane barriers. Drugs with an extremely low partition coefficient will have limited bioavailability because they cannot pass these membranes [27].

The drawbacks of conventional lipid-based delivery techniques have led to the development of polymer-lipid hybrid (PLH) systems as a workable substitute. The solubilization power of lipid-based nanocarriers is combined with the stabilizing properties of polymeric excipients in PLH systems. Polymers provide a variety of biopharmaceutical advantages for oral drug administration in lipid-based systems because of their ability to 1. preserve lipid colloids, 2. finely control the physico-chemical features, and 3. selectively alter delivery channels. Biodegradable polymers have been used to create PLH systems together with natural, semi-synthetic, and synthetic polymers with various physicochemical properties and bioactivities. The thoughtful selection of additives and production techniques of PLH systems enable improved pharmacokinetic performance in contrast to the antecedent lipid-based drug delivery systems. Numerous studies have shown that PLH systems can increase the oral bioavailability of bioactive compounds, peptides and proteins, nucleic acids, and poorly soluble and permeable vaccines. They have promise and the potential to be used in therapeutic settings [28].

Much emphasis has been placed on the mucoadhesive DDS. Oral administration of a mucoadhesive dendrimer (nanocarrier) appears to be a unique and superior method for oral drug delivery. Typically, 1. a mucoadhesive will enter tissue or the mucous membrane surface (interpenetration), and 2. a mucoadhesive will establish intimate contact with a membrane (wetting and swelling phenomenon). This nanocarrier-based method has the capacity to improve cellular interaction through precise formulation and delivery of the dual drug for a synergistic effect. Using chitosan as a model, Gonçalves et al. (2014) investigated the efficacy of chitosan-based nanocarriers for stomach administration of medicines in the treatment of *Helicobacter pylori*. Because of their ability to stick to the mucosal surface, remain there for an extended period, and allow the medicine to diffuse to the site of infection, these nanocarriers guarantee the bioactives' total safety even in an acidic environment [29]. Mucoadhesive drug delivery using modified polyamidoamine (PAMAM) dendrimers were described by Yandrapu et al. in 2013. The cationic mucin layer reacts quickly to the anionic dendrimer. With molecular dimensions between 1 and 100 nm, dendrimers are advantageous because they are less likely to be taken up by the reticuloendothelial system (RES) [30].

For water-insoluble bioactive chemicals, the issue of restricted bioavailability can be addressed by employing nanocarrier systems based on lipids for oral administration. Using emulsifiers or surfactants as excipients in lipid nanoparticles can boost bioavailability. Self-emulsifying drug delivery systems (SEDDs), nanoemulsions, microemulsions, solid lipid nanoparticles (SLNs), liposomes, and nanostructured lipid carriers (NLCs) are lipid-based innovative drug delivery systems that encapsulate bioactive substances and enhance their oral solubility and bioavailability [31,32].

Nanoemulsions are a type of emulsion composed of small oil droplets spread in a water-based medium and stabilized by an emulsifying agent. The resulting emulsion is kinetically stable, retaining its isotropic clarity and absence of turbidity even after lengthy storage. The size of a droplet is measured to be between 20 and 200 nanometers. In contrast to SEDDs, nanoemulsions are generated by direct assembly rather than self-assembly. Nanoemulsions have oil cores that can be loaded with bioactives to improve oral administration. Estrasorb, Flexogan, and Restasis are only a few examples of nanoemulsion formulations of poorly water-soluble medications authorized by the US Food and Drug Administration. Nanoemulsions have several benefits over conventional food systems, not the least of which is their ability to encapsulate vitamins and minerals without adverse side effects. Other advantages include rapid gastrointestinal (GI) digestion, excellent physical stability, simple texture modification, and the ability to encapsulate lipophilic compounds. The stable nanoemulsions were produced using both high-energy and low-energy emulsification. In addition to microfluidics, membrane emulsification, and ultrasonic and high-pressure homogenization, high-energy techniques include microfluidics. The phase inversion temperature method, the emulsion inversion point method, and spontaneous emulsification are examples of these low-energy emulsification processes [33].

NLCs, also known as second-generation lipid nanoparticles, comprise various lipids, emulsifiers, and water. Due to the incorporation of liquid lipids, which reduces particle size, the danger of gelation, and drug leakage during storage by distorting the formation of perfect lipid crystals, the drug loading capacity increases. With the aid of NLCs, the encapsulated bioactives can be absorbed orally due to their selective absorption through lymphatic transport or Peyer's patches. By altering the ratio of liquid to solid lipids, drug release from NLCs may be precisely regulated. Their manufacture utilizes multiple emulsions, sonication, microemulsion, phase inversion, solvent injection, high-pressure homogenization, solvent evaporation, solvent injection, and emulsification-solvent diffusion. In the past, NLCs were utilized to enhance the oral bioavailability of a variety of drugs. Studies have described the usage of NLCs to circumvent solubility, permeability, stability, and toxicity issues. Several modified NLCs have been studied to make mucus adhesives and mucus-penetrating particles and enhance targeting. Because they facilitate the active transport of drug-loaded NLCs through the intestinal membrane, peptidic ligands have a wider variety of uses in oral delivery [34].

Submicron medication delivery methods, called nanocapsules, are another reliable DDS with an oily or aqueous core surrounded by a thin polymer membrane. As a delivery system for bioactive compounds, nanocapsules provide several benefits. They shield the enclosed medications from the elements and allow for a measured release. One of the most promising strategies for lymphatic targeting, nanocapsules have the potential for achieving differentiated properties with a straightforward production procedure. When delivered, nanocapsules coated with hydrophobic polymers may be rapidly taken up by lymphatic cells due to the particle's universal recognition as a foreign entity [35]. Prego et al. (2006) produced chitosan-polyethylene glycol (PEG) nanocapsules for peptide delivery via the GIT. Using chitosan nanocapsules enhanced and extended the oral absorption of peptides. The Caco-2 model cell demonstrated that chitosan's PEGylation attenuated the nanocapsules' cytotoxicity. In an *in-vivo* study, chitosan-PEG nanocapsules were found to improve and extend intestinal absorption of salmon calcitonin. Furthermore, they found that the nanocapsules' *in-vivo* efficacy was affected by the PEGylation level. By altering the degree of chitosan PEGylation, it is possible to produce nanocapsules with good stability, minimal cytotoxicity, and increased absorption [36].

Active targeting comprises integrating a targeting ligand onto the surface of the nanocarrier to increase uptake by diseased cells through target recognition of the ligand. By increasing selective drug accumulation at inflamed areas of the colon, this technique can improve the therapeutic effectiveness and reduce adverse reactions. As targeting moieties, monoclonal antibodies and peptides are preferred options due to their high specificity and potential mucopenetrative qualities. Oral targeted drug delivery can be based on an extensive range of moiety types. Due to the various hurdles in the GI system that limit oral administration of antibodies and peptide-based formulations, such as stomach acid and enzymes, nanodelivery approaches may require different formulation designs. Targeted delivery methods can be developed based on the surface receptor's ability to internalize. The basis of this pharmacological technique is that interactions between the targeting moiety and certain receptors expressed selectively at inflamed sites might increase the bioadhesion of the drug formulation to specific cells and the amount of endocytosis. In biological environments, the chemistry of ligand conjugation and its practical application are two issues that must be considered. To this end, it is essential to analyze the stability of the ligand or the nonspecific binding of proteins as the ligand moves through the circulation toward the target site. Recently, several targeting ligands for oral colon-specific drug delivery strategies have been studied. Zhang et al. (2007) developed galactosylated trimethyl chitosan-cysteine (GTC) nanoparticles for the oral delivery of mitogen-activated protein kinase kinase kinase (Mapk4) siRNA (siMapk4), a crucial upstream regulator of TNF-α production. Studies on animals and in test tubes indicate that siRNA can successfully inhibit TNF-production and distribute itself selectively in ulcerative colitis [37].

Nanoscale crystals of a drug are created solely from the molecule itself and are unceremoniously called drug nanocrystals. Typically, surfactants or polymeric steric stabilizers are added to maintain their stability. Diameters of nanocrystals are often less than 1 micrometer and, more commonly, fewer than 500 nanometers. Nanocrystals can be made using either a top-down or a bottom-up approach. These crystals are filled with a complete dose of the active substance for usage against liposomes, polymeric nanoparticles, nanoemulsions, lipid nanoparticles, etc. Both liquid and solid dosage forms are conceivable (tablets and capsules). Megace ES (megestrol), Emend (aprepitant), Tricor (fenofibrate), Triglide (fenofibrate), and Rapamune are only a handful of the several oral formulations available for clinical use (rapamycin). Increased solubility and saturation rates and improved cell membrane adhesion enable nanocrystals to attain bioavailability acceptable for therapeutic usage. Nanocrystals containing coenzyme Q10 were developed by Piao et al. (2011). In the rat study, the oral bioavailability of nanocrystals was 2.5 times higher than that of coarse suspensions, and the improved solubility of CoQ10 was linked to the development of nanocrystals [38]. Increased bioavailability by oral administration of drug nanocrystals is only conceivable if the molecule shows dissolution rate-limited bioavailability. However, little research has been conducted in this area, and when paired with other injectable techniques, this strategy can significantly extend dosing choices.

The carbon nanotube (CNT) is an allotrope of carbon atoms that may be used as a nanocarrier. With a high aspect ratio, a diameter as small as 1 nm, and a length of several microns, CNTs may be considered graphene sheets wrapped into a seamless cylinder with an open or closed end. SWCNTs are CNTs made from a single graphene sheet, whereas MWNTs are CNTs formed from multiple graphene sheets (MWNTs). Since their discovery by Iijima in 1991, these carbon allotropes have generated considerable interest due to their distinctive physical and chemical properties. The potential use of CNTs in a vast array of sectors, ranging from electronics and sensors to nanocomposite materials with outstanding strength and low weight, makes their bioapplications viable. CNT-based drug delivery offers enormous promise for application in treating oral cancer. Bhirde et al. showed in 2009 that using a drug-SWCNT bioconjugate to kill cancer cells was more successful than using nontargeted bioconjugates. Attaching the anticancer drug cisplatin and the epidermal growth factor (EGF) to SWCNTs enables them to target head and neck squamous cell carcinoma cells (HNSCC) preferentially [39].

In light of their immense potential applications in areas as diverse as targeted medication administration, magnetic separation, biotechnology, and diagnostic imaging, metallic nanocarriers, including silver, gold, and iron oxide, constitute a significant source of contemporary concern. This type of nanocarrier can be coupled with targeted moieties since it can be made and manipulated to have numerous chemical functional groups. With their inertness, low toxicity, simple production, and high accumulation in tumors and inflamed tissues via the EPR effect, surface functionalization, etc., nanocarriers based on gold offer a potential platform for oral drug administration. According to research published by Lai et al. (2006), thioridazine was microencapsulated using gold nanoparticles. Like alkane thiols, the dialkyl sulfide thioridazine can efficiently adsorb on gold. Gold nanoparticles have been included in microencapsulation experiments to boost encapsulation efficiency. Furthermore, gold nanoparticles may operate as a diffusion barrier to the release of thioridazine when encapsulated and combined with thioridazine in microcapsules. Acute oral toxicity studies on albino rats using a gold nanoparticle solution of 50 nm showed no symptoms of gross toxicity or deleterious effects, as described by the author [40].

9.5 PATHOLOGICAL STIMULI-RESPONSIVE NANO-THERANOSTICS

As effective carriers for pharmaceuticals, genes, and antigens, nanoparticles in the form of dendrimers, nanogels, and polymeric micelles have been intensively researched. Nanomaterials with a redox response have emerged as effective biomaterials. Developing biological systems that are redox-responsive is helped by polymers with labile groups. Poly(b-aminoesters), polyanhydrides, and poly(lactic/glycolic acid) are typical redox-responsive polymers because they include acid-labile moieties. Thiol groups, platin conjugation, thioether, disulfide, and diselenide are the most widely used redox-responsive compounds for controlled drug release applications.

9.5.1 REACTIVE OXYGEN SPECIES (ROS) SENSITIVE NANO-THERANOSTICS

The aerobic metabolic process generates reactive oxygen species. They have an additional electron that may be exploited to create radicals, ions, or molecules (**Table 9.2**) [41]. The effects of superoxide, hydrogen peroxide, and hydroxyl radicals on cancer pathogenesis in the setting of cancer cells are well documented. Higher amounts

TABLE 9.2

List of Reactive Oxygen Species Reproduced with permission from A. Singh, M. Amiji (2018) [41].

Free Oxygen Radical ROS	Non-radical ROS
Superoxide O_2^{-}	Hydrogen peroxide H_2O_2
Hydroxyl radical $^{\cdot}OH$	Singlet oxygen $^1O_2$
Nitric oxide $NO^{\cdot}$	Ozone/trioxygen O_3
Peroxyl radicals $ROO^{\cdot}$	Organic hydroperoxides $ROOH$
Alkoxyl radicals $RO^{\cdot}$	Hypochloride $HOCl$
Sulfonyl radicals $ROS^{\cdot}$	Peroxynitrite $ONO^{\cdot}$
Thiyl peroxyl radicals $RSOO^{\cdot}$	Nitrosoperoxycarbonate anion $O=NOOCO_2$
	Nitrocarbonate anion $O_2NOCO_2^{\cdot}$
	Dinitrogen dioxide N_2O_2
	Nitronium NO^+
	Highly reactive lipid or carbohydrate derived carbonyl compounds

of ROS can be caused by increased metabolic and oxidase activity, mitochondrial dysfunction, peroxisome activity, improved cellular receptor signaling, and oncogene activity. In most malignancies, elevated ROS stimulates cell growth/proliferation, differentiation, protein synthesis, glucose metabolism, cell survival, and inflammatory signaling pathways. H_2O_2 can serve as a secondary messenger in cellular signaling and regulate the activity of proteins [41]. Superoxide radicals are produced in the inner mitochondrial membrane as a consequence of the electron transport chain and through the activation of NADPH oxidases (NOX). Superoxide is converted to hydrogen peroxide by SOD enzymes in the mitochondrial matrix or by Cu/ZnSOD in the cytoplasm. A cytosol Fenton reaction can generate hydroxyl radicals from either hydrogen peroxide or superoxide.

The high ROS vulnerability of tumor cells is exploited by ROS-responsive materials or linkers for nano-drug delivery systems to improve drug transport and induce targeted release. Many different medication delivery systems that can react to reactive oxygen species have been created and studied. They rely heavily on two fundamental chemical processes: induced solubility switch and degradation. Typically, these systems work by destabilizing nanosystems and releasing medicines upon oxidation of a specific atom (e.g., S, Se) or oxidative breakage of carbon-heteroatom bonds (e.g., C-S) in the presence of H_2O_2. In this way, drug release occurs as a result of carrier disassembly, cleavage-induced carrier degradation, and cleavage of the linker between the carrier and the drug. The capacity of the ROS-responsive material to respond to the ROS level seen in a healthy body is still a necessity [42]. Except for H_2O_2, almost all reactive oxygen species (ROS) are highly short-lived in biological environments due to their significant reactivity with biomolecules within cells. ROS can undergo smooth interconversions in ideal microenvironments, enhancing complex processes.

It is feasible to use the high quantities of ROS observed in cancer cells to cure cancer. O_2^{-}, $^1O_2$, and $^{\cdot}OH$ are reactive oxygen species, but their high reactivity, low concentrations, and short half-lives in biological systems make them difficult to exploit in cancer therapy. As a result of its stability and high concentration, H_2O_2 is utilized extensively in cancer treatment. The ability of H_2O_2 to generate highly reactive $\cdot$OH via the Fenton and Fenton-like reactions in combination with transition metal ions has contributed significantly to the development of CDT in recent years. Under acidic conditions, H_2O_2 and iron (Fe^{2+} and Fe^{3+}) trigger the Fenton reaction in cancer cells. In addition to Fe, Fe-like reactions may be carried out using transition metals Mn, Cu, Ni, and Co. To create a synergistic effect on cancer, the H_2O_2-based CDT therapy is always combined with other treatments, such as PTT, PDT, and chemotherapy. Our team employed Fe_3S_4 tetragonal nanosheets to achieve MRI-guided simultaneous PTT and CDT (TNSs). The rapid release of Fe ions in an acidic environment boosted the Fenton reaction in combination with heat generation, producing a high-efficiency photothermal effect with PTT/CDT synergistic therapy. In the presence of H_2O_2, cell death was significantly enhanced in the TNSs/H_2O_2 and TNSs/H_2O_2/NIR groups, demonstrating the superiority of CDT over TNSs and NIR. In addition, the considerable inhibitory effect found in the tumor diameters of mice treated with Fe3S4 TNSs alone is a result of the CDT impact with a high level of $\cdot$OH production by the Fenton reaction. CDT primarily depends on H_2O_2 levels, yet redox agents in cancer cells should reduce its effectiveness. Diverse techniques, including GSH depletion, the photodynamic treatment (PDT) effect, and the stimulation with medicines such as glucose oxidase, NAD(P)H:quinone oxidoreductase-1, and dihydroartemisinin, were employed to increase H_2O_2 levels in cancer cells (DHA) [43].

9.5.2 ENZYME-SENSITIVE CARBON-BASED NANO-THERANOSTICS

Enzymes are essential to several biological processes. In pathological situations, enzyme expression is likely to differ from the norm. Monitoring variations in enzyme expression is one of the most popular methods used in modern medicine for evaluating diseases. Alkaline phosphatase activity is significantly up in a variety of bone malignancies, whereas g-glutamyl transpeptidase levels are elevated in a variety of cancers, including liver cancer, cervical cancer, and ovarian cancer. Utilizing enzyme expression levels and drug activation for targeted imaging of tumor cells is, therefore, a viable strategy. Using substrates to construct highly selective enzyme probes is a versatile and efficient strategy. Since enzyme substrates, fluorophores, and chemotherapeutic drugs may be incorporated into a single, minute molecule, theranostic reagents can give increased specificity for enzyme detection and drug release upon activation [44].

Lu et al. 2021 created a novel albumin-binding prodrug (Mal-glu-SN38) that uses a self-immolation linker to connect a glucuronide trigger with an albumin-binding group. Mal-glu-SN38, when administered intravenously, establishes a covalent connection with human serum albumin *in-vivo* by Michael addition, extending its half-life in circulation. Because tumor tissue preferentially absorbs albumin, the concentration of Mal-glu-SN38 rises in the microenvironment of the tumor. Mal-glu-SN38 strictly releases SN38 when it detects a high concentration of -glucuronidase in tumor tissue, allowing for imaging monitoring of tumor tissue while exhibiting cytotoxicity; this combines diagnosis and treatment. As a result of Mal-glu-SN38's targeting effect and prolonged half-life, tumors in the HCT116 xenograft model shrunk or vanished following treatment [45].

Resistance to anticancer drugs is a big worry; however, Sharma et al. (2018) demonstrated another instance of a prodrug C1 with lower resistance [46]. The prodrug C1 is composed of triphenylphosphonium (TPP), doxorubicin (Dox), and dichloroacetic acid (DCA). The prodrug functions by activating the mitochondrial TPP enzyme. DCA may reprogram metabolism, inhibit drug-resistance-related pyruvate dehydrogenase (PDH) and pyruvate dehydrogenase kinase (PDK), and decrease the development of tumor cells by lowering their generation of glycolytic by-products by entering mitochondria. By creating an amide link between DCA and Dox, the release period of the medicine might be prolonged. The released Dox enters the mitochondria and, ultimately, the nucleus, where it exerts its anticancer effects. By producing a variety of control molecules, the researchers could assess the properties of the prodrug. The prodrug has strong anticancer activity in both human cancer cells and xenograft tumor models resistant to Dox.

9.5.3 OTHER BIOLOGICAL STIMULI-RESPONSIVE NANO-THERANOSTICS

Nano-theranostics based on additional biomolecules associated with tumors, such as ATP, H2S, and NO, have also been developed. ATP is an essential biomolecule in metabolism, the primary energy source for every live cell in the body. The extracellular concentration of ATP in the TME is $100-500 \times 10^{-6}$ M, which is 10^3-10^4 fold higher than that in normal tissues ($10-100 \times 10^{-9}$ M) and is necessary to sustain the rapidly developing tumor. Thus, it is vital to image ATP in cancer cells to investigate its pathogenic roles. Tumors might be diagnosed with greater accuracy, and new avenues for treating the disease could be discovered with ultrasensitive monitoring of extracellular ATP. Using a UV light-activatable DNA aptamer probe and lanthanide-doped UCNPs, Li et al. developed a luminescence-activated DNA nanodevice for ATP detection in live cells [47]. DNA complementary to the aptamer strand first fixed it in place. This complementary DNA included a group that could be activated by UV light. The photoactivatable-inhibitor carrying the quencher then binds to an aptamer strand conjugated to the Cy3 fluorophore, resulting from the closeness between Cy3 and the quencher, a known phenomenon as FRET occurs, resulting in a decreased FL intensity. The nanodevice is UV light-activatable because the photocleavable (PC) inhibitor and aptamer hybrid cannot respond with ATP until the PC-inhibitor is photolysis. After being exposed to UV light, the PC group breaks down and releases little snippets of DNA that the PC-inhibitor has a more challenging time adhering to than before. The dissolved PC-inhibitor is then released from the aptamer strand in the presence of ATP, leading to a dramatic uptick in FL intensity. Therefore, the UCNPs in the Apt-Act/UCNPs nanodevice serves as the UV-activatable light and cause the DNA probe to be remotely activated by NIR irradiation penetrating deeply into tissue. The nano-theranostics drug performed well for NIR-activated ATP imaging in both live cells and *in-vivo* [48].

Concentrations of H_2S between 0.3 and 3.4 mmol/L have an essential role in colon cancer and its related diseases. Due to this, several H_2S probes and treatments for the detection of colon cancer have been developed [49]. Cu_2O has been utilized as an

H$_2$S-stimulated turn-on theranostic with diagnostic and therapeutic characteristics to react with H$_2$S generated naturally by the body. Cu$_2$O lacks NIR absorption, so it cannot be utilized as a PTT. However, copper sulfide is formed when Cu$_2$O reaches the colon tumor site and reacts with endogenous H$_2$S; this molecule has a high NIR absorption and may be employed for PAI and PTT [48].

9.6 SUMMARY

The unique physicochemical properties of nano-theranostics have made significant strides in the past decade, presenting an excellent opportunity to enhance the identification and treatment efficacy of malignant tumors. Drug loading, imaging, and complimentary combination therapy are several applications of this innovative technology. In addition, stimulus-responsive nanomaterials that may be noninvasively modulated by exogenous/endogenous stimuli, resulting in on-demand tumor theranostics, have garnered considerable interest. This chapter has described several nanomaterials and discussed how they respond to external or internal stimuli. These delicate nanoconstructs make possible the capacity to diagnose, plan, and administer therapy. Unfortunately, there are still difficulties to overcome before semiconductor nanoparticles may be employed to treat cancers using theranostics. Despite this, stimulus-responsive nanomaterials will have broader biomedical applications and greater clinical translational value for tumor-specific theranostics due to the rapid development of nanotechnology, the inheritance of medical engineering, and the invention of new medical engineering techniques. In numerous *in-vitro* biomedical applications, such as *in-vitro* diagnostics, sensors, and probes, the toxicity of carbon-based nanoparticles is not the primary concern. As our knowledge improves and better nanoparticles are synthesized, more variety of intelligent nanoparticles may be utilized extensively in biomedicine.

REFERENCES

[1] T. Takagi, A concept of intelligent materials, J. Intell. Mater. Syst. Struct. 1 (1990) 149–156. doi:10.1177/1045389X9000100201.

[2] M. Aflori, Smart nanomaterials for biomedical applications—a review, Nanomater. (Basel). 11 (2021) 396. doi:10.3390/nano11020396.

[3] V.P. Torchilin, Fundamentals of stimuli-responsive drug and gene delivery systems, in: Stimuli-Responsive Drug Delivery Systems, Royal Society of Chemistry (2018): pp. 1–32. https://pubs.rsc.org/en/content/chapter/bk9781788013536-00001/978-1-78801-113-6.

[4] H. Fatima, M.Y. Naz, S. Shukrullah, H. Aslam, S. Ullah, M.A. Assiri, A review of multifunction smart nanoparticle based drug delivery systems, Curr. Pharm. Design. 28 (n.d.) 2965–2983.

[5] V. Torchilin, Multifunctional and stimuli-sensitive pharmaceutical nanocarriers, Eur. J. Pharm. Biopharm. 71 (2009) 431–444. doi:10.1016/j.ejpb.2008.09.026.

[6] K. Kuperkar, D. Patel, L.I. Atanase, P. Bahadur, Amphiphilic block copolymers: Their structures, and self-assembly to polymeric micelles and polymersomes as drug delivery vehicles, Polym. 14 (2022) 4702. doi:10.3390/polym14214702.

[7] H. Liu, T. Prachyathipsakul, T. M. Koyasseril-Yehiya, S. P. Le, S. Thayumanavan, Molecular bases for temperature sensitivity in supramolecular assemblies and their applications as thermoresponsive soft materials, Mater. Horizons. 9 (2022) 164–193. doi:10.1039/D1MH01091C.

[8] D. Dorniani, B. Saifullah, F. Barahuie, P. Arulselvan, M.Z.B. Hussein, S. Fakurazi, L.J. Twyman, Graphene oxide-gallic acid nanodelivery system for cancer therapy, Nanoscale Res. Lett. 11 (2016) 491. doi:10.1186/s11671-016-1712-2.

[9] A.D. Sontakke, R. Fopase, L.M. Pandey, M.K. Purkait, Development of graphene oxide nanoscrolls imparted nano-delivery system for the sustained release of gallic acid, Appl Nanosci. 12 (2022) 2733–2751. doi:10.1007/s13204-022-02582-8.

[10] S.P. Dunuweera, R.M.S.I. Rajapakse, R.B.S.D. Rajapakshe, S.H.D.P. Wijekoon, M.G.G.S.N. Thilakarathna, R.M.G. Rajapakse, Review on targeted drug delivery carriers used in nanobiomedical applications, Curr. Nanosci. 15 (n.d.) 382–397. doi:10.2174/157 3413714666181106114247.

[11] S. Ghosh, P. Jayaram, S.P. Kabekkodu, K. Satyamoorthy, Targeted drug delivery in cervical cancer: Current perspectives, Eur. J. Pharmacol. 917 (2022) 174751. doi:10.1016/j. ejphar.2022.174751.

[12] A. Tewabe, A. Abate, M. Tamrie, A. Seyfu, E. Abdela Siraj, Targeted drug delivery— from magic bullet to nanomedicine: Principles, challenges, and future perspectives, J. Multidiscip. Healthc. 14 (2021) 1711–1724. doi:10.2147/JMDH.S313968.

[13] M.P. Patel, R.R. Patel, J.K. Patel, Chitosan mediated targeted drug delivery system: A review, J. Pharm. Pharm. Sci. 13 (2010) 536–557. doi:10.18433/J3JC7C.

[14] E. Bhargav, N. Madhuri, K. Ramesh, A. Manne, V. Ravi, Targeted drug delivery-a review, World J. Pharm. Pharm. Sci. 3 (2013).

[15] Thakur, A. Roy, S. Chatterjee, P. Chakraborty, P. Mahata, Recent Trends in Targeted Drug Delivery, SM Group (2015): p. 29. doi:10.13140/RG.2.1.2443.9762.

[16] M.K. Jaiswal, A. Pradhan, R. Banerjee, D. Bahadur, Dual pH and temperature stimuli-responsive magnetic nanohydrogels for thermo-chemotherapy, J. Nanosci. Nanotechnol. 14 (2014) 4082–4089. doi:10.1166/jnn.2014.8662.

[17] P. Mondal, N.S. Samanta, A. Kumar, M.K. Purkait, Recovery of H2SO4 from wastewater in the presence of NaCl and KHCO3 through pH responsive polysulfone membrane: Optimization approach, Polym. Tes. 86 (2020) 106463. doi:10.1016/j. polymertesting.2020.106463.

[18] P.A. Lund, D. De Biase, O. Liran, O. Scheler, N.P. Mira, Z. Cetecioglu, E.N. Fernández, S. Bover-Cid, R. Hall, M. Sauer, C. O'Byrne, Understanding how microorganisms respond to acid pH is central to their control and successful exploitation, Front. Microbiol. 11 (2020). https://www.frontiersin.org/articles/10.3389/fmicb.2020.556140 (accessed December 2, 2022).

[19] M.R. Aguilar, J.S. Román, Smart Polymers and Their Applications, Woodhead Publishing, Cambridge (2019).

[20] X. Li, B.-Y. Zheng, M.-R. Ke, Y. Zhang, J.-D. Huang, J. Yoon, A Tumor-pH-responsive supramolecular photosensitizer for activatable photodynamic therapy with minimal in vivo skin phototoxicity, Theranostics. 7 (2017) 2746–2756. doi:10.7150/thno.18861.

[21] K.-Y. Ju, J. Kang, J. Pyo, J. Lim, J. Ho Chang, J.-K. Lee, pH-Induced aggregated melanin nanoparticles for photoacoustic signal amplification, Nanoscale. 8 (2016) 14448–14456. doi:10.1039/C6NR02294D.

[22] M. Constantin, S. Bucătariu, I. Stoica, G. Fundueanu, Smart nanoparticles based on pullulan-g-poly(N-isopropylacrylamide) for controlled delivery of indomethacin, Int. J. Biol. Macromol. 94 (2017) 698–708. doi:10.1016/j.ijbiomac.2016.10.064.

[23] I. Bonadies, F. Di Cristo, A. Valentino, G. Peluso, A. Calarco, A. Di Salle, pH-Responsive resveratrol-loaded electrospun membranes for the prevention of implant-associated infections, Nanomater. 10 (2020) 1175. doi:10.3390/nano10061175.

[24] Y. Cao, P. Rewatkar, R. Wang, S.Z. Hasnain, A. Popat, T. Kumeria, Nanocarriers for oral delivery of biologics: Small carriers for big payloads, Trends Pharmacol. Sci. 42 (2021) 957–972. doi:10.1016/j.tips.2021.08.005.

[25] J.-Y. Zhang, X.-X. Liu, J.-Y. Lin, X.-Y. Bao, J.-Q. Peng, Z.-P. Gong, X. Luan, Y. Chen, Biomimetic engineered nanocarriers inspired by viruses for oral-drug delivery, Int. J. Pharm. 624 (2022) 121979. doi:10.1016/j.ijpharm.2022.121979.

[26] U. Agrawal, R. Sharma, M. Gupta, S.P. Vyas, Is nanotechnology a boon for oral drug delivery? Drug Discov. Today. 19 (2014) 1530–1546. doi:10.1016/j.drudis.2014.04.011.

[27] M. Mozafari, Nanoengineered Biomaterials for Advanced Drug Delivery, Elsevier, Cambridge (2020).

[28] S. Maghrebi, C.A. Prestidge, P. Joyce, An update on polymer-lipid hybrid systems for improving oral drug delivery, Expert Opin. Drug Deliv. 16 (2019) 507–524. doi:10.1080/17425247.2019.1605353.

[29] I.C. Gonçalves, P.C. Henriques, C.L. Seabra, M.C.L. Martins, The potential utility of chitosan micro/nanoparticles in the treatment of gastric infection, Expert Rev. Anti Infect. Ther. 12 (2014) 981–992. doi:10.1586/14787210.2014.930663.

[30] S.K. Yandrapu, P. Kanujia, K.B. Chalasani, L. Mangamoori, R.V. Kolapalli, A. Chauhan, Development and optimization of thiolated dendrimer as a viable mucoadhesive excipient for the controlled drug delivery: An acyclovir model formulation, Nanomed. Nanotechnol. Biol. Med. 9 (2013) 514–522. doi:10.1016/j.nano.2012.10.005.

[31] L. Zhang, S. Wang, M. Zhang, J. Sun, Nanocarriers for oral drug delivery, J. Drug Target. 21 (2013) 515–527. doi:10.3109/1061186X.2013.789033.

[32] K. Kohli, S. Chopra, D. Dhar, S. Arora, R.K. Khar, Self-emulsifying drug delivery systems: An approach to enhance oral bioavailability, Drug Discov. Today. 15 (2010) 958–965. doi:10.1016/j.drudis.2010.08.007.

[33] N.V. Solodkov, J. Shim, J.C. Jones, Self-assembly of fractal liquid crystal colloids, Nat. Commun. 10 (2019) 198. doi:10.1038/s41467-018-08210-w.

[34] N. Poonia, R. Kharb, V. Lather, D. Pandita, Nanostructured lipid carriers: Versatile oral delivery vehicle, Future Sci. OA. 2 (2016) FSO135. doi:10.4155/fsoa-2016-0030.

[35] M.-J. Park, P. Balakrishnan, S.-G. Yang, Polymeric nanocapsules with SEDDS oil-core for the controlled and enhanced oral absorption of cyclosporine, Int. J. Pharm. 441 (2013) 757–764. doi:10.1016/j.ijpharm.2012.10.018.

[36] C. Prego, D. Torres, E. Fernandez-Megia, R. Novoa-Carballal, E. Quiñoá, M.J. Alonso, Chitosan–PEG nanocapsules as new carriers for oral peptide delivery: Effect of chitosan pegylation degree, J. Con. Rel. 111 (2006) 299–308. doi:10.1016/j.jconrel.2005.12.015.

[37] S. Zhang, B. Zhao, H. Jiang, B. Wang, B. Ma, Cationic lipids and polymers mediated vectors for delivery of siRNA, J. Con. Rel. 123 (2007) 1–10. doi:10.1016/j.jconrel.2007.07.016.

[38] H. Piao, M. Ouyang, D. Xia, P. Quan, W. Xiao, Y. Song, F. Cui, In vitro–in vivo study of CoQ10-loaded lipid nanoparticles in comparison with nanocrystals, Int. J. Pharm. 419 (2011) 255–259. doi:10.1016/j.ijpharm.2011.07.016.

[39] A.A. Bhirde, V. Patel, J. Gavard, G. Zhang, A.A. Sousa, A. Masedunskas, R.D. Leapman, R. Weigert, J.S. Gutkind, J.F. Rusling, Targeted killing of cancer cells in vivo and in vitro with EGF-directed carbon nanotube-based drug delivery, ACS Nano. 3 (2009) 307–316. doi:10.1021/nn800551s.

[40] M.-K. Lai, C.-Y. Chang, Y.-W. Lien, R.C.-C. Tsiang, Application of gold nanoparticles to microencapsulation of thioridazine, J. Con. Rel. 111 (2006) 352–361. doi:10.1016/j.jconrel.2005.12.017.

[41] A. Singh, M. Amiji (Eds.), Stimuli-Responsive Drug Delivery Systems, The Royal Society of Chemistry, Cambridge (2018). doi:10.1039/9781788013536-00109.

[42] S. Joshi-Barr, C. de Gracia Lux, E. Mahmoud, A. Almutairi, Exploiting oxidative microenvironments in the body as triggers for drug delivery systems, Antioxid. Redox. Signal. 21 (2014) 730–754. doi:10.1089/ars.2013.5754.

[43] X. Yu, M. Lu, Y. Luo, Y. Hu, Y. Zhang, Z. Xu, S. Gong, Y. Wu, X.-N. Ma, B.-Y. Yu, J. Tian, A cancer-specific activatable theranostic nanodrug for enhanced therapeutic efficacy via amplification of oxidative stress, Theranostics. 10 (2020) 371–383. doi:10.7150/thno.39412.

[44] X. Rong, C. Liu, X. Li, H. Zhu, K. Wang, B. Zhu, Recent advances in chemotherapy-based organic small molecule theranostic reagents, Coord. Chem. Rev. 473 (2022) 214808. doi:10.1016/j.ccr.2022.214808.

[45] Y. Huang, L. Wang, Z. Cheng, B. Yang, J. Yu, Y. Chen, W. Lu, SN38-based albumin-binding prodrug for efficient targeted cancer chemotherapy, J. Con. Rel. 339 (2021) 297–306. doi:10.1016/j.jconrel.2021.09.040.

[46] A. Sharma, M.-G. Lee, H. Shi, M. Won, J.F. Arambula, J.L. Sessler, J.Y. Lee, S.-G. Chi, J.S. Kim, Overcoming drug resistance by targeting cancer bioenergetics with an activatable prodrug, Chem. 4 (2018) 2370–2383. doi:10.1016/j.chempr.2018.08.002.

[47] J. Zhao, J. Gao, W. Xue, Z. Di, H. Xing, Y. Lu, L. Li, Upconversion luminescence-activated DNA nanodevice for ATP sensing in living cells, J. Am. Chem. Soc. 140 (2018) 578–581. doi:10.1021/jacs.7b11161.

[48] X. Hu, E. Ha, F. Ai, X. Huang, L. Yan, S. He, S. Ruan, J. Hu, Stimulus-responsive inorganic semiconductor nanomaterials for tumor-specific theranostics, Coord. Chem. Rev. 473 (2022) 214821. doi:10.1016/j.ccr.2022.214821.

[49] L. An, X. Wang, X. Rui, J. Lin, H. Yang, Q. Tian, C. Tao, S. Yang, The in situ sulfidation of Cu2O by endogenous H2S for colon cancer theranostics, Angew. Chem. Int. Ed. 57 (2018) 15782–15786. doi:10.1002/anie.201810082.

10 Toxicological Studies of Carbon-Based Nanocarriers

10.1 AN OVERVIEW OF TOXICOLOGICAL STUDIES

The growing needs of various fields, including industry, medicine, agriculture, and electronics, have led to the rapid development of nanotechnology [1]. Among nanotechnology products, carbon-based nanomaterials hold great promise due to their unique properties, which make them suitable for a wide range of applications, such as drug delivery and others [2]. Carbon nanomaterials come in different forms, such as carbon nanotubes (CNTs), carbon black nanoparticles, fibers, fullerenes, and other related structures [3]. For instance, carbon black (CB) nanoparticles have a grape-like morphology consisting of highly fused spherical particles and are considered traditional carbonaceous nanomaterials. Additionally, carbon black is a quasi-graphitic form of pure elemental carbon and is a significant contributor to ambient air pollution [4]. Carbonaceous nanomaterials come in various forms, each with a unique shape. C-fullerenes, for instance, have symmetrical closed-cage structures that resemble a soccer ball and consist of 60 carbon atoms [5]. On the other hand, CNTs are fibrous materials with needle-like shapes and high aspect ratios, sharing similarities with asbestos fibers. They exist in two primary forms, single-wall CNTs (SWCNTs) and multiwall CNTs (MWCNTs), and can take on various derived structures such as horns, loops, and peapods. Horn-shaped single-wall carbon nanohorns (SWCNHs) with cone angles of approximately 20° are synthesized by laser ablation and are essentially metal-free with high purity [6]. Another type of carbonaceous nanomaterial, nanographite (NG) or graphite nanoplatelets, is a two-dimensional sheet of sp^2-bonded carbon atoms, just one atom thick.

Graphene is the most essential element of the graphene-based nanomaterials (GBNs) family, which also comprises few-layer graphene (FLG), graphene oxide (GO), reduced GO (rGO), and nano GO (NGO). Although FLG is commonly referred to as graphene, it is composed of 2–10 stacked layers of graphene and was initially developed as a by-product of the synthesis of graphene [7]. Graphene is formed of a monolayer nanosheet with oxygenated functional groups, including hydroxyl, carboxyl, and epoxide groups, all over its edges and surface in its oxidized state, known as GO. Utilizing chemical and thermal processing in reducing conditions, GO can be reduced to rGO, which has a lower oxygen content. NGO, sometimes known as graphene nanosheets on occasion, is the term for GO having a lateral dimension of less than 100 nm.

DOI: 10.1201/9781003358114-10

The distinctive physicochemical characteristics of graphene have sparked an unprecedented surge in its interest among scientists since it was discovered in 2004 [7,8]. Many studies and demonstrations of the application of graphene in nanoelectronics, material science, and engineering have lately been conducted. [9,10]. Nevertheless, GO, a type of graphene that has undergone oxidation, has lately come to light as having significant potential in the biomedical field. Graphene and GBN have already investigated a variety of biological applications, including drug transport, tissue engineering, biosensing, disease diagnostics, cancer targeting, photothermal therapy (PTT), etc., despite this recent surge in interest [11,12].

Similarly, the carbon and graphene quantum dots, in addition to structurally modified forms of graphene such as nanoscrolls, nano-onions, and nanorods, are also part of the discussion in biomedical applications owing to their superior surface characteristics, colloidal stability, higher surface area, aspect-ratio, and drug loading capacity. Overall, it was observed that the carbon-based nanocarriers had demonstrated their potential for biomedical applications, including drug delivery, bioimaging and biosensing, tissue engineering, and gene therapy. However, the main issue impeding the widespread use of these nanocarriers is their "toxicity." Researchers typically struggle to balance the negative effects caused by carbon-based nanomaterials' toxicity with the compound's possible therapeutic effects. Thus, choosing an experimental paradigm for *in-vivo* or *in-vitro* conditions is essential for determining the toxicity of these nanomaterials. Till now, numerous studies have investigated the toxicological aspects of carbon-based nanocarriers, including graphene, GO, CNTs, fullerene, and quantum dots. This chapter mainly focuses on the toxicological aspects of these nanocarriers.

10.2 NANO-TOXICOLOGY OF CARBONACEOUS MATERIALS

Nanoscale naturally occurring and manufactured carbonaceous materials can be found in various sizes ranging from 1 to 100 nm. They can be emitted during specific combustion processes, like the combustion of methane and propane [13]. Several studies have assessed the health effects of exposure to carbon nanomaterials in occupational and environmental settings [14]. Research into the effects of air pollution and mineral dust particles has revealed that inhaling particles smaller than 100 nm in size can result in lung injury by generating reactive oxygen species (ROS), cell damage, and inflammation [15]. *In-vitro* models for cytotoxicity evaluation in animal studies have been developed to eliminate a few variables to obtain better experimental outcomes. Various cell types have been studied to evaluate the harmful effects of carbon nanoparticles, with macrophages being the most studied as the first line of defense against foreign particles. Previous studies have reported multiple toxic effects of carbon nanomaterials, such as DNA damage, ROS generation, mitochondrial dysfunction, lysosomal damage, and eventual cell death [16].

The dissimilarities in the physicochemical characteristics or configurations of carbon nanomaterials, as well as the types of cells under consideration and the techniques employed for particle dispersion, could be some of the factors that lead to varying outcomes regarding the cytotoxicity of materials based on carbon. Although carbon-based nanomaterials have been found to be toxic to cells, their immunological effects have been extensively investigated. The immune system, which is responsible for detecting foreign agents and initiating immune responses, is composed of innate and adaptive immune systems. The innate immune system is the first line of defense, employing the complement system and phagocytic cells. In contrast, the adaptive immune system utilizes specific, long-lasting mechanisms mediated by T and B lymphocytes [17]. Concerning the immunological effects of carbon-based nanomaterials, the activation of pulmonary macrophages and the induction of inflammation have been thoroughly examined. Furthermore, the potential entry of nanoparticles (NPs) into various parts of the human body, such as the lungs, cardiovascular system, liver, and even the brain, through inhalation, has led to the characterization of other harmful effects of carbon nanomaterials *in-vivo* [18]. The toxicity of NPs toward biological systems may stem from their small size, large surface area, and reactivity [19]. For instance, studies have shown that single-wall carbon nanotubes (SWCNTs) can cause acute and chronic pulmonary pathologies and damage the blood chemistry, liver, and cardiovascular system [20]. It is noteworthy that ultrafine particles have the ability to cross the alveolar-capillary barrier and enter the bloodstream. When SWCNTs are injected intravenously, they can penetrate the blood-brain barrier and reach the brain, as evidenced by research [21]. Additionally, the interaction between CNTs and the components of the immune system should be given special consideration. Although a significant amount of research has been conducted in the last ten years to reveal the immunological characteristics of carbon-based nanomaterials, there are still numerous unanswered questions due to the intricate nature of the immune defense mechanisms.

10.2.1 TOXICITY OF GRAPHENE AND GRAPHENE OXIDE-BASED NANOMATERIALS

10.2.1.1 Graphene—*In-Vitro* Mammalian Cell Toxicity

A study conducted on neuronal PC12 cells using the MTT assay and the LDH release assay to evaluate mitochondrial toxicity and cell membrane integrity found that the shape of graphene and SWCNT influenced their biological activities [22]. The research findings showed that when PC12 cells were exposed for 24 hours, the metabolic activity decreased in a way that was dependent on the dose; it was observed that graphene induced higher toxicity at low concentrations but lower toxicity at high concentrations compared to SWCNT. Graphene tested at the highest concentration (100 mg/mL) led to a significant increase in LDH release and reactive oxygen species (ROS) generation. Moreover, the activation of caspase 3 suggested that graphene caused a time-dependent rise in apoptosis when administered at a concentration of 10 mg/mL. Yuan et al. (2011) conducted a study to compare the potential cytotoxicity of graphene and SWCNT on the human hepatoma HepG2 cell line at the proteome level [23]. To analyze the cellular functions of HepG2 cells exposed to graphene and SWCNT, the researchers utilized the isobaric-tagged relative and absolute quantification-coupled two-dimensional liquid chromatography-based mass spectrometry (iTRAQ-2D LC-MS/MS) approach. In general, exposure to 1 mg/mL of either nanomaterial led to the altered expression of 37 proteins linked to metabolic pathways, cytoskeleton formation, redox regulation, and cell growth. Notably, graphene caused more moderate changes in protein levels compared to SWCNT.

A noteworthy discovery was that the expression of calcium-binding proteins exhibited different patterns when exposed to graphene and SWCNT, implying that their mechanisms of action were distinct.

Subsequently, graphene pristine in nature was discovered for ROS increase and induced apoptosis in murine RAW 264.7 macrophages, which are crucial effector cells of the innate immune system [24]. This was thought to be due to the depletion of mitochondrial membrane potential (MMP) and the activation of the mitochondrial pathway triggered by ROS. According to this research, the involvement of both mitogen-activated protein kinases and transforming growth factor-b (TGF-b) related signaling pathways was associated with the toxicity of macrophages treated with pristine graphene. The effect of graphene platelets on human glioblastoma U87 and U118 cells was investigated, with a focus on cell morphology, mortality, viability, membrane integrity, and the type of cell death [25]. Graphene platelets were found to localize near the cells but did not penetrate them. Treatment with 100 µg/mL of graphene platelets for 24 hours caused approximately 50% of the cells to die, lose membrane integrity, and undergo apoptosis. Additionally, when exposed to layered graphene platelets with one to ten layers at concentrations ≥5 µg/cm², immortalized human acute monocytic leukemia cells (THP-1) showed a significant increase in LDH release, indicating loss of membrane integrity. The exposure to graphene platelets also resulted in a decrease in reduced glutathione levels and an increase in the expression of various cytokines, including monocyte chemotactic protein-1, interleukin-1, macrophage inflammatory protein-1R, and IL-1b.

10.2.1.2   Graphene oxide—*In-vitro* mammalian cell toxicity

In-vitro toxicity studies have extensively investigated GO as a member of GFNs. Although the initial comprehensive study on GO toxicity did not show any apparent effects on cellular uptake or mortality, viability, morphology, and membrane integrity in adenocarcinomic human alveolar basal epithelial (A549) cells, exposure to GO was found to induce oxidative stress even at a low concentration of 10 mg/mL [26]. However, this is one of the few instances in which GO exhibited negative cytotoxicity in mammalian cells. A few months later, Hu et al. (2011) reported that GO caused concentration-dependent cytotoxicity in the same cell line, which could be significantly reduced by incubation with 10% fetal bovine serum, owing to GO's high protein adsorption capacity [27]. Subsequently, a wide range of human and animal cell lines, encompassing immortalized and normal cell lines, stem cells, immune cells, and blood components, have been explored to appraise the toxicity, genotoxicity, and underlying mechanisms of GO.

The toxicity of GO has been studied in immortalized cells, specifically in the HepG2 cell line. Lammel et al. (2013) examined the cytotoxicity of GO at concentrations ranging from 1 to 16 µg/mL using four assays: 5-carboxyfluorescein diacetate-acetoxymethyl ester (CFDA-AM), Alamar blue assay, neutral red uptake assay, and fluorescamine assay [28]. The CFDA-AM assay showed a dose-dependent decrease in fluorescence intensity, beginning at 4 µg/mL, indicating damage to the plasma membrane. The strong physical interaction between GO and the phospholipid bilayer was responsible for the loss of structural integrity of the plasma membrane, as per findings. It was further observed through TEM and scanning electron micrographs that GO could penetrate the plasma membrane, causing changes in cell morphology and an increase in the count of apoptotic cells. Moreover, the increased ROS levels at concentrations as low as 1 µg/mL and dose-dependent depletion of the MMP suggested that impaired mitochondrial function may result in intracellular ROS formation. The authors concluded that plasma membrane damage and oxidative stress are crucial factors in GO-induced cytotoxicity based on the modes of action assessed.

In another study, Yuan et al. (2012) utilized iTRAQ-2D LC-MS/MS to evaluate the cytotoxicity of GO and oxidized SWCNT in HepG2 cells, aiming to characterize cellular function [29]. Similar to their prior research, treatment with 1 µg/mL of both GO and oxidized SWCNT led to changes in protein expression involved in metabolic pathways, redox regulation, cytoskeleton formation, and cell growth, with GO inducing fewer alterations in expression than oxidized SWCNTs. A study compared the cytotoxicity of GO-1 and its repeated $KMnO_4$-H_2SO_4 oxidation products, GO-2 and GO-3, in HeLa cells using the MTT assay, revealing that GO treatment only caused a slight reduction in proliferation rate and slightly perturbed cell cycle, and led to an increase in intracellular ROS levels. GO was found to be less cytotoxic in HepG2 cells. The lateral sizes of GO-1, GO-2, and GO-3 were reported to be 205.8 nm, 146.8 nm, and 33.78 nm, respectively [30]. At concentrations ranging from 20 to 100 µg/mL, GO-1 induced considerable cytotoxicity, while GO-2 and GO-3 exhibited higher cell viability with enhanced cellular uptake in HeLa cells, indicating that larger GO sizes inflicted more damage to the cell membrane compared to smaller GOs, according to a study. Another study also found dose-dependent toxicity of GO in HeLa cells, albeit with a lower cell uptake ratio than CNT and nanodiamonds [31]. Moreover, GO toxicity was observed in human neuroblastoma SH-SY5Y cells at concentrations ≥80 µg/mL [32].

GO toxicity has also been reported in BEAS-2B human lung cells as well as in the HBI.F3 human neural stem cell line. In BEAS-2B cells, the MTT assay showed a significant decrease in cell viability in a concentration- and time-dependent manner at concentrations ranging from 10 to 100 µg/mL, along with an increase in both early and late apoptotic cells compared to the control [33]. Similarly, HBI.F3 cell viability decreased with increasing GO nano pellet concentration (25–200 µg/mL), as verified by both the MTT assay and differential pulse voltammetry, which is a microscopic imaging tool [34].

Compared to previous research, GO was found to have minimal toxicity in spontaneously arising human retinal pigment epithelium (ARPE-19) cells. Various methods, including optical micrography, LDH assay, the CCK-8 assay, and apoptosis assay, were used to measure toxicity in terms of viability, cell morphology, and membrane integrity [35]. According to a study, the cells were not affected by the addition of up to 100 mg/mL GO for 72 hours, but some changes in cell morphology were observed after seven days of culture with GO. The release of LDH by less than 8% of cells at all concentrations suggested minimal damage to the cell membrane. Therefore, the study indicates that GO has favorable biocompatibility with retinal pigment epithelium cells and causes only minor effects on cell viability and morphology.

10.2.2 TOXIC EFFECTS OF CARBON NANOTUBES

Due to their unique physicochemical properties, CNTs have proven useful in many biomedical applications. The population has also been exposed to more CNTs and CNT-based nanocomposites as a result of improvements in their use across a range of industries. Although CNTs have several uses, "their toxicity" is the main issue preventing their widespread use. Researchers frequently struggle to balance the negative effects caused by CNTs' toxicity with the possible therapeutic effects of these materials. To determine the toxicity of this nanomaterial, it is essential to choose an experimental paradigm, whether it be *in-vitro* or *in-vivo* [36]. Various variables, including size, surface charge, administration method, dosage concentration, and exposure duration, influence the toxicity of CNTs. In addition to the previously mentioned parameters, the incubating circumstances, such as the exposure dosage, culture period, and type of cell, also directly affect the toxicity of CNTs [37]. For their *in-vivo* biological uses, CNTs must first undergo cytotoxicity testing. The main outcomes of *in-vitro* experiments focused on cell uptake, cell viability, and ROS.

The cytotoxicity of carbon nanomaterials is closely associated with their size, shape, dosage, and surface characteristics. In line with this, Zhang et al. (2012) investigated the absorption and toxicity of HeLa cells by MWCNTs, nanodiamonds (ND), and graphene oxide (GO) [31]. Cellular absorption ratios for the three kinds of carbon nanomaterials were in the order ND > MWCNTs > GO. However, there was a poor correlation between the cytotoxicity of these compounds and the cellular uptake ratios. MWCNTs were taken up by cells more readily than GO, but no differences in their cytotoxicity were found. ND displayed more excellent biocompatibility with MWCNTs and GO. SWCNTs are thought to be more hazardous than MWCNTs, according to studies showing that the mass basis and dosages substantially impact the cytotoxicity of CNTs. The cell survival of HepG2 fibroblasts exposed to SWCNTs and graphene was examined by Yuan et al. (2011) [29]. As a result of activating P53-mediated degradation, the results showed that SWCNTs had a higher level of cytotoxicity, may have been able to produce oxidative stress, and finally triggered apoptosis [29].

Validating the biocompatibility of CNTs requires toxicological analysis *in-vivo* after cytotoxicity investigation. Biomedical studies typically use animal models, such as mice, zebrafish, and rats, to fully understand nanomaterials' dynamic behaviors and biocompatibility *in-vivo*. Some researchers have functionalized CNTs using biocompatible polymers and other biosafety chemicals to boost the biocompatibility of CNTs [36]. Positron emission tomography was used by Liu et al. (2007) to examine the *in-vivo* bioavailability of SWCNTs coupled with more accommodative and hydrophilic PEG [38]. The PEG-functionalized SWCNTs showed prolonged blood circulation times and low reticuloendothelial system absorption. Mice did not have any adverse side effects, such as fatigue or weight loss, and no clear toxicity-related conditions were found. SWCNTs were known to have a high level of cytotoxicity in the past; however, Xue et al. (2016) found that aggregated SWCNTs significantly lessened the behavioral and neurochemical effects of methamphetamine in mice [39]. Notably, at the dosage levels employed in the study, neither the striatum nor the midbrain displayed any signs of neuronal toxicity or the mice's normal behaviors, including eating, drinking, and moving around.

The tendency for oxidative stress, generation of free radicals, accumulation of peroxidative products, DNA fragmentation, and inflammation continue to be obstacles to the widespread use of CNTs in the treatment of neurological illnesses, despite repeated attempts to make them more biocompatible. The fundamental issue with employing CNTs as an intrinsic medicine for treating neurological disorders is their safety, particularly regarding brain ejection and disintegration. The functionalization of CNTs merits considerable research to increase the brain's breakdown and expulsion of CNTs.

10.2.3 Toxicology of Graphene Quantum Dots

To measure and evaluate the toxicity of living organisms, both *in-vitro* and *in-vivo* experiments are typically conducted in a laboratory setting shown in **Figure 10.1**. *In-vitro* tests utilize living cells from organisms as the test subjects. They are commonly referred to as "cytotoxicity" tests [40]. Conversely, *in-vivo* tests are performed on entire living organisms as the test subjects. The toxicity of GQDs, including both raw and doped varieties (such as nGQDs and bGQDs), has been investigated using both *in-vitro* and *in-vivo* methods. A variety of human and animal cells have been utilized in *in-vitro* testing. HeLa cells (cervical cancer cells) and A549 cells (lung carcinoma cells) are among the most extensively studied cell types, while MCF-7 cells (breast cancer cells), red blood cells, and stem cells have also been examined. In terms of *in-vivo* testing, mice, zebrafish, *Caenorhabditis elegans*, and green gram sprouts have all been used in these studies.

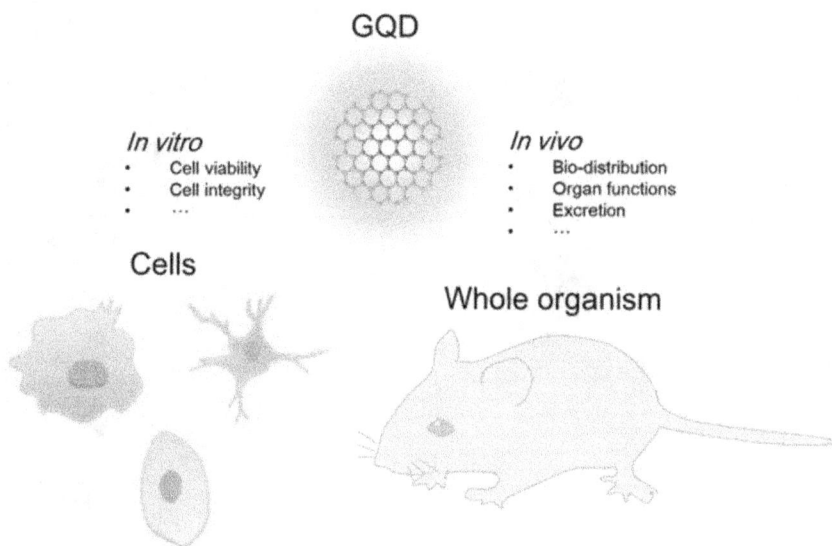

FIGURE 10.1 Schematic Explanation of *In-Vitro* and *In-Vivo* Tests [Reprinted with permission from *Wang et al. (2016)*] [40].

10.2.3.1 *In-Vitro* Toxicity Analysis of GQDs

In an *in-vitro* test, cell viability is commonly used to determine cytotoxicity (or *in-vitro* toxicity). Widely used assays such as MTT, LDH, or ATP are utilized to assess cell viability. The test substance is added to the cell culture, and the number of living cells before and after a specific incubation time (e.g., 24 hours) is measured. The ratio between these two numbers represents cell viability. In addition to cell viability, researchers also observe other indicators such as cell membrane damage, morphological changes, and the release of certain chemicals (such as lactate dehydrogenase (LDH), adenosine triphosphate (ATP), and lipid extracts) due to cell damage. **Figure 10.2** depicts the typical results of these cytotoxicity tests, which reveal that cell viability and the release of common chemicals from cells (such as LDH) are concentration-dependent [40]. As the concentration of GQDs increases, cell viability gradually decreases while chemical releases gradually increase. Wu et al. (2013) conducted an *in-vitro* toxicity assessment of graphene oxide (GO) and GQDs on MGC-803 (human gastric cancer) and MCF-7 cells (human breast cancer) using MTT assays. Their study demonstrated that GO is significantly more cytotoxic than GQDs [41].

Additionally, Nurunnabi et al. (2013) conducted a comparison of GQD cytotoxicity among three cancer cell lines: KB (epidermal cancer cells), MDA-MB231, and

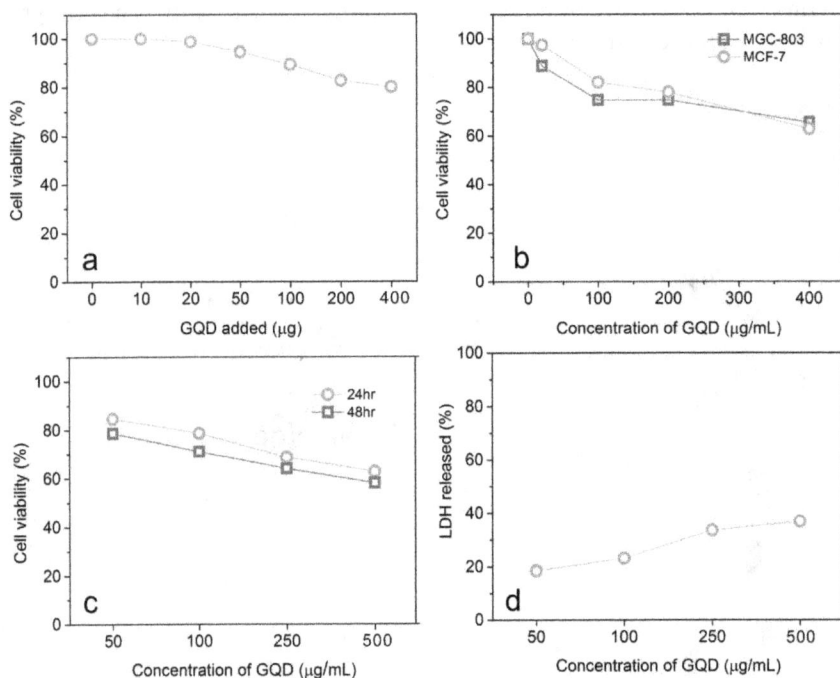

FIGURE 10.2 Examples of Results of *In-Vitro* Tests: (a) Cell Viability for MG-63 Cells, (b) Cell Viability of MCF-7 Cells and MGC-803 Cells, (c), and (d) Cell Viability and LDH Release of A549 Cancer Cells. [Reprinted with permission from *Wang et al. (2016)*] [40].

A549 [42]. Using yellow-emitting GQDs synthesized by Zhang et al. (2012), it is possible to image stem cells that are difficult to label with current technology [43]. In toxicity tests, the stem cells retained over 80% viability after being cultured with GQDs at a concentration of 100 mg mL^{-1} for 3 days. These results suggest that their GQDs exhibit low cytotoxicity and are a promising biocompatible agent for labeling stem cells. In addition to testing common GQDs, the cytotoxicity of chemically doped GQDs was also examined in studies such as those conducted by [44]. In their study, Wang et al. (2015) investigated the cytotoxicity of graphene oxide (GO) and nitrogen-doped GQDs on red blood cells (RBCs) [45]. They assessed hemolytic activity, morphological changes, and the release of ATP in RBCs after being separately exposed to GO and nGQDs. Their results showed that GO caused significant hemolysis and released ATP, whereas nGQDs did not cause similar damage to the RBCs. This indicates that nGQDs exhibit much lower cytotoxicity than GO. Hai et al. (2015) synthesized boron-doped GQDs and evaluated their biocompatibility with HeLa cells in their study [46]. In general, based on the majority of *in-vitro* toxicity tests conducted on different types of cells and GQDs, GQDs appear to have low cytotoxicity. However, evidence also suggests that the presence of the reactive oxygen species (ROS) mechanism, known to be a toxicity mechanism for other nanomaterials, is not entirely absent in GQDs [47]. Recent research on macrophages further demonstrated that GQDs could induce apoptosis and autophagy, possibly due to the generation of ROS.

Moreover, the study indicated that ROS's effect depends on the concentration of GQDs. It is worth mentioning that GQDs possess an intrinsic peroxidase-like catalytic activity, which can enhance the antibacterial performance of H$_2$O$_2$ for wound infections treatment [48]. Despite this, Wu et al. compared the intracellular reactive oxygen species (ROS) generated by GQDs and GO and found that the level of ROS induced by their GQDs is lower than that of GO [49]. However, this may not be adequate to eliminate concerns about cytotoxicity when dealing with certain types of GQDs or cells, particularly in situations with an extremely low tolerance for toxicity.

10.2.3.2 *In-Vivo* Toxicity Analysis of GQDs

To evaluate the *in-vivo* behavior of GQDs, a typical experiment involves injecting a specific dosage of GQDs into a living organism, such as a mouse, and monitoring its biodistribution, organic accumulation, and excretion over a period of time, typically 24 hours. Wu et al. (2013) were the first to report *in-vivo* work on GQDs, demonstrating their potential for *in-vivo* imaging of mice using bottom-up synthesized GQDs, but did not investigate their toxicity [41]. The first systematic *in-vivo* toxicity study was conducted by Nurunnabi et al. (2013), who examined the *in-vivo* imaging, biodistribution, and ex vivo organic imaging of cancer-bearing mice treated with GQDs synthesized from carbon fiber exfoliation [42]. The *in-vivo* imaging results indicate that GQDs could be detected in the skin tumor site 12 hours after injection but not in deeper organs, suggesting their potential for superficial tissue imaging (e.g., skin cancer detection). However, 24 hours after injection, no fluorescence signal was detected at the tumor site or any other part of the mouse's body (**Figure 10.3a**) [40]. The ex vivo imaging of extracted organs such as the kidney, liver, and heart revealed that GQDs were distributed throughout the entire body via the circulatory

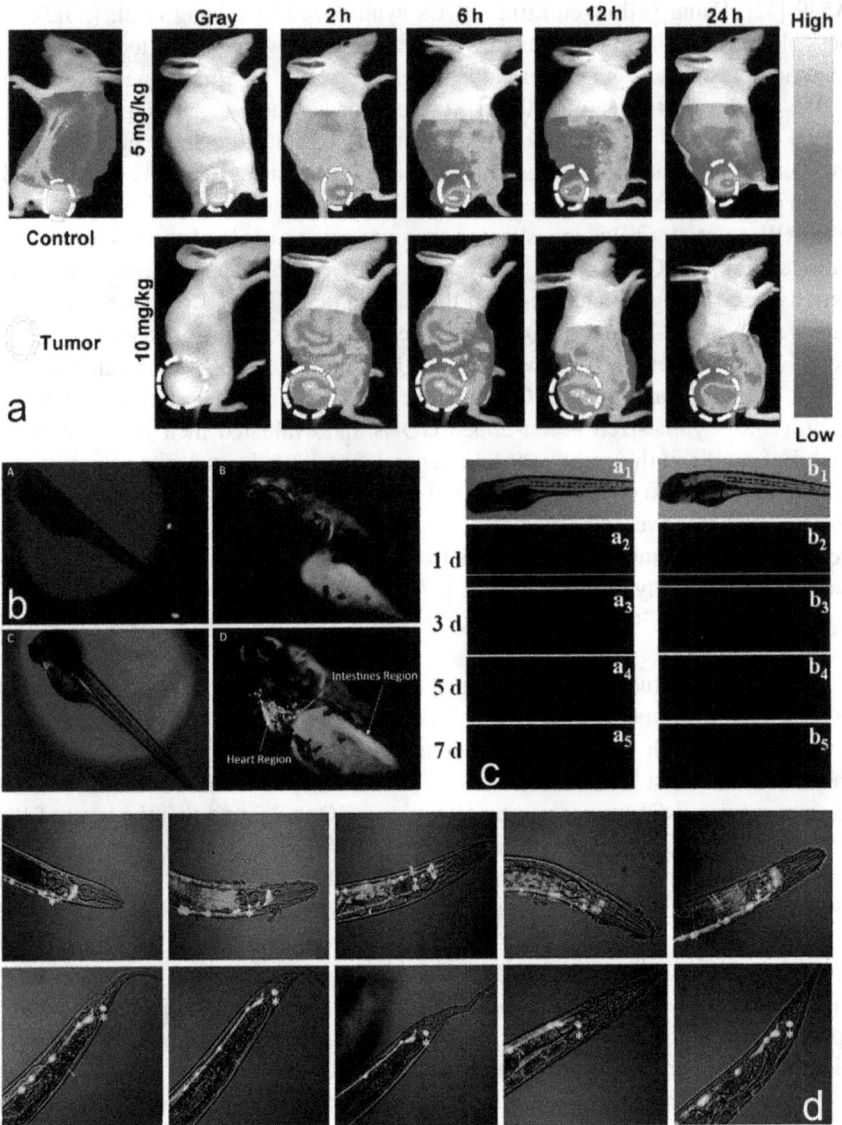

FIGURE 10.3 Example of *in-vivo* toxicity tests: (a) mice, (b) and (c) zebrafish, (d) *Caenorhabditis elegans*. [Reprinted with permission from *Wang et al. (2016)*] [40].

system within the first 12 hours, with accumulation varying in different organs. For instance, during the early stage (two hours), GQDs mainly accumulate in the liver and heart. The liver accumulation decreased gradually, and after 12 hours, a significant increase in kidney accumulation was observed. Generally, the fluorescence signal of GQDs weakened at 24 hours compared to 12 hours, indicating that GQDs can be easily eliminated through the excretory system. Using a rat model, the authors also conducted a comprehensive analysis of complete blood count, serum biochemistry, and histological analysis of tissues. The results showed no significant difference between the GQDs-injected group and the control group within 22 days, indicating low *in-vivo* toxicity of the GQDs.

Additionally, recent *in-vivo* studies were conducted with zebrafish models by Wang et al. (2013), who investigated the effect of GQDs on the development of zebrafish embryos [50]. They found that their GQDs mainly accumulated in the intestines and heart of the zebrafish, as shown in **Figure 10.3b** [40]. The concentration of GQDs was found to determine their impact on zebrafish embryos during development. The growth of embryos was monitored at varying concentrations of GQDs (50, 100, and 200 mg), and it was observed that concentrations exceeding 50 mg mL^{-1} caused negative effects on the embryos, such as decreased hatch and heart rate, increased mortality, and disfigurement. Another study on zebrafish embryos showed that GQDs had difficulty entering the circulation system and could be excreted within seven days. This suggests that the impact of GQDs on zebrafish is concentration-dependent, and their removal from the body is facilitated by the excretory system **(Figure 10.3c)** [40,41]. The biocompatibility of GQDs was found to be excellent at a concentration lower than 2 mg mL^{-1}, as there was no discernible difference between the test group and the control group. Moreover, the possibility of using functionalized GQDs for *in-vivo* imaging of apoptotic cells to study the apoptosis process was demonstrated. The contradictory results of the two studies on the *in-vivo* toxicity for zebrafish could be attributed to the different types of GQDs used in their research. The former study used GQDs synthesized from cutting graphene oxide, while the latter utilized GQDs synthesized from hydrothermal treatment of leaf extracts. This implies that GQDs produced through different methods exhibit distinct toxicity characteristics. Furthermore, research was also conducted on plants. Li et al. (2014) conducted growth experiments on green gram sprouts to compare the *in-vivo* toxicity of GQDs with three other carbon materials, including carbon quantum dots (CQDs), graphene oxides (GO), and single-wall carbon nanotubes (SWCNTs) [51]. The study results indicated that GQDs exhibited the lowest toxicity among the four materials.

10.2.4 Toxicological Aspects of Fullerenes

10.2.4.1 Toxicokinetic

Toxico-kinetic studies are thought to be important for identifying potential target organs for fullerene toxicity after inhalation and dermal or oral exposure. Overcoming several barriers is necessary to allow fullerenes to be absorbed from the exposure site and distributed to secondary targets, and if this happens, they can produce toxic effects throughout the body.

10.2.4.1.1 Absorption

Yamago et al. (1995) found that orally administered radio-labeled 14C fullerene derivatives (tri-methylene methane) were not efficiently absorbed by rats and mice for a period of 160 hours but were rather eliminated in the feces within 48 hours [52]. Nevertheless, minute quantities were detected in urine, indicating that certain fullerenes were able to cross the intestinal barrier. Folkmann et al. (2009) proposed that fullerenes are absorbed after oral exposure because oxidative damage in the liver and lungs was dose-dependent after oral exposure via gavage [53]. The significance of these findings is unclear, as the solvent corn oil demonstrated the same effect and the presence of fullerenes in these organs was not demonstrated.

Fullerenes (in nano and microparticulate form) were not detected in blood after inhalation by rats in a study by Baker et al. (2008), indicating that they do not translocate from their respiratory exposure site [54]. The calculated pulmonary deposition fractions for the C_{60} fullerene nanoparticle (55 nm, 2.22 mg/m^3) group (14.1%) were 50% higher than for the microparticle (0.93 lm, 2.35 mg/m^3) group (9.3%). However, the half-life of fullerene nanoparticles, which was 26 days, was comparable to that of fullerene microparticles (29 days), indicating that the removal of fullerene from the lungs involves similar elimination processes, like mucociliary clearance and macrophage absorption. Rats were subjected for 130 and 145 days, respectively, in the study, which corresponds to the nano- and microparticle exposure times required to establish steady-state lung loads. In a modified Bronaugh's diffusion chamber, Kato et al. (2009) evaluated C_{60} dissolved in squalane (Lipo-Fullerene, LF-SQ) for skin permeability for 24 hours, and they discovered that C_{60} was undetectable on the epidermis and dermis for administration at low doses (2.23 and 22.3 ppm C_{60} in LF-SQ) [55]. Although C_{60} was not found in the dermis of a human skin biopsy after injection at concentrations as high as 223 ppm, it was found to infiltrate into the epidermis. The authors concluded that systemic circulation toxicity need not be taken into account for C_{60} dissolved in LF-SQ.

A fullerene-substituted peptide can pass through the epidermal layers via passive diffusion, as demonstrated by Rouse et al. in 2007 [56]. The rate at which these particles go into the dermis is accelerated by mechanical stresses, such as those brought on by a repetitive flexing motion (such as while walking barefoot, for example).

10.2.4.1.2 Distribution, Metabolism, and Elimination

Due to the low absorption, little information has been found regarding the distribution of fullerenes after inhalation, oral, or cutaneous absorption. Under situations of lung particle overload and associated inflammatory state, translocation of some nanoparticles from the respiratory tract to secondary organs has been demonstrated via uptake into pulmonary lymphatics and blood circulation [15]. Following intra-tracheal instillation (3.3 mg/kg) and inhalation exposure (0.12 mg/m^3), a recent study conducted as part of the NEDO project revealed limited systemic translocation of fullerenes to the brain (0.17% of lung concentration) and other organs in rats [57]. C_{60} (agglomerated to a size of about 1 micron) did not spread from the lung to other tissues until 168 hours after being administered through intra-tracheal instillation at doses of 1 or 5 mg/kg [58]. One milligram per cubic meter of fullerenes (20 nm) was inhaled for six hours, but no distribution to the liver or spleen, and only minute levels in the kidneys were discovered. The fact that C_{60} had poor pulmonary clearance and a relationship between its disposition and that of ^{13}C indicates that C_{60} is not being digested.

Alveolar macrophages in the lungs have been shown to phagocytose fullerenes [59]. Thus, macrophages perform their function in the host's defense; yet after consuming fullerenes, oxidative or inflammatory processes may be triggered (which requires consideration). Electron microscopic analysis revealed that phagocytosed fullerenes in alveolar macrophages generated finely scattered granules but were not converted to organelles or nuclei.

Following intraperitoneal administration, Gharbi et al. (2005) noted a robust macrophagic response and fullerene accumulation (2.5–5 g/kg C_{60}) within Kupffer cells in the liver [60]. Other cell types, including keratinocytes, epithelial cells, and eye lens cells, have also been shown to internalize fullerenes in-vitro, frequently with fatal and damaging effects [56].

It is evident that there is probably only a tiny amount of fullerene absorption after exposure through physiologically significant routes. In particular, fullerenes tend to stay in the lungs and gut, where they can be removed through alveolar macrophages, the mucociliary escalator, feces, and urine. According to the kind (functionalization) of fullerene, the solvent employed, and the characteristics of the skin, there is probably little to no absorption of fullerenes via the skin. Due to the scarcity of data, the study is currently unable to draw broad conclusions about the absorption, distribution, metabolism, and excretion profile of fullerenes and their derivatives.

10.2.4.2 Acute and Repeated Dose Toxicity

During an observation period of up to 14 days following oral administration of a single dose of 2000 mg/kg fullerite (a combination of C_{60} and C_{70}), no mortality or other indicators of toxicity in terms of behavior or body weight were seen in rats [61]. Following a single oral treatment of rats with 2500 mg/kg of polyalkylsulfonated (water soluble) C_{60}, Chen et al. (1998) revealed no effects, and as a result, it was determined that the substance was not acutely hazardous [62]. Based on these two investigations, acute no-observed adverse-effect levels (NOAELs) for fullerite (a combination of C_{60} and C_{70}) and polyalkylsufonated (water soluble) C_{60} are proposed to be 2000 mg/kg and 2500 mg/kg, respectively. Nevertheless, because only one dose was evaluated in each study, and no effects were noted, the actual acute oral NOAEL is likely more significant. Fullerenes have relatively low acute oral toxicity; however, there is no evidence of their long-term effects from repeated oral intake.

The exposure method that is thought to be most responsible for the issue surrounding (airborne) nanoparticles is inhalation. The deposition of discrete NP in the respiratory tract, where nanoparticles might have local impacts, is determined by the particle size (aerodynamic diameter). Compared to an equivalent mass of bigger particles, ultrafine nanometric particles have been found to cause greater inflammation and to be more tumorigenic. Although it has been demonstrated that some nanoparticles in the lungs are transferred to other organs in the body, no generalizations can be drawn [15].

When Fischer 344 rats were exposed to fullerenes via nasal inhalation at concentrations of 2.22 mg/m³ (nanoparticle, 55 nm diameter) and 2.35 mg/m³ (microparticle, 0.93 mm diameter) for 3 h/day for ten consecutive days, with toxicological assessments carried out up to seven days after exposure, neither inflammatory potential nor toxicity in the lung was observed. Rats exposed to nanoparticles had higher C_{60} lung particle loads than rats exposed to microparticles [54]. Rats exposed to nanoparticles had significantly higher protein concentrations in their bronchoalveolar lavage fluid

(BALF). Necroscopy revealed no visible lesions, either large or small (e.g., no lesions in the liver or heart). Serum chemistry alterations in the hematology department were minimal. Although alveolar macrophages internalized C_{60}, no cellular infiltration (a sign of an inflammatory reaction) was seen within the lung. The investigation did not reach the steady-state lung loads, which were estimated to last 130 and 145 days for nano and microparticles, respectively. The authors concluded that longer-term investigations might reveal toxicological findings connected to exposure. Male Wistar rats were exposed to 0.12 mg/m^3 fullerenes (4.1–104 particles/cm^3, 96 nm diameter, specific surface area 0.92 m^2/g) for six hours each day, five days a week, for four weeks in a study on sub-acute inhalation [59]. Throughout the 28-day inhalation exposure period and the up to three-month observation period that followed, there was no discernible inflammation or tissue damage [63]. The histological results of the inhalation and intra-tracheal instillation studies did not reveal the presence of a foreign body granuloma.

Several *in-vitro* dermal models have been used to study the effects of fullerene on skin cells. Keratinocytes were demonstrated to internalize fullerenes; however, the nature of the reactions seen varied. Scrivens et al. (1994) found no effects on cell proliferation at doses between 20 nM and 2 M; however, Bullard-Dillard et al. (1996) found that C_{60} caused a reduction in cell proliferation that was noticeable at high concentrations (2 M) and over a prolonged length of time (eight days) [64,65]. In HEK keratinocytes, exposure to phenylalanine-derivatized C_{60} (up to 0.4 mg/mL) increased the production of pro-inflammatory mediators such as IL-8, IL-6, and IL-1 and caused dose-dependent cytotoxicity through necrotic mechanism [66]. One investigation found that the particles did not enter the cells directly but indirectly through the intercellular gaps between skin cells [56]. According to Sayes et al. (2005), the type and degree of functionalization affected the lethal potential (initiated by lipid peroxidation) of various kinds of derivatized fullerenes to human dermal fibroblasts (HDF), HepG2 hepatocytes, and normal human astrocytes (NHA) [67].

In several experiments, Aoshima et al. (2009) looked into the possible toxicity of highly purified fullerenes (HPF: a combination of C_{60} and C_{70}, fullerite, 99.5% purity) to the skin and eyes. In a test for contact phototoxicity, 25% HPFs applied to guinea pigs' clipped-free skin for 50 minutes while they were subjected to long-wavelength UV light (11.2 J/cm^2) did not show any phototoxic potential up to 72 hours later [68]. In a human patch test, HPFs (0.01 g on a Finn Chamber) exposed under occlusive conditions did not cause skin reactions one or 24 hours later [68].

Due to their slow systemic absorption (no absorption within 24 hours), fullerenes may not have acute systemic toxicological effects [69]. However, depending on the mode of application (solvent), fullerenes have been found to penetrate deeply into the stratum corneum and also reach the viable epidermis. Ito et al. (2010) reported that fullerene has a ROS-reducing effect and verified that the co-application of ascorbate and fullerene protected mouse skin from UV radiation *in-vivo* [70]. They also reported that applying 1 w/w% fullerene reduced UV-B-induced erythema (skin redness caused by capillary congestion) *in-vivo*. No toxicity was observed in comparison to the control when fullerene was applied to UV-irradiated live mouse skin, and erythema, the ROS index, and the apoptosis index all decreased.

10.2.4.3 Irritation/Corrosivity

Highly purified fullerene (HPF) have been studied for their ability to cause eye irritation, primary and cumulative skin irritation, skin sensitization, skin photo-sensitization, contact phototoxicity, and clinical patch tests. In a Draize test (GLP), 0.5 g HPFs (in 0.3 mL propylene glycol (PG)) did not cause primary irritation to rabbit skin 24 hours after exposure, and evaluation at 0–48 hours after removal of the patches also revealed no such irritation. A cumulative skin-irritation test tracked clinical symptoms for eight and 15 days after regularly applying 20 mg HPFs in 0.2 mL PG. It was determined that HPFs did not cause cumulative cutaneous irritation in rabbits. When subjected to long-wavelength UV radiation (11.2 J/cm^2) for 50 minutes, 25% HPFs applied to guinea pigs' clipped-free skin did not exhibit any phototoxic potential for up to 72 hours after UV exposure. In a patch test model used to evaluate the irritating skin potential of fullerene soot in 30 volunteers (who reported irritation and allergy susceptibilities) after a 96-hour exposure time, Huczko et al. (2008) found no negative results [71].

The potential eye toxicity of HPF was investigated using a Draize rabbit eye-irritation test [68]. 0.1 g HPFs instilled into rabbit eyes did not elicit a response over the observation period of up to four days, while the group that had their eyes cleaned briefly experienced moderate irritation (after 24 h). Fullerene soot dispersion did not cause any toxicity in the eye for up to 72 hours, according to Huczko et al. (2008) [71]. According to the existing studies, the fullerene kinds evaluated did not have an irritating effect on the skin or eyes.

10.2.4.4 Sensitization

In a skin sensitization test, HPFs were injected intradermally at concentrations of 50% (w/v) during the induction phase and 25% during the challenge phase (as described by the author Aoshima et al., 2009 in compliance with Guidelines for Toxicity Studies of Drugs) [68]. In a skin-photosensitization test, the same HPF concentrations were used, but the application areas were also exposed to 10 J/cm^2 of long-wavelength UV light for 30–31 minutes. In guinea pigs, there was no skin sensitizing potential and no skin photo-sensitization potential (up to 48 hours after challenge and UV radiation, respectively). A local lymph node assay (LLNA) utilizing HPFs found no sensitivity in the same paper [68]. A C_{60} fullerene derivate coupled to bovine thyroglobulin (in Freund's adjuvant) after intraperitoneal injection in mice caused antigenic behavior by encouraging the production of IgG isotype fullerene-specific antibodies (Chen et al., 1998a). Erlanger et al. (2001) built on the findings by demonstrating that anti-C_{60} antibodies could interact with single-wall carbon nanotubes, which were observed using atomic force microscopy [72]. The results suggested that C_{60} derivatives might function as immune response modifiers by acting as sensitizing agents.

10.2.4.5 Mutagenicity

To look into the DNA damage brought on by fullerene exposure, several genotoxicity tests, mostly *in-vitro*, have been carried out. Studies on the bacterial reverse muta-genicity of all fullerene types (C_{60}, fullerite, fullerene derivatives, and lipo-fullerene) were negative, except for one study in which the mutagenic effects were obvious under visible light [73]. Because prokaryotes cannot perform endocytosis and the nanomaterials may not be able to diffuse across the bacterial cell wall, bacterial mutagenicity-based assays may not be suitable for detecting genotoxicity caused by nanomaterials in this context. As a result, this lack of uptake may result in false negative results [74].

Following intra-tracheal instillation of C_{60}, Totsuka et al. (2009) demonstrated a dose-dependent increase in micronuclei *in-vitro* as well as DNA damage and mutations in the lung (alkaline assay and mutations) [75]. The authors concluded that while oxidative DNA damage may occasionally play a role in the mutagenicity of small particles, the genotoxic potency was not always correlated with size since microsized Kaolin (4.8 um) also had similar effects. Compared to the exposure that workers are typically exposed to at work, the applied particle doses in this study were exceptionally high (0.2 mg/mouse).

C_{60} tested negative in comet assays, a chromosomal aberration test *in-vitro*, a micronucleus test *in-vivo*, and other tests [76]. Fullerite, a blend of colloidal C_{60} and C_{70}, showed no chromosomal abnormality up to large doses, while aqueous solutions of colloidal C_{60} were genotoxic [61]. Vigorously antioxidative compounds called fullerenols ($C_{60}(OH)_{24}$) may even guard against genotoxic consequences. They were demonstrated to reduce the frequency of micronuclei and chromosomal abnormalities in cells damaged by mitomycin C in *in-vitro* experiments [77]. The protective impact was more potent at lower levels, suggesting a correlation with the antioxidative effects at low fullerene concentrations. However, the antioxidative benefits can change to a pro-oxidative response at larger doses.

10.2.4.6   Carcinogenicity

The derivatives of fullerene may have therapeutic potential for the treatment of cancer. Fullerenes have been shown to have antitumor effects *in-vivo* and *in-vitro* depending on derivatization, dispersion, and exposure to light in some investigations. It would seem that fullerene accumulation in tumors is possible because of the hyperpermeability of the tumor vasculature and its extremely low organ toxicity. Light exposure appears to have an increased capacity to destroy tumors [78].

Three different functionalized fullerene materials ($Gd@C_{82}(OH)_{22}$, $C_{60}(OH)_{22}$, and $C_{60}(C(COOH)_2)_2$) were shown to have ROS-scavenging abilities by Yin et al. (2008), who also concluded that these fullerene derivatives might be useful *in-vivo* cytoprotective and therapeutic agents [79]. A gadolinium-based metallofullerol with potential for application in chemotherapy, $Gd@C_{82}(OH)_{22}$, has been shown to prevent the growth of malignant tumors in mice after intraperitoneal treatment, and this was because of its ROS scavenging activity [80]. The ability of water-soluble $C_{60}(OH)_{20}$ nanoparticles to induce immune cells to produce more cytokines, particularly TNF-a, which is essential for the cellular immune system's ability to destroy aberrant cells, was established by Liu et al. in 2009 [81]. They discovered that $C_{60}(OH)_{20}$ effectively and almost without side effects inhibited the growth of tumors in mice (low cytotoxicity inducing neither cell death nor affecting the viability of lymphocytes and macrophages).

A single intraperitoneal injection of crocidolite asbestos, long multiwall carbon nanotubes (MWCNTs), or fullerenes (C_{60}) was used in a carcinogenicity investigation in p53(+/-) mice [82]. Because they are unable to repair genotoxic damage and/or purge damaged cells by apoptosis, p53 defective animals are not only extraordinarily vulnerable to (genotoxic) carcinogens but also to reactive oxygen species (ROS)-related carcinogenesis. No peritoneal adhesion, fibrous thickening, or tumor induction was present in the fullerenes group. On the serosal surface, there were only a few little black plaques. The two substances that had the highest potential to cause cancer were long MWCNT and asbestos. The relatively brief exposure time is a flaw in the study that affects our capacity to form a conclusion about the absence of fullerene carcinogenic consequences. Due to the significant mortality rate in MWCNT-treated animals, it is crucial to mention that extremely high concentrations (3 mg/animal in 1 mL suspension) were utilized, and the trial was stopped at week 25 for all treatment groups.

10.3 REMEDIATION STRATEGIES

Carbon nanomaterials have unique physical, chemical, and electronic properties that make them useful in a wide range of applications. However, their small size and high surface area can also result in toxicity and adverse health effects when they come into contact with living organisms. Here are some strategies for remediation of the toxic effects of carbon nanomaterials:

1. Surface functionalization: one approach to reducing the toxicity of carbon nanomaterials is to modify their surface chemistry through functionalization. This can involve attaching biocompatible molecules or polymers to the surface of the nanomaterials to reduce their reactivity and prevent them from interacting with biological molecules in harmful ways.
2. Encapsulation: another strategy is to encapsulate the carbon nanomaterials in a protective coating that can prevent them from interacting with biological systems. This can be achieved through the use of liposomes, polymers, or other materials that can form a barrier around the nanomaterials.
3. Removal of impurities: carbon nanomaterials can be contaminated with impurities that can contribute to their toxicity. Purification techniques, such as filtration or chemical treatment, can remove these impurities and improve the biocompatibility of the nanomaterials.
4. Biological degradation: some microorganisms have the ability to degrade carbon nanomaterials, converting them into less toxic forms. Researchers are exploring the use of biological systems, such as bacteria and fungi, for the biodegradation of carbon nanomaterials.
5. Safe handling and disposal: proper handling and disposal of carbon nanomaterials can also help reduce their potential for toxicity. This includes using appropriate protective equipment when working with the materials and disposing of them to minimize the risk of environmental contamination.

Overall, a multidisciplinary approach is needed to address the potential toxicity of carbon nanomaterials. This includes continued research into the mechanisms of toxicity and the development of new remediation strategies.

10.4 SUMMARY

This chapter mainly focuses on the toxicology studies of the different carbon-based nanomaterials such as graphene oxide, carbon nanotubes, graphene quantum dots, and fullerenes. It provides an extensive outlook of the toxic effects of various carbon nanomaterials when exposed through oral, dermal entities. This chapter also focuses on the immunological effects of carbon nanomaterials apart from their toxicological discussions. Various cells have been utilized for *in-vitro* and *in-vivo* studies to showcase the toxic nature of various carbon nanomaterials. To prevent various toxic and harmful effects caused by carbon nanomaterials, such as DNA damage, ROS generation, mitochondrial dysfunction, lysosomal damage, and eventual cell death, remediation strategies are also discussed in this chapter to provide an idea about the future prospect of study in order to tackle such problems.

REFERENCES

[1] P.C. Ray, H. Yu, P.P. Fu, Toxicity and environmental risks of nanomaterials: Challenges and future needs, J Env. Sci Heal. C Env. Carcinog. Ecotoxicol. Rev. 27 (2009) 1–35. doi:10.1080/10590500802708267.

[2] A. Hirsch, The era of carbon allotropes, Nat Mater. 9 (2010) 868–871. doi:10.1038/nmat2885.

[3] R.H. Hurt, M. Monthioux, A. Kane, Toxicology of carbon nanomaterials: Status, trends, and perspectives on the special issue, Carbon N. Y. 44 (2006) 1028–1033. doi:10.1016/j.carbon.2005.12.023.

[4] A. Figarol, J. Pourchez, D. Boudard, V. Forest, C. Akono, J.M. Tulliani, J.P. Lecompte, M. Cottier, D. Bernache-Assollant, P. Grosseau, In vitro toxicity of carbon nanotubes, nano-graphite and carbon black, similar impacts of acid functionalization, Toxicol. Vitr. 30 (2015) 476–485. doi:10.1016/j.tiv.2015.09.014.

[5] C.M. Long, M.A. Nascarella, P.A. Valberg, Carbon black vs. black carbon and other airborne materials containing elemental carbon: Physical and chemical distinctions, Env. Pollut. 181 (2013) 271–286. doi:10.1016/j.envpol.2013.06.009.

[6] S. Zhu, G. Xu, Single-walled carbon nanohorns and their applications, Nanoscale. 2 (2010) 2538–2549. doi:10.1039/c0nr00387e.

[7] K.S. Novoselov, A.K. Geim, S.V. Morozov, D. Jiang, Y. Zhang, S.V. Dubonos, I.V. Grigorieva, A.A. Firsov, Electric field effect in atomically thin carbon films, Sci. 306 (2004) 666–669. doi:10.1126/science.1102896.

[8] A.K. Geim, Graphene: Status and prospects, Sci. 324 (2009) 1530–1534. doi:10.1126/science.1158877.

[9] X. Huang, Z. Yin, S. Wu, X. Qi, Q. He, Q. Zhang, Q. Yan, F. Boey, H. Zhang, Graphene-based materials: Synthesis, characterization, properties, and applications, Small. 7 (2011) 1876–1902. doi:10.1002/smll.201002009.

[10] L. Dai, Functionalization of graphene for efficient energy conversion and storage, Acc. Chem. Res. 46 (2013) 31–42. doi:10.1021/ar300122m.

[11] M. Teimouri, A.H. Nia, K. Abnous, H. Eshghi, M. Ramezani, Graphene oxide–cationic polymer conjugates: Synthesis and application as gene delivery vectors, Plasmid. 84–85 (2016) 51–60. doi:10.1016/j.plasmid.2016.03.002.

[12] C. Spinato, C. Ménard-Moyon, A. Bianco, Chemical functionalization of graphene for biomedical applications, Funct. Graphene. 9783527335 (2014) 95–138. doi:10.1002/9783527672790.ch4.

[13] B.J. Panessa-Warren, J.B. Warren, S.S. Wong, J.A. Misewich, Biological cellular response to carbon nanoparticle toxicity, J Phys Condens Matter. 18 (2006) S2185. doi:10.1088/0953-8984/18/33/s34.

[14] D.B. Warheit, B.R. Laurence, K.L. Reed, D.H. Roach, G.A.M. Reynolds, T.R. Webb, Comparative pulmonary toxicity assessment of single-wall carbon nanotubes in rats, Toxicol Sci. 77 (2004) 117–125. doi:10.1093/toxsci/kfg228.

[15] G. Oberdörster, E. Oberdörster, J. Oberdörster, Nanotoxicology: An emerging discipline evolving from studies of ultrafine particles, Env. Heal. Perspect. 113 (2005) 823–839. doi:10.1289/ehp.7339.

[16] D. Cui, F. Tian, C.S. Ozkan, M. Wang, H. Gao, Effect of single wall carbon nanotubes on human HEK293 cells, Toxicol. Lett. 155 (2005) 73–85. doi:10.1016/j.toxlet.2004.08.015.

[17] J. Meng, X. Li, C. Wang, H. Guo, J. Liu, H. Xu, Carbon nanotubes activate macrophages into a M1/M2 mixed status: Recruiting naïve macrophages and supporting angiogenesis, ACS Appl. Mater. Interfaces. 7 (2015) 3180. doi:10.1021/am507649n.

[18] G. Oberdörster, Z. Sharp, V. Atudorei, A. Elder, R. Gelein, W. Kreyling, C. Cox, Translocation of inhaled ultrafine particles to the brain, Inhal. Toxicol. 16 (2004) 437. doi:10.1080/08958370490439597.

[19] O. Moss, V. Wong, When nanoparticles get in the way: Impact of projected area on in vivo and in vitro macrophage function, Inhal Toxicol. 18 (2006) 711–716. doi:10.1080/08958370600747770.

[20] A. Erdely, T. Hulderman, R. Salmen, A. Liston, P.C. Zeidler-Erdely, D. Schwegler-Berry, V. Castranova, S. Koyama, Y.A. Kim, M. Endo, P.P. Simeonova, Cross-talk between lung and systemic circulation during carbon nanotube respiratory exposure: Potential biomarkers, Nano Lett. 9 (2009) 36–43. doi:10.1021/nl801828z.

[21] S.T. Yang, W. Guo, Y. Lin, X.Y. Deng, H.F. Wang, H.F. Sun, Y.F. Liu, X. Wang, W. Wang, M. Chen, Y.P. Huang, Y.P. Sun, Biodistribution of pristine single-walled carbon nanotubes in vivo†, J. Phys. Chem. C. 111 (2007) 17761–17764. doi:10.1021/jp070712c.

[22] T. Zhang, M. Tang, L. Kong, H. Li, T. Zhang, S. Zhang, Y. Xue, Y. Pu, Comparison of cytotoxic and inflammatory responses of pristine and functionalized multi-walled carbon nanotubes in RAW 264.7 mouse macrophages, J Hazard Mater. 219 (2012) 203–212. doi:10.1016/j.jhazmat.2012.03.079.

[23] J. Yuan, H. Gao, C.B. Ching, Comparative protein profile of human hepatoma HepG2 cells treated with graphene and single-walled carbon nanotubes: An iTRAQ-coupled 2D LC–MS/MS proteome analysis, Toxicol. Lett. 207 (2011) 213–221. doi:10.1016/J. TOXLET.2011.09.014.

[24] Y. Li, Y. Liu, Y. Fu, T. Wei, L. Le Guyader, G. Gao, R.S. Liu, Y.Z. Chang, C. Chen, The triggering of apoptosis in macrophages by pristine graphene through the MAPK and TGF-beta signaling pathways, Biomaterials. 33 (2012) 402–411. doi:10.1016/j. biomaterials.2011.09.091.

[25] A. Schinwald, F.A. Murphy, A. Jones, W. MacNee, K. Donaldson, Graphene-based nanoplatelets: A new risk to the respiratory system as a consequence of their unusual aerodynamic properties, ACS Nano. 6 (2012) 736–746. doi:10.1021/nn204229f.

[26] Y. Chang, S.T. Yang, J.H. Liu, E. Dong, Y. Wang, A. Cao, Y. Liu, H. Wang, In vitro toxicity evaluation of graphene oxide on A549 cells, Toxicol. Lett. 200 (2011) 201–210. doi:10.1016/J.TOXLET.2010.11.016.

[27] W. Hu, C. Peng, M. Lv, X. Li, Y. Zhang, N. Chen, C. Fan, Q. Huang, Protein corona-mediated mitigation of cytotoxicity of graphene oxide, ACS Nano. 5 (2011) 3693–3700. doi:10.1021/nn200021j.

[28] T. Lammel, P. Boisseaux, M.L. Fernández-Cruz, J.M. Navas, Internalization and cytotoxicity of graphene oxide and carboxyl graphene nanoplatelets in the human hepatocellular carcinoma cell line Hep G2, Part. Fibre Toxicol. 10 (2013) 1–21. doi:10.1186/1743-8977-10-27/FIGURES/12.

[29] J. Yuan, H. Gao, J. Sui, H. Duan, W.N. Chen, C.B. Ching, Cytotoxicity evaluation of oxidized single-walled carbon nanotubes and graphene oxide on human hepatoma HepG2 cells: An iTRAQ-coupled 2D LC-MS/MS proteome analysis, Toxicol. Sci. 126 (2012) 149–161. doi:10.1093/TOXSCI/KFR332.

[30] H. Zhang, C. Peng, J. Yang, M. Lv, R. Liu, D. He, C. Fan, Q. Huang, Uniform ultrasmall graphene oxide nanosheets with low cytotoxicity and high cellular uptake, ACS Appl. Mater. Interfaces. 5 (2013) 1761–1767. doi:10.1021/AM303005J/SUPPL_FILE/AM303005J_SI_001.PDF.

[31] X. Zhang, W. Hu, J. Li, L. Tao, Y. Wei, A comparative study of cellular uptake and cytotoxicity of multi-walled carbon nanotubes, graphene oxide, and nanodiamond, Toxicol. Res. (Camb). 1 (2012) 62–68. doi:10.1039/C2TX20006F.

[32] M. Lv, Y. Zhang, L. Liang, M. Wei, W. Hu, X. Li, Q. Huang, Effect of graphene oxide on undifferentiated and retinoic acid-differentiated SH-SY5Y cells line, Nanoscale. 4 (2012) 3861–3866. doi:10.1039/C2NR30407D.

[33] N.V.S. Vallabani, S. Mittal, R.K. Shukla, A.K. Pandey, S.R. Dhakate, R. Pasricha, A. Dhawan, Toxicity of graphene in normal human lung cells (BEAS-2B), J. Biomed. Nanotechnol. 7 (2011) 106–107. doi:10.1166/JBN.2011.1224.

[34] S.M. Kang, T.H. Kim, J.W. Choi, Cell chip to detect effects of graphene oxide nanopellet on human neural stem cell, J. Nanosci. Nanotechnol. 12 (2012) 5185–5190. doi:10.1166/JNN.2012.6378.

[35] L. Yan, Y. Wang, X. Xu, C. Zeng, J. Hou, M. Lin, J. Xu, F. Sun, X. Huang, L. Dai, F. Lu, Y. Liu, Can graphene oxide cause damage to eyesight? Chem. Res. Toxicol. 25 (2012) 1265–1270. doi:10.1021/TX300129F/ASSET/IMAGES/LARGE/TX-2012-00129F_0008.JPEG.

[36] C. Xiang, Y. Zhang, W. Guo, X.J. Liang, Biomimetic carbon nanotubes for neurological disease therapeutics as inherent medication, Acta Pharm. Sin. B. 10 (2020) 239–248. doi:10.1016/J.APSB.2019.11.003.

[37] R. Jha, A. Singh, P.K. Sharma, N.K. Fuloria, Smart carbon nanotubes for drug delivery system: A comprehensive study, J. Drug Deliv. Sci. Technol. 58 (2020) 101811. doi:10.1016/J.JDDST.2020.101811.

[38] Z. Liu, W. Cai, L. He, N. Nakayama, K. Chen, X. Sun, X. Chen, H. Dai, In vivo biodistribution and highly efficient tumour targeting of carbon nanotubes in mice, Nano-Enabled Med. Appl. (2020) 403–429. doi:10.1201/9780429399039-14.

[39] X. Xue, J.Y. Yang, Y. He, L.R. Wang, P. Liu, L.S. Yu, G.H. Bi, M.M. Zhu, Y.Y. Liu, R.W. Xiang, X.T. Yang, X.Y. Fan, X.M. Wang, J. Qi, H.J. Zhang, T. Wei, W. Cui, G.L. Ge, Z.X. Xi, C.F. Wu, X.J. Liang, Aggregated single-walled carbon nanotubes attenuate the behavioural and neurochemical effects of methamphetamine in mice, Nat. Nanotechnol. 11 (2016) 613–620. doi:10.1038/nnano.2016.23.

[40] S. Wang, I.S. Cole, Q. Li, The toxicity of graphene quantum dots, RSC Adv. 6 (2016) 89867–89878. doi:10.1039/C6RA16516H.

[41] X. Wu, F. Tian, W. Wang, J. Chen, M. Wu, J.X. Zhao, Fabrication of highly fluorescent graphene quantum dots using l-glutamic acid for in vitro/in vivo imaging and sensing, J. Mater. Chem. C. 1 (2013) 4676–4684. doi:10.1039/C3TC30820K.

[42] M. Nurunnabi, Z. Khatun, K.M. Huh, S.Y. Park, D.Y. Lee, K.J. Cho, Y.K. Lee, In vivo biodistribution and toxicology of carboxylated graphene quantum dots, ACS Nano. 7 (2013) 6858–6867. doi:10.1021/NN402043C/SUPPL_FILE/NN402043C_SI_001.PDF.

[43] M. Zhang, L. Bai, W. Shang, W. Xie, H. Ma, Y. Fu, D. Fang, H. Sun, L. Fan, M. Han, C. Liu, S. Yang, Facile synthesis of water-soluble, highly fluorescent graphene quantum dots as a robust biological label for stem cells, J. Mater. Chem. 22 (2012) 7461–7467. doi:10.1039/C2JM16835A.

[44] R. Li, Y. Liu, Z. Li, J. Shen, Y. Yang, X. Cui, G. Yang, Bottom-up fabrication of single-layered nitrogen-doped graphene quantum dots through intermolecular carbonization arrayed in a 2D plane, Chem. A Eur. J. 22 (2016) 272–278. doi:10.1002/CHEM.201503191.

[45] T. Wang, S. Zhu, X. Jiang, Toxicity mechanism of graphene oxide and nitrogen-doped graphene quantum dots in RBCs revealed by surface-enhanced infrared

absorption spectroscopy, Toxicol. Res. (Camb). 4 (2015) 885–894. doi:10.1039/C4TX00138A.

[46] X. Hai, Q.X. Mao, W.J. Wang, X.F. Wang, X.W. Chen, J.H. Wang, An acid-free microwave approach to prepare highly luminescent boron-doped graphene quantum dots for cell imaging, J. Mater. Chem. B. 3 (2015) 9109–9114. doi:10.1039/C5TB01954K.

[47] H. Sun, F. Zhang, H. Wei, B. Yang, The effects of composition and surface chemistry on the toxicity of quantum dots, J. Mater. Chem. B. 1 (2013) 6485–6494. doi:10.1039/C3TB21151G.

[48] H. Sun, N. Gao, K. Dong, J. Ren, X. Qu, Graphene quantum dots-band-aids used for wound disinfection, ACS Nano. 8 (2014) 6202–6210. doi:10.1021/NN501640Q/SUPPL_FILE/NN501640Q_SI_001.PDF.

[49] C. Wu, C. Wang, T. Han, X. Zhou, S. Guo, J. Zhang, C. Wu, T. Han, X. Zhou, S. Guo, C. Wang, J. Zhang, Insight into the cellular internalization and cytotoxicity of graphene quantum dots, Adv. Healthc. Mater. 2 (2013) 1613–1619. doi:10.1002/ADHM.201300066.

[50] A. Wang, K. Pu, B. Dong, Y. Liu, L. Zhang, Z. Zhang, W. Duan, Y. Zhu, Role of surface charge and oxidative stress in cytotoxicity and genotoxicity of graphene oxide towards human lung fibroblast cells, J. Appl. Toxicol. 33 (2013) 1156–1164. doi:10.1002/JAT.2877.

[51] X. Li, Z. Zhou, D. Lu, X. Dong, M. Xu, L. Wei, Y. Zhang, The effect of pristine carbon-based nanomaterial on the growth of green gram sprouts and pH of water, Nanoscale Res. Lett. 9 (2014) 1–6. doi:10.1186/1556-276X-9-583/FIGURES/4.

[52] S. Yamago, H. Tokuyama, E. Nakamura, K. Kikuchi, S. Kananishi, K. Sueki, H. Nakahara, S. Enomoto, F. Ambe, In vivo biological behavior of a water-miscible fullerene: 14C labeling, absorption, distribution, excretion and acute toxicity, Chem. Biol. 2 (1995) 385–389. doi:10.1016/1074-5521(95)90219-8.

[53] J.K. Folkmann, L. Risom, N.R. Jacobsen, H. Wallin, S. Loft, P. Møller, Oxidatively damaged DNA in rats exposed by oral gavage to C60 fullerenes and single-walled carbon nanotubes, Environ. Health Perspect. 117 (2009) 703–708. doi:10.1289/EHP.11922.

[54] G.L. Baker, A. Gupta, M.L. Clark, B.R. Valenzuela, L.M. Staska, S.J. Harbo, J.T. Pierce, J.A. Dill, Inhalation toxicity and lung toxicokinetics of C60 fullerene nanoparticles and microparticles, Toxicol. Sci. 101 (2008) 122–131. doi:10.1093/TOXSCI/KFM243.

[55] S. Kato, H. Aoshima, Y. Saitoh, N. Miwa, Biological safety of lipofullerene composed of squalane and fullerene-C60 upon mutagenesis, photocytotoxicity, and permeability into the human skin tissue, Basic Clin. Pharmacol. Toxicol. 104 (2009) 483–487. doi:10.1111/J.1742-7843.2009.00396.X.

[56] J.G. Rouse, J. Yang, J.P. Ryman-Rasmussen, A.R. Barron, N.A. Monteiro-Riviere, Effects of mechanical flexion on the penetration of fullerene amino acid-derivatized peptide nanoparticles through skin, Nano Lett. 7 (2007) 155–160. doi:10.1021/NL062464M/SUPPL_FILE/NL062464MSI20061121_080543.PDF.

[57] N. Shinohara, M. Gamo, J. Nakanishi, Risk Assessment of Manufactured Nanomaterials: Fullerene (C60) (2009). http://www.aist-riss.jp/main/modules/product/nano_rad.html (accessed March 9, 2023).

[58] X. Yuan, X. Zhang, L. Sun, Y. Wei, X. Wei, Cellular toxicity and immunological effects of carbon-based nanomaterials, Part. Fibre Toxicol. 16 (2019) 1–27. doi:10.1186/S12989-019-0299-Z.

[59] K. Fujita, Y. Morimoto, A. Ogami, T. Myojyo, I. Tanaka, M. Shimada, W.N. Wang, S. Endoh, K. Uchida, T. Nakazato, K. Yamamoto, H. Fukui, M. Horie, Y. Yoshida, H. Iwahashi, J. Nakanishi, Gene expression profiles in rat lung after inhalation exposure to C60 fullerene particles, Toxicol. 258 (2009) 47–55. doi:10.1016/J.TOX.2009.01.005.

[60] N. Gharbi, M. Pressac, M. Hadchouel, H. Szwarc, S.R. Wilson, F. Moussa, [60]Fullerene is a powerful antioxidant in vivo with no acute or subacute toxicity, Nano Lett. 5 (2005) 2578–2585. doi:10.1021/NL051866B/SUPPL_FILE/NL051866BSI20051102_091207.PDF.

[61] T. Mori, H. Takada, S. Ito, K. Matsubayashi, N. Miwa, T. Sawaguchi, Preclinical studies on safety of fullerene upon acute oral administration and evaluation for no mutagenesis, Toxicol. 225 (2006) 48–54. doi:10.1016/J.TOX.2006.05.001.

[62] H.H.C. Chen, C.H.I. Yu, U.H. Ueng, S. Chen, B.J. Chen, J. Kuen, J. Huang, L.Y. Chiang, Acute and subacute toxicity study of water-soluble polyalkylsulfonated C, in rats*, Toxicol. Pathol. 26 (1998) 143–151.

[63] Y. Morimoto, M. Hirohashi, A. Ogami, T. Oyabu, T. Myojo, K.I. Nishi, C. Kadoya, M. Todoroki, M. Yamamoto, M. Murakami, M. Shimada, W.N. Wang, K. Yamamoto, K. Fujita, S. Endoh, K. Uchida, N. Shinohara, J. Nakanishi, I. Tanaka, Inflammogenic effect of well-characterized fullerenes in inhalation and intratracheal instillation studies, Part. Fibre Toxicol. 7 (2010) 1–18. doi:10.1186/1743-8977-7-4/FIGURES/12.

[64] W.A. Scrivens, J.M. Tour, K.E. Creek, L. Pirisi, Synthesis of 14C-labeled Ceo, its suspension in water, and its uptake by human keratinocytes, J. Chem. Soc. Chem. Commun. 116 (1994) 55. https://pubs.acs.org/sharingguidelines (accessed March 9, 2023).

[65] R. Bullard-Dillard, K.E. Creek, W.A. Scrivens, J.M. Tour, Tissue sites of uptake of14C-labeled C60, Bioorg. Chem. 24 (1996) 376–385. doi:10.1006/BIOO.1996.0032.

[66] J.G. Rouse, J. Yang, A.R. Barron, N.A. Monteiro-Riviere, Fullerene-based amino acid nanoparticle interactions with human epidermal keratinocytes, Toxicol. Vitr. 20 (2006) 1313–1320. doi:10.1016/J.TIV.2006.04.004.

[67] C.M. Sayes, A.M. Gobin, K.D. Ausman, J. Mendez, J.L. West, V.L. Colvin, Nano-C60 cytotoxicity is due to lipid peroxidation, Biomater. 26 (2005) 7587–7595. doi:10.1016/j.biomaterials.2005.05.027.

[68] H. Aoshima, Y. Saitoh, S. Ito, S. Yamana, N. Miwa, Safety evaluation of highly purified fullerenes (HPFs): Based on screening of eye and skin damage, J. Toxicol. Sci. 34 (2009) 555–562. doi:10.2131/JTS.34.555.

[69] X.R. Xia, N.A. Monteiro-Riviere, J.E. Riviere, Skin penetration and kinetics of pristine fullerenes (C60) topically exposed in industrial organic solvents, Toxicol. Appl. Pharmacol. 242 (2010) 29–37. doi:10.1016/J.TAAP.2009.09.011.

[70] S. Ito, K. Itoga, M. Yamato, H. Akamatsu, T. Okano, The co-application effects of fullerene and ascorbic acid on UV-B irradiated mouse skin, Toxicol. 267 (2010) 27–38. doi:10.1016/J.TOX.2009.09.015.

[71] A. Huczko, H. Lange, E. Calko, Short communication: Fullerenes: Experimental evidence for a null risk of skin irritation and allergy, Fuller. Sci. Technol. 7 (2008) 935–939. doi:10.1080/10641229909351390.

[72] B.F. Erlanger, B.-X. Chen, M. Zhu, L. Brus, Binding of an anti-fullerene IgG monoclonal antibody to single wall carbon nanotubes, Nano Lett. 1 (2001) 465–467. doi:10.1021/nl015570r.

[73] N. Sera, H. Tokiwa, N. Miyata, Mutagenicity of the fullerene C60-generated singlet oxygen-dependent formation of lipid peroxides, Carcin. 17 (1996) 2163–2169. doi:10.1093/CARCIN/17.10.2163.

[74] N. Singh, B. Manshian, G.J.S. Jenkins, S.M. Griffiths, P.M. Williams, T.G.G. Maffeis, C.J. Wright, S.H. Doak, NanoGenotoxicology: The DNA damaging potential of engineered nanomaterials, Biomater. 30 (2009) 3891–3914. doi:10.1016/J.BIOMATERIALS.2009.04.009.

[75] Y. Totsuka, T. Higuchi, T. Imai, A. Nishikawa, T. Nohmi, T. Kato, S. Masuda, N. Kinae, K. Hiyoshi, S. Ogo, M. Kawanishi, T. Yagi, T. Ichinose, N. Fukumori, M. Watanabe, T. Sugimura, K. Wakabayashi, Genotoxicity of nano/microparticles in in vitro micronuclei, in vivo comet and mutation assay systems, Part. Fibre Toxicol. 2009 61.6 (2009) 1–11. doi:10.1186/1743-8977-6-23.

[76] N. Shinohara, K. Matsumoto, S. Endoh, J. Maru, J. Nakanishi, In vitro and in vivo genotoxicity tests on fullerene C60 nanoparticles, Toxicol. Lett. 191 (2009) 289–296. doi:10.1016/J.TOXLET.2009.09.012.

[77] D. Jović, V. Jaćević, K. Kuča, I. Borišev, J. Mrdjanovic, D. Petrovic, M. Seke, A. Djordje-
      vic, The puzzling potential of carbon nanomaterials: General properties, application, and
      toxicity, Nanomater. (Basel). 10 (2020) 1–30. doi:10.3390/nano10081508.
[78] Y. Tabata, Y. Murakami, Y. Ikada, Photodynamic effect of polyethylene gly-
      col–modified fullerene on tumor, Japanese J. Cancer Res. 88 (1997) 1108–1116.
      doi:10.1111/J.1349-7006.1997.TB00336.X.
[79] J.J. Yin, F. Lao, J. Meng, P.P. Fu, Y. Zhao, G. Xing, X. Gao, B. Sun, P.C. Wang, C. Chen,
      X.J. Liang, Inhibition of tumor growth by endohedral metallofullerenol nanoparticles
      optimized as reactive oxygen species scavenger, Mol. Pharmacol. 74 (2008) 1132–1140.
      doi:10.1124/MOL.108.048348.
[80] C. Chen, G. Xing, J. Wang, Y. Zhao, B. Li, J. Tang, G. Jia, T. Wang, J. Sun, L. Xing,
      H. Yuan, Y. Gao, H. Meng, Z. Chen, F. Zhao, Z. Chai, X. Fang, Multihydroxylated
      [Gd@C82(OH)22]n nanoparticles: Antineoplastic activity of high efficiency and low
      toxicity, Nano Lett. 5 (2005) 2050–2057. doi:10.1021/NL051624B/SUPPL_FILE/
      NL051624BSI20050906_043223.PDF.
[81] Y. Liu, F. Jiao, Y. Qiu, W. Li, Y. Qu, C. Tian, Y. Li, R. Bai, F. Lao, Y. Zhao, Z. Chai,
      C. Chen, Immunostimulatory properties and enhanced TNF- α mediated cellular
      immunity for tumor therapy by C60(OH)20 nanoparticles, Nanotechnol. 20 (2009).
      doi:10.1088/0957-4484/20/41/415102.
[82] A. Takagi, A. Hirose, T. Nishimura, N. Fukumori, A. Ogata, N. Ohashi, S. Kitajima,
      J. Kanno, Induction of mesothelioma in p53+/– mouse by intraperitoneal application of
      multi-wall carbon nanotube, J. Toxicol. Sci. 33 (2008) 105–116. doi:10.2131/JTS.33.105.

11 Challenges and Opportunities of Carbon-Based Nanomaterials as Nanocarriers

11.1 THE GLOBAL DEMAND FOR NANOPHARMACEUTICALS— JOURNEY FROM LAB TO SHOPS

The worldwide nanomedicine market was worth $1.71 billion in 2020 and is expected to reach $4 billion by 2030, growing at a compound annual growth rate (CAGR) of 9.2% between 2021 and 2030 [1]. In layman's analogy, nanomedicine is the medical subfield that uses information about nanotechnology to improve health. Nanomedicine is the application of nanoscale materials, such as biocompatible nanoparticles and smart nanocarriers, which also includes the diagnosis, transport, sensing, and actuation of therapeutics inside living organisms.

Nanomaterials have physicochemical properties that differ from their bulk chemical counterparts due to their minute size. Due to these qualities, new routes for pharmaceutical research and development have become available. There is a possibility that the nano formulation's physicochemical features will enable it to overcome biological barriers, toxicity, and persistence in the environment and the human body. In the pharmaceutical sector, nanoparticles can be created from the top down or the bottom up. With the help of mechanical or chemical energy, top-down processes reduce huge volumes of material to smaller quantities. On the other hand, the bottom-up technique uses atomic or molecular species as the starting point for a chain reaction that ultimately produces bigger precursor particles.

The path of a nanopharmaceutical from the laboratory to the market includes research and development, preclinical testing, clinical trials, and regulatory approval. After a nanopharmaceutical has been produced and proved safe and effective in animal research, it must undergo human clinical trials to establish its safety and efficacy in a broader population. If the medicine is effective in these studies, it can be submitted for regulatory approval to the FDA in the United States or the European Medicines Agency (EMA) in Europe [2]. In contrast to conventional therapeutics, the early and late stages of the development of therapeutical nanoparticles are fraught with several obstacles. These issues are primarily linked to nanoparticles' hierarchical and heterogeneous morphology, which makes it such that even a seemingly minor change

DOI: 10.1201/9781003358114-11

in one aspect might significantly affect the particle's pharmacokinetics or therapeutic efficacy. Common issues include, for example, the failure to maintain a tight particle size distribution. For most applications, particles less than 200 nm are desirable. With a broad normal distribution, the average particle size must be impractically small if the population of particles bigger than 200 nm is to be restricted. Consequently, it is desirable to use a manufacturing technique that results in a confined size distribution.

In addition, the nanoparticle's experimental and production phases may provide various unexpected challenges. In many instances, the synthesis techniques for making nanoparticles must be rethought entirely, as a methodology that is efficient in the lab is ineffective in a factory. In a factory, the nanoparticle structural variation must be lower, the production quantity must be significantly large, and the synthesis must be more sterile than in a laboratory. Even if a particle is functional, all these problems may make its manufacture uneconomical. Due to the tendency of nanoparticles to aggregate and degrade in solution over time, any commercially marketable particle must be stable in both environments. Moreover, the difficulty in establishing the toxicity of nanoparticles over a microscopic molecule offers additional regulatory challenges. Thus, the duration and cost of clinical testing are significantly increased. Due to these limitations, it is crucial to consider scalability and reproducibility from the outset of the development process in order to avoid problems down the line [3]. The average period for research and approval of a new medicine is about 12 years, and the average cost of development is over $2.6 billion. One can agree that the process of taking a nanopharmaceutical from the lab to stores may be lengthy and expensive.

Once a nanopharmaceutical has been authorized, it may be produced and supplied to pharmacies and other retail locations. However, the expense of research and development, clinical trials, and regulatory approval can be considerable, making nanopharmaceuticals more expensive than conventional medications. As more nanotechnology-based medications are created and authorized for use, the demand for nanopharmaceuticals is anticipated to continue to increase in the future years. **Figure 11.1** illustrates the phases of the development of nanotherapeutics [4].

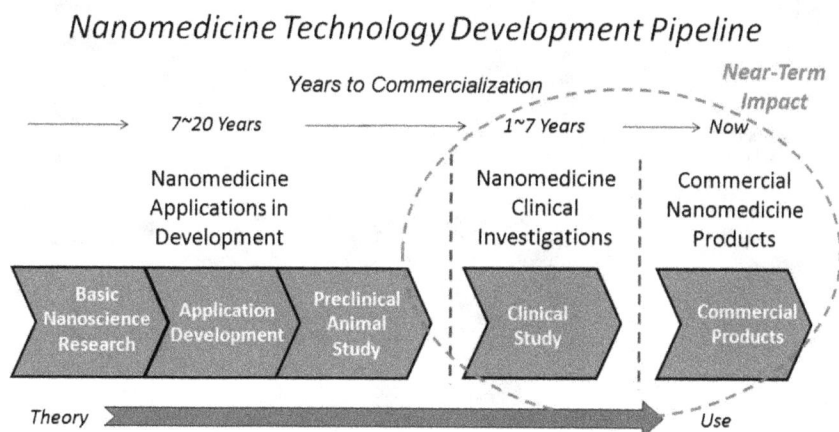

FIGURE 11.1 Pathways by Which a Chemical Compound Is Developed into a Pharmaceutical. [Reprinted with permission from *Etheridge et al. (2013)*] [4].

11.2   A GLIMPSE OF THE FUTURE FOR CARBON-BASED NANOCARRIERS FOR DRUG DELIVERY

In the medical area, carbon-based materials have a restricted number of applications. Carbon nanomaterials (CNMs) are a remarkable innovation in nanotechnology that continues to make news in the scientific and technological sectors. Due to their diversity, which includes carbon nanotubes (CNTs), graphene quantum dots (GQDs), graphene oxide (GO), fullerene, carbon nanofibers (CNFs), and carbon sheets, CNMs are readily exploitable for biological purposes (CS) [5]. **Figure 11.2** shows the plethora of CNMs. Sumio Iijima discovered in 1991 that the carbon arc discharge produced multiwall CNTs, and he and Donald Bethune were later able to generate single-wall CNTs [6]. CNMs are carbon allotropes, but their nanoscale dimensions imply a different structural structure. Graphene, fullerenes, carbon fibers, amorphous carbon, and carbon nano-onions are examples of CNMs. Unlike carbon nanotubes and fibers, graphene has a two-dimensional (2D) structure. CNM has demonstrated promise in a variety of biological applications, including medication delivery, biosensors, cancer therapy, tissue engineering, disease and infection detection, and diagnostic imaging [7]. CNM toxicity is still a problem, limiting its biological use. CNM toxicity is influenced by numerous factors, including the substance's shape, size, and chemical composition, as well as the individuals' susceptibility to the substance, the rate at which they ingest it, the rate at which their cells absorb it, and the mechanism of cytoplasmic and nuclear interference. Due to adulteration, some CNMs may be hazardous. The addition of metal ions to CNM synthesis increases their cytotoxicity. Researchers have demonstrated that cancer cells that consume CNMs perish due to DNA and lipid damage brought on by an increase in reactive oxygen species (ROS). Exposure to graphene materials increases ROS,

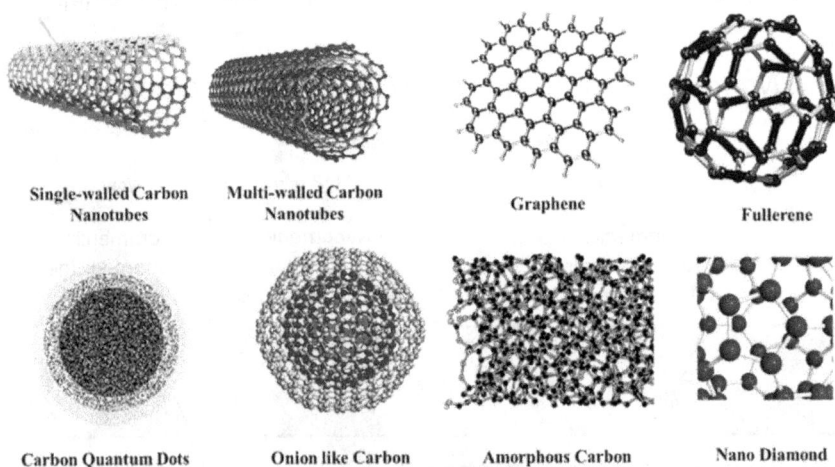

Single-walled Carbon Nanotubes   Multi-walled Carbon Nanotubes   Graphene   Fullerene

Carbon Quantum Dots   Onion like Carbon   Amorphous Carbon   Nano Diamond

FIGURE 11.2 The Various Kinds of Carbon Nanomaterials Available as Nanocarriers for Administering Medication. [Reprinted with permission from *Brindhadevi et al. (2023)*] [5].

which affects macrophage function, destroys mitochondrial membranes, and eventually results in cell death [8].

The solubility, safety, and biodegradability of CNMs can be enhanced by modifying their surface functionalization. The slower clearance and extended retention in the body improve the efficacy of pharmaceutical delivery. Cationic and anionic functionalization can increase the toxicity of CNMs beyond that of unfunctionalized CNMs when added to CNMs. It has been claimed that the surface functionalization of amino acids, medications, small molecules, peptides, and proteins can enhance the solubility and efficiency of CNMs. Various interaction mechanisms, including ionic, covalent, and van der Waal forces, are employed to tag target-specific molecules on CNMs [5]. This modification results in the transmission of several traits and characteristics with potential medical applications. Contact with active compounds or drugs can modify the surface functional groups required for drug loading and grafting onto the appropriate morphologies of CNMs. To improve their physical, chemical, and biological properties for usage in biomedical applications, it is imperative to explore the unique characteristics of CNM.

Furthermore, with its uncontrolled release, the traditional pill has been replaced by medication delivery techniques with greater bioavailability and fewer side effects. Ongoing research is being conducted on more precise, controllable, and user-friendly ways of pharmaceutical administration. At the forefront of research are drug delivery methods for future viruses, safety, symbiotic delivery systems, gender-sensitive delivery systems, affordability, greener drug delivery systems, and systems that achieve unmet clinical needs.

11.2.1 Overcoming the Blood-Brain Barrier

The blood-brain barrier (BBB) is a selectively permeable membrane that acts as a barrier between the bloodstream and the central nervous system, protecting the brain from harmful substances. However, this barrier also makes it difficult for drugs to reach the brain, limiting the effectiveness of many treatments for neurological diseases. In terms of years of healthy life lost due to disability, neurological disorders rank #1 globally. Glioblastoma multiforme is among the deadliest neoplasms and is one of the rare diseases that may end in death shortly after diagnosis. Asia has the most fatality rate, with a median survival time of seven to 15 months following diagnosis [9]. The traditional and initial line of defense against brain tumors is surgical resection. However, glioblastoma is distinctive in that it infiltrates and develops aggressively in the blood arteries of the surrounding brain parenchyma, making complete surgical ablation difficult. Aging populations are disproportionately affected by neurological disorders. Neurodegenerative diseases, such as dementia, epilepsy, and other seizure-inducing disorders, Parkinson's disease and other movement disorders, mental issues, stroke, and transient ischemic attack, necessitate immediate study into therapies and prevention [10].

The limited solubility of neurotherapeutics via the oral route and their bioavailability being hindered by two barriers, the BBB and the blood-cerebrospinal fluid barrier (BCSF), significantly restrict the treatment and management options for neurological illnesses. The blood-brain barrier divides the brain's circulatory system from its nerve tissues, making it extraordinarily difficult to deliver therapeutic agents to the brain's site of action. In chemotherapy, drugs are used to induce cell death in brain cancer patients; however, drug delivery is hindered by several factors, including tumor heterogeneity, hypoxic tumor environment, the presence of glioma stem cells, aberrant signaling pathways, and most importantly, the existence of the BBB, resulting in high recurrence rates, overall resistance to therapy, and devastating neurological deterioration. In the past two decades, advanced intelligent drug delivery systems have enabled more effective treatment of neurological disorders and malignancies such as schizophrenia, migraine, Parkinson's, Alzheimer's, and brain tumors. Nanotherapeutics is an emerging field that aims to overcome the BBB by using nanoscale particles to deliver drugs directly to the brain. This approach has shown promising results in preclinical studies, as the small size of these particles allows them to bypass the BBB and target specific cells within the brain. Recently, nanoscale drug carriers have been utilized to boost the therapeutic effectiveness of therapeutic medications with no or little side effects, as listed in **Table 11.1** [9]. The distribution of drugs to the brain presents several obstacles. However, many pharmaceutical nanocarriers may be utilized to develop successful drug delivery systems with desirable properties.

Enclosing the medicinal substance in the nanocarrier can improve its solubility and stability. Nanocarriers containing a chemical capable of interacting with the targeted receptor expressed on the targeted cell's surface can inhibit cancer cells from absorbing the drug [11]. Due to their new physicochemical properties and lower toxicity, carbon nano-onions (CNOs) have shown promise [9,12]. CNOs have a

TABLE 11.1

List of Medications Administered with Nanocarriers or Functionalized Nanocarriers. [Reprinted with permission from *Majumder et al. (2021)*] [9].

Drug	Nanocarrier	Functionalization	Uses
Doxorubicin	SWCNT	PEG	Reduced toxicity
	MWCNT	Folic acid	Active targeting
	Human serum albumin	Amino/acid group	Antineoplastic
	PLLA-b-PEG	Folic acid	Solid tumors
	Polymer-lipid hybrid	Lipid	
	Poly (DEAP-Lys)-b-PEG - b-PLLA	Poly(lysine)	
Paclitaxel	SWCNT	PEG	Increased circulation period
	Trimyristin	Sterically stabilized	Ovarian, lung, and breast cancer
	PEG-PE	Lipid	Various cancers
Cisplatin	SWCNT		Reduced toxicity
Methotrexate	MWCNT	Folic acid	Controlled toxicity
Estrogen	PLGA	Alendronate	Bone-osteoporosis
Oligonucleotide	PEG or PE particles	Transferrin	Brain-gene
siRNA	PE	RGD peptides	Vasculature cancer
Retinoic acid	PLA	Galactose	Hepatocytes

multilayered fullerene structure. Since nanoparticles (NPs) of range 20 nm or less are permitted to pass through it, the size of CNOs between 1 and 15 nm promotes barrier permeability mainly through the transient opening of tight junctions or fusing with membrane bilayers and ion-pairing [13]. The BBB is the most significant barrier in brain-targeted delivery because it restricts the bioaccumulation of drugs at the target site. The BBB comprises several cell types: neurons, astrocytes, pericytes, and brain capillary endothelial cells [14].

Nanomedicines with high lipophilicity are ideal for drug administration to the brain because they can more readily traverse the BBB. Because of their unique optical, thermal, magnetic, and physicochemical properties—including their tiny size, huge specific surface area, and high chemical reactivity—materials with sizes between 10 nm and 100 nm are now the focus of BBB-crossing applications [15]. Another example is magnetic nanoparticles, which can be guided through the BBB using a magnetic field. Under the influence of a magnetic field, magnetic nanoparticles (MNPs) can enter human cells and tissues, making them useful for diagnostic purposes. These MNPs may be directed to and kept in diseased tissue with an external magnetic field, allowing for the differentiation of cancerous cells from normal cells in the body [16]. In medicine, polymer-coated iron oxide nanoparticles are employed for a variety of applications, including medication administration, magnetic resonance imaging (MRI), and hyperthermia due to their nontoxicity and biocompatibility. They do better than metallic inorganic nanoparticles like cobalt, nickel, and others. Magnetic susceptibility (χ) is defined as the ratio of induced magnetization (M) to an applied magnetic field (H) and is used to categorize the magnetic characteristics of various materials. Those with no magnetic moment and a slight negative magnetic susceptibility are called diamagnetic.

In contrast, those with a random or parallel magnetic moment and a slight negative magnetic susceptibility are called paramagnetic, and those with a magnetic moment parallel to H and a significant negative magnetic susceptibility are called ferromagnetic or ferrimagnetic [17]. After being functionalized with the polymer coating, MNPs can efficiently load additional pharmaceuticals due to the presence of multiple functional groups on the polymer surface. Additionally, this increases the half-life of MNPs, which decreases their toxicity to cells. Surface functionalization can utilize natural and synthetic polymers, lipid molecules, and functional ligands for selective or receptor-mediated targeting [18]. This method has been tested in preclinical studies for treating brain tumors and has shown promising drug delivery and efficacy results.

In conclusion, nanotherapeutics can revolutionize the treatment of neurological diseases by allowing drugs to bypass the BBB and directly target the brain. While further research is needed to fully realize this approach's potential, the results have been promising, and nanotherapeutics may play a vital role in the future of neurological disease treatment.

11.2.2 ADVANCES IN OCULAR THERAPIES

The human eye consists of two segments: the anterior and posterior segments. The cornea, conjunctiva, aqueous chamber, iris, ciliary body, and lens comprise the anterior section of the eye, also known as the anterior segment. Because the front of the eye is easily accessible, eyedrops administered topically are standard therapy for anterior eye diseases. Due to the corneal barrier, quick tear film turnover, and rapid tear drainage, topical eyedrops are unreliable due to their poor ocular absorption. The posterior region of the eye consists of the vitreous body, retina, and choroid [19]. Eyedrop-delivered drugs have a very low concentration in the retina and vitreous humor because they must travel a great distance and overcome many ocular obstacles to reach the back of the eye. Due to the presence of the blood-retinal barrier (BRB), medications cannot be successfully transported to the eye via the systemic route; instead, very high doses are required, which might cause undesired systemic side effects. As they may transport drugs directly to the back of the eye, vitreous humor and intravitreal (IVT) injections are now frequently employed in clinics to treat acute eye diseases. Therapeutic success needs frequent IVT injections because vitreous humor turnover allows quick clearance of unutilized medications following IVT injections. It has been demonstrated that patients who require frequent IVF injections may be less cooperative with their therapy, pay larger financial expenditures, and be at increased risk for injection-related complications [20]. To reduce the strain on patients and improve treatment efficacy, IVT drug delivery devices with extended drug release characteristics are required. Subconjunctival (SCT), subtenon, and peribulbar injections are examples of periocular delivery that are less invasive than IVT injections but can still carry drugs to the back of the eye. To reach the retina and vitreous, medications must first pass through the sclera, choroid, and retinal pigment epithelium (RPE) of the eye. Due to these drug transport obstacles in the ocular tissue layers, effective drug concentrations cannot be delivered to the retina following periocular administration [21]. Suprachoroidal administration is a promising method for delivering drugs to the back of the eye since it circumvents the sclera, a significant diffusion barrier encountered by periocular drug delivery [22]. Suprachoroidal medicine delivery poses the risk of retinal hemorrhage and detachment, necessitating the use of specialist equipment (such as microneedles) to ensure the drug reaches the retina in a safe and regulated way [20].

Others may increase the solubility of hydrophobic medications in an aqueous solution, offer prolonged drug release with less toxicity and greater efficacy, increase drug retention duration, and enhance drug penetration through ocular barriers. Nanomedicines found for ocular drug administration include liposomes, polymeric nanoparticles, micelles, and dendrimers, to name a few. Liposomes' aqueous core comprises phospholipids, cholesterol, and lipid-conjugated polymers. The aqueous core of liposomes can be loaded with hydrophilic drugs, whereas lipid bilayers can be loaded with lipophilic drugs [23]. It is possible to modify polymeric nanoparticles to store a significant number of drugs for prolonged, controlled release. Dendrimers are spherical, nanostructured (3–20 nm) polymers with minimal polydispersity. The functional groups on the surface of dendrimers might be utilized to attach pharmaceuticals, or the medications could be enclosed within the dendrimer core. Dendrimers' manufacturing, surface chemistry, and conjugation strategy can be modified to maximize drug loading and release [24]. Micelles are self-assembled spherical vesicles with a hydrophilic corona and a hydrophobic core that can solubilize and stabilize hydrophobic drugs [25].

Nanomedicine for the eye has been created using cutting-edge nanofabrication techniques such as particle replication in a non-wetting template (PRINT) and the hydrogel template approach [26,27]. The PRINT process is a nanofabrication method that uses roll-to-roll manufacturing to produce monodispersed NPs and microparticles of a specific size, shape, and modulus [26]. Using PRINT technology to create NPs requires three steps: first, constructing micro molds with precise micro- or nano-cavities; second, molding therapeutic substances into the cavities; and finally, releasing NPs from the mold after they have hardened. Manufacturing particles with repeatable form, size, and surface modification on a large scale using a continuous process, the physiochemical properties of PRINT particles could be modified by modifying matrix composition or post-functionalization [20]. PRINT has been shown to function with a variety of biocompatible polymers and pharmaceuticals, such as nucleic acids, proteins, and antibodies. For controlled drug delivery to the eye, PRINT technology has produced ocular formulations such as subconjunctival (SCT) implants, intracameral (IC) implants, intravitreal (IVT) implants, nano- and micro-suspensions, and other similar forms. AR13503, a potent inhibitor of Rho kinase and protein kinase C (PKC), may one day be used to treat retinal neovascularization. The biodegradable polymers PLGA/PDLA/poly(ester amide) (PEA) were produced into a rod shape and appropriately sized for injection with a 27 gauge needle utilizing PRINT technology (80). AR13503 implants utilizing PRINT technology demonstrated *in-vitro* drug release for more than 60 days. In 2019, clinical trials for the PRINT-based AR13503 implant to treat diabetic macular edema (DME) and wet age-related macular degeneration (AMD) will commence. The PRINT method has been proven effective for the GMP production of kilogram quantities of NPs [20].

The hydrogel template method permits the production of vast quantities of uniform nanoparticles and microparticles, which are then transported by the template itself. Nanowafers are ultrathin, translucent lenses that contain nano-drug reservoirs. They are fabricated utilizing hydrogel template technology. Generation of the PVA template with well-fabricated arrays, e-beam lithography was used to form a pattern on a silicon wafer, and then PVA solution was poured over the pattern. Nanowafers were produced by pouring solutions of medicinal substances into a PVA mold. By adjusting the capacity of the drug reservoirs, drug loading and particle size may be regulated. The ocular surface can be implanted directly with nanowafers for extended drug release. In contrast to standard contact lenses, which must be removed to avoid bacterial infection, nanowafers are made from dissolvable PVA and may dissolve away automatically.

11.2.3 IMPROVEMENTS IN CANCER TREATMENTS

In the global South, cancer has emerged as the major cause of mortality. Carbon nanoparticles are at the forefront as an efficient medicine delivery technology for cancer diagnosis and treatment. CNMs are the ideal delivery mode for transferring pharmaceutical substances to the site of action, avoiding degradation of the molecules loaded. In addition, it helps retain the potency of the molecule at its site of action while simultaneously reducing its off-target effect and boosting its overall efficacy. CNMs of many types release anticancer medicines in a regulated and sustained manner to prevent the multiplication of cancer cells. CNMs have been loaded with several anticancer drugs, including doxorubicin (DOX), betulinic acid (BA), methotrexate (MTX), gemcitabine (GEM), etoposide (ETO), paclitaxel (PTX), chelerythrine (CPT), camptothecin (CPT), carboplatin (CPM), cisplatin (CIS), platinum (II), and platinum (IV) [28].

Due to their toxicity and insolubility, only graphene sheets, carbon quantum dots, and carbon nanotubes have been effectively exploited for cancer treatment and diagnostics. These CNMs are less toxic than other metallic nanoparticles and may be functionalized with a variety of ligands to facilitate the conjugation of anticancer drugs within or on their structure. They used a range of polymers, including PEG and chitosan, ligand-specific attachment sites readily accessible by tumor cells that have been functionalized. The drug doxorubicin can be bound to graphene through hydrogen bonds to oxygenated functional groups, allowing for time-controlled drug release. Genetic material may be adsorbed onto graphene through interaction between the nucleic acid base and the polyaromatic basal plane of graphene nanomaterials. This enables the transfer of single-stranded nucleic acid resistant to destruction by variables like temperature, pH, and enzymes.

There was a developing concern with the elimination or toxicity of CNMs, but this issue has been rectified, thanks to the use of organic components in the synthesis of CNMs. If research into boosting target specificity and pharmaceutical loading capacity is conducted, it is possible to construct treatment programs with a longer duration. Recent research has demonstrated that CNMs carrying siRNA effectively destroy cancer cells. More effective delivery methods, such as CQDs, may be developed with the help of the research and development of innovative anticancer drugs and agents. In addition, it is possible to obtain 100% efficacy against cancer cells by loading numerous drugs onto a single CNM [5].

11.3   VIRAL NANOPARTICLES AS DRUG DELIVERY SYSTEMS

The growth of nanotechnology over the last several decades has opened new opportunities in the world of medical research, notably in the area of medicine administration. Traditional drug carriers have been constructed from liposomes and lipids, synthetic and natural polymers, and inorganic nanoparticles [29]. Nanoparticles for medication delivery must be biocompatible, biodegradable, and have a low degree of toxicity to have a substantial therapeutic impact [30]. However, the toxicity and low delivery effectiveness of a number of synthetic carriers demand the development and deployment of alternate delivery techniques. There is an urgent need to introduce novel pharmaceutical delivery strategies to the research and development pipeline because there is no "perfect solution." Protein-based nanoparticles, such as protein cages and viruses, are examples of an emerging class of novel drug carriers [31]. Protein cages are instances of self-assembled supramolecular structures composed of their component protein monomers. Their constituent elements are not infectious by definition. Virus-like particles (VLPs) are analogous, but they vary in that they are created by carefully assembling the viral coat proteins. Viruses are sturdy structures that can withstand external forces and resist degeneration, but they are also sensitive to signals in their surrounding cellular environment, allowing them to release their genome when instructed to do so.

Within the category of viruses, two subcategories can be identified. These are known as VLPs and viral nanoparticles (VNPs). It is widely believed that VLPs, the genome-free equivalents of VNPs, do not induce infection. Due to the possibility that viral genomes may or may not be present, they may impart unique immunostimulatory patterns. This study examines VLP and VNP plant viruses in addition to bacteriophages. In some situations, we also explore the application of different protein cages and highlight a few viral nanotechnologies for mammalian cells. Since the self-assembly of repetitive protein subunits forms viral capsids, they possess a high degree of polyvalence. Viruses may infect a variety of cell types. Plant viruses are typically non-enveloped organisms that can have a spherical/icosahedral or filamentous/tubular shape. Plant viruses are also capable of morphing over time. Viruses are considered natural nucleic acid carriers because they protect and deliver their payload, the principal characteristic exploited for medication distribution [32,33]. Infusion, encapsulation, absorption, or conjugation of drug cargo to the inner and external surfaces of the coat protein interfaces, combinations of chemical procedures, and attachment to the different functional groups given by the protein structure can be utilized. These operations can occur on either side of the protein. This versatility enables a vast array of possibilities, including reversible binding of active chemicals, protection inside proteinaceous matrices, and selective targeting to the site where the action will occur [29].

Due to their morphological uniformity, biocompatibility, water solubility, facile functionalization, and high absorption efficiency, natural delivery carriers, and VNP-based carriers, in particular, provide a number of significant advantages. Nanomedical approaches for drug delivery or imaging must also utilize biological properties to construct clever nanosized cages with high stability, appropriate pharmacokinetics, cell targeting, and effective cell penetration. Since plant viruses seldom exhibit tissue tropisms, secondary functions such as cell surface receptor binding, targeting ability, membrane crossing, and nuclear penetration might be added into a nanoparticle formulation (synthetic or natural) [34].

Even though no plant- or bacteriophage-based nanomedicine has yet been approved for clinical use, several systems are now undergoing investigation, and a few are on the verge of entering translational development. Among the plant VLP and VNP-based nanotechnology platforms being explored for varied nanomedical applications are tobacco mosaic virus (TMV), cowpea mosaic virus (CPMV), cowpea chlorotic mottle virus (CCMV), physalis mottle virus (PhMV), and potato virus X (PVX). Notable bacteriophages include MS2, P22, Q, and M13. One may encounter viruses ranging in length from less than 30 nm to more than 1 micron, as illustrated in **Figure 11.3** [29]. Utilizing biochemistry and guided evolution, viral nanocarriers for medication delivery, imaging, and theranostic applications have been produced, and their use has been growing. In this chapter, we discuss the diagnostic and therapeutic potential of VNPs and VLPs in a variety of biomedical settings, including antimicrobial, cancer, protein/peptide, and gene therapies; monotherapy and combination therapies against cancer; vaccines against infectious diseases, cancer, and other diseases; nanocarriers for imaging modalities; and theranostics with photothermal therapy (PTT).

Currently, chemotherapy is the treatment of choice for cancer. However, maximum-tolerated pharmaceutical dosages are frequently employed in cancer therapy, which

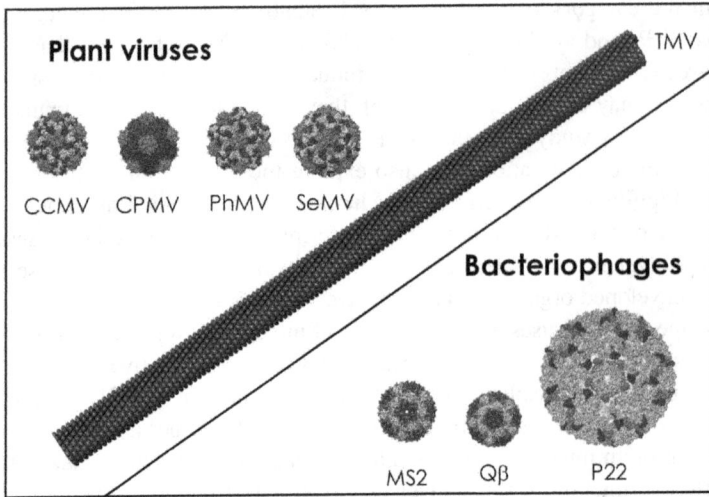

FIGURE 11.3 Scaled Images of Various Plant VLPs and Bacteriophages. [Reprinted with permission from *Chung et al. (2020)*] [29].

might result in severe side effects and limited clinical use. The limited clinical use is due to the high rates of medication resistance and recurrence, rapid drug clearance, and non-targeted delivery [35]. The development of drug delivery strategies that provide targeted and intracellular distribution, increase active drug accumulation in tumor tissues, and minimize the doses required to produce therapeutic effects may ameliorate these challenges and enhance treatment outcomes.

VLPs possess several characteristics that make them appropriate for the targeted delivery of pharmaceuticals to their intended locations of action. In an early study, MS2 VLPs modified with a targeting peptide (SP94) were used to selectively transport chemotherapeutic drugs (DOX, cisplatin, and 5-FU) to human hepatocellular carcinoma (HCC) cells [36]. These modified VLPs induced selective cytotoxicity *in-vitro*, even at extremely low doses, and demonstrated high avidity and selectivity for HCC with limited uptake by healthy cells. DOX-loaded VLPs were 20 times more effective in killing HCC cells than free DOX (IC$_{50}$ values of 10–15 nM) [29].

Platinum-based anticancer medications, employed in the treatment of about 50% of cancer patients undergoing chemotherapy, have been widely supplied utilizing plant virus-based nanoparticles [37]. Since platinum-based drugs such as cisplatin and drug candidate phenanthriplatin (phenPt) may be quickly loaded into the TMV cavities via a charge-driven reaction or by creating stable covalent adducts, TMV provides an interesting platform for the effective administration of these drugs. Compared to free cisplatin, TMV-cisplatin VNP complexes were more readily taken up by cancer cells and showed more cytotoxicity [38]. VNPs containing cisplatin were modified with mannose and lactose moieties on their external surface for targeted drug delivery. In MCF-7 and HepG2 cancer cell lines, the targeted and drug-loaded TMV demonstrated higher cytotoxicity through the specific recognition between mannose and galectin and lactose and the asialoglycoprotein receptor on the cell membranes. Functionalizing TMV and CPMV with mitoxantrone (MTO) is another example of a medication delivery application involving plant VNPs. However, like other anti-neoplastic drugs, MTO has serious cardiac side effects despite its excellent efficacy against most malignancies (it is a topoisomerase II inhibitor) [29].

Mitoxantrone-mediated functionalization of TMV and CPMV is another example of a drug delivery application employing plant VNPs. Despite its effectiveness against the vast majority of cancers, MTO, like other anti-neoplastic medicines, has severe cardiac adverse effects (it is a topoisomerase II inhibitor). We demonstrated that MTO-TMVs were more effective than controls when administered subcutaneously into a null mouse model of MDA-MB-231 triple-negative breast cancer [39]. At a tumor volume of 100 mm³, MTO-TMV was injected intratumorally (i.t.). We also utilized passive diffusion to load MTO into the internal cavity of CPMV and found that MTO-CPMV displayed enhanced cytotoxic effects *in-vitro* when paired with tumor necrosis factor-related apoptosis-inducing ligand (TRAIL) [40]. To particularly target non-lymphoma, the antimitotic drug valine-citrulline monomethyl auristatin E (vcMMAE) was applied to the outside of Hodgkin's TMV VNPs. Internalization into endolysosomal components has been established by studies of particle ingestion, suggesting that proteases most likely mediate drug release.

11.4   NANOBOTS: THE FUTURE OF NANOSIZED THERAPEUTICS

The miniature robotic systems have proven their worth in the previous decade, allowing for accurate diagnostics and therapeutic interventions inside a system as complicated as the human body. Because of their capacity for autonomous navigation, nanobots may be thought of as a broad class of locomotive artificial molecular robots. These nanocarriers can power themselves, making them a viable option for real-time picture monitoring that is also sufficiently biocompatible [41,42].

In the past, passive and active targeting were the norm when using nanomaterials in biological applications like silica and lipid-polymer-based carriers. However, these approaches are constrained in clinical applications by the nonspecific targeting impact of the passive approach and the low targeting ratio of the active approach [43]. More refined nanobots for use in future biomedical technology will allow these restrictions to be lifted. The success of these materials can be attributed to the advanced level of bioengineering that can be performed on their surfaces. Clinical applications of these nano-systems are still in the early stages of development, but completing clinical trials and breaking into the worldwide market is a crucial component of the research and development process [42].

The fundamental idea behind the motion of nano-machines is to convert energy into motion by scavenging fuel from the system, like chemical catalysis (i.e., the generation of O_2 or H_2), or by harnessing power from ultrasound, electrical, or magnetic fields, or by applying the aforementioned combinational approach. Nanosurgery, which is computationally executed in the host; targeted medication administration; bioimaging; and bio-isolation are all critical uses of designed nanobots. Compared to traditional nano-systems, which use passive transport through diffusion or external pressures and macroscopic powered devices in nanoactuators, this one has the key advantages of self-power and self-navigation. Nanobots have proven their worth in recent years by overcoming the obstacles as previously mentioned and enabling accurate navigation in the intricate biological environment [42].

Once implanted, nanobots' movement can only be controlled and monitored in real time by electric/magnetic fields or acoustic systems exterior to the body. Therefore, it is crucial to plan carefully and bioengineer application-specific nanobots that can be safely given and delivered to their final destination. One of the primary goals of nanorobotics has always been to have access to regulate its motion [44]. Furthermore, motors with varying shapes, material composition, and energy conversion are required to permit their assigned responsibilities under optimal settings with consistent biocompatibility across a wide range of biological activities or intended functions.

The design of nanobots is influenced by delivery tasks, such as nanobot movement along a user-defined path or a theoretically/experimentally optimized path, execution tasks, such as delivering drugs, killing diseased cells, or cleaning up pollution, and exit tasks, such as recycling or in-situ degradation [45]. Chemical or fuel-driven nanobots are separated from fuel-free nanobots, which are propelled by magnetic or electric forces, light, or ultrasound [42]. Sauvage, Stoddard, and Feringa were awarded the Nobel Prize for their ground-breaking and comprehensive work on molecular motors [46]. A group of molecules with characteristics like those of synthetic muscle, lift, and axle has been created. Catenanes and rotaxanes are two examples of this novel chemical family that is gaining extensive use in nanorobotics to achieve finely controlled molecular mobility. In addition, Balzani et al. demonstrated that a rotaxane-based synthetic motor with a length of 5 nanometers may be continuously fed by sunlight and exhibited autonomous movement when exposed to light [47]. The research revealed that the stable synthetic structure lasted for 1000 cycles while generating 10^{-17} W of power per molecule. In addition, the researchers claimed that their method was effective up until the point at which solar energy was created. Researchers have discovered new approaches to solve concerns like biocompatibility, motility, and Brownian motion since then. Various propulsion methods and fuel-dependent and fuel-free systems for supplying nanodevices with energy are also researched [48]. Propulsion is a crucial aspect of nanobots, as it determines their ability to move and perform tasks in complex environments. There are several methods that have been developed for the propulsion of nanobots, including:

- Chemical propulsion.
- Electromagnetic propulsion.
- Photophoretic propulsion.
- Thermophoretic propulsion.
- Biological or bio-hybrid propulsion.

Chemical propulsion involves using a chemical reaction to generate a flow of fluid that propels the nanobot. Nanobots may employ fuel degraded on catalytic surfaces (such as platinum or other metals) to generate gas bubbles [49]. On the surface of a catalyst, for example, H_2O_2 generates a high concentration of O_2 gas, which coalesces to produce enormous bubbles with a critical nucleation radius, R_0. Even though buoyancy force and surface adhesion are at conflict, the surrounding dissolved O_2 continues to seep into the bubble and assist its growth. When the bubble reaches the detachment radius, it is released, generating a change in momentum that serves as the nanobots' propulsion force. This mechanism's advantages include a quick system that consistently reaches its target at high power levels. This method is well suited for navigating through fluids and is used in applications such as environmental monitoring and drug delivery. A recent study reported utilizing a bottle-shaped nanodevice to provide antibiotics to eradicate *Helicobacter pylori* (H. *pylori*), which causes stomach cancer. This is an example of synthetic nanodevice research based on the notion of H_2O_2 breakdown [50]. Another study by Diez et al. produced doxorubicin-loaded multifunctional platinum-mesoporous silica nanomotors to treat cancer (DOX). Preparing DOX-loaded nanobots with a high catalytic surface area enhanced propulsion, enabling GSH-induced targeted dispersion via bubble propulsion [51]. Small Brownian contributions were observed, however, due to the collision-induced motion of the nanobots. Despite their excellent mobility and propulsion, the reaction products of nano propellers powered by fossil fuels were shown to be toxic to living tissue [42]. So, to address the issue, recent developments in nanobot technology have demanded the use of biocompatible fuel sources, such as enzyme and silver, manganese, and iron-based catalytic surfaces [52,53]. Using enzyme-powered nanobots made from UiO-66 type metal-organic frameworks (MOFs) to separate rhodamine B from water samples is a unique method, as proven by Yang et al. [54]. MOFs are favored nanomotor systems because of their enormous surface area, programmable pore size, and changeable surface functionality [55].

Electromagnetic propulsion encompasses using electromagnetic fields to propel the nanobot. For example, a magnetic field can propel a nanobot equipped with magnetic material. This method is well suited for navigating through liquids and has medical imaging and environmental monitoring applications. The classification of magnetic field-induced propulsion depends on whether the magnetic field is rotating or oscillating [56,57]. Fabrication and external force must be regulated since these nanobots' physical shape and locomotion mode substantially impact their construction and movement. The concept is new in terms of targeted distribution and imaging, despite the paucity of study in this field. Iron-coated Mg nanoparticles based on Janus nanobots were generated in a recent work published in Nature Portfolio's *Communications Chemistry*, confirming the practicality of this technique [42]. In this research, $Mg\text{-}Fe_3O_4$ nanoparticles were thiol-chemically connected with glutathione (GSH)-Cy5-PAMAM-NH2-G4 (G4) dendrimers. Antibodies against epithelial cell adhesion molecule (EpCAM) were added for specificity. The study involves the utilization of Au-single link with DOX content. The team of Karaca et al. fabricated nickel nanowires that were altered with an anti-miRNA-21 probe consisting of FAM-ssDNA. The motion of these nanowires was achieved through a synergistic effect of magnetic and acoustic propulsion [58]. Under 22 mT magnetic fields, the calculated speed of nanobots in a microfluidic channel was 15 m s^{-1}, and under the expression of both magnetic and acoustic fields, the speed increased to 120 m s^{-1}, with the frequency of the applied field governing the latter. As a bonus, this nanomotor showed intriguing biosensing and therapeutic uses against cancer cells; however, adding mi-RNA to the device, which might have boosted its sensitivity but required a sophisticated environment, would have raised its cost.

Photophoretic propulsion comprises using light to propel the nanobot. For example, a nanobot can be designed with a light-absorbing material that creates a force when exposed to light. This method is well suited for navigating gaseous environments and has applications in environmental monitoring and drug delivery. In fuel-free propulsion, light is often used to slow down ready nanomotors, giving the operator more leeway to direct the system's motion by adjustments to the light's intensity, polarization, frequency, and time of flight [42]. Light-induced power, also known as single-beam gradient forces, photothermal, or photocatalytic propulsion [59], is the process behind the optical propulsion of nanobots. In recent years, nanomotors equipped with phototaxis properties have shown promise as a viable strategy for future biological applications due to their light-driven motion.

Light-induced electrophoretic mobility is similar to the electrophoretic mobility mentioned previously; the key distinction is the incorporation of photocatalysis into the nanobots' motion. Devices are propelled forward by creating photo-catalytically-induced asymmetric chemical gradients surrounding the nanostructure. He et al. first created a light-responsive ZnO-Pt Janus micromotor that could align itself in the direction of light illumination and exhibit negative phototaxis at speeds of up to 32 ms^{-1} in water [60]. ZnO is a semiconducting material with a large band gap that permits electron transport from the valance band to the conduction band when exposed to UV light, where valence band holes oxidize water to form H$^+$ ions. As this happens, H$_2$ is being reduced from H$^+$ by photogenerated electrons that have shifted to the Pt side, where the Fermi level is lower. Due to the proposed photocatalytic and photoelectric capabilities, hole-induced ZnO oxidation resulted in the formation of Zn^{+2} via a photo-corrosion process. The dipole-induced local electric field created by the unequal distribution of H$^+$ and Zn^{+2} ions drives the negatively charged ZnO/Pt Janus micromotor toward the ZnO end through self-electrophoresis. However, a paper published in *Nano Research* showed the relevance of photothermally produced temperature differential in nanobot movement for biomedical applications [61]. Lipase-loaded, spiky-shelled carbon@silica nanobots were created for triglyceride breakdown in NIR light in this work. Advantages of employing carbon yolk and spiky shell construction of nanomotor include strong absorption in the NIR region, which can be tuned by etching time and temperature, and high loading of lipase. Diffusion of the nanobots via self-thermophoresis and triglyceride degradation in ten minutes was achieved due to the asymmetric distribution of carbon yolk inside the silica nanobots, which created a temperature gradient. A recent work reportedly created liquid metals-based nanobots with the benefits of biodegradability, low vapor pressure, transformable characteristics, and minimal toxicity to further minimize the system's toxicity and boost photocatalytic performance [62]. Light may be used to cause liquid crystals to expand and contract, altering the fluidity of the material and allowing the structure to move [42,63]. Using urease as their driving force, Xu et al. created liquid metal (LM) nanobots based on a GaInSn alloy that was grafted with the antibiotic cefixime trihydrate (CT) [62]. Two approaches were used to determine the system's motion, which were as follows: Under a concentration gradient, nanobots freely diffused toward the high urea concentration due to the urease-induced chemotactic characteristics. Under NIR illumination, the morphology of LM@PDA changed, and fragments of CT-PDA were released into the biological system due to its excellent photothermal conversion capabilities. This was because the interaction between the (GaO)OH component and the surrounding water produced local heat and reactive oxygen species (ROS), hence facilitating antibacterial photothermal treatment and dual-mode ultrasonic (US) and photoacoustic (PA) imaging signals. Additionally, Zheng et al. created a Janus nanobot composed of gold-modified Gadolinium [Gd(III)] doped mesoporous silica nanoparticles (Au@Gd-MSN) for MR imaging of tumor cells [64].

Thermophoretic propulsion is another method that utilizes temperature gradients to propel the nanobot. For example, a nanobot can be designed to move toward a heat source, where it can consume energy to perform its intended function. This method has applications in areas such as medical imaging and energy conversion. Gold nanoparticles have garnered significant attention owing to their outstanding photothermal characteristics [65]. Yang et al. produced Au-BP7@SP Janus nanohybrids with active motion thermophoresis and improved photothermal effect [66]. By turning mechanical energy into thermal energy, the compelling momentum of these Janus particles will effectively increase the temperature of the cells treated with NIR radiation, therefore eliminating malignant cells in two days. Without damaging the surrounding healthy tissue, these particles may efficiently pinpoint the site of the tumor, considerably enhancing the treatment efficacy and reducing the risk of adverse side effects. This research has demonstrated that the efficient mobility of Janus nanoparticles is associated with photothermal cancer therapy, which can pave the way for a novel cancer treatment strategy utilizing Janus nanoparticles.

Since the discovery of nanobots in 2002, the connected fields of propulsion techniques, motion control, and anticipated functionality have expanded at a rapid rate. Recent study has uncovered the function of microbes and biological cellular components, such as cilia and flagella, in the self-propulsion of nanobots, which has the potential for treatments and diagnostics [42,67]. In general, these hybrid biomotors are formed of microorganisms, such as E. coli, Bacillus spp., or magnetotactic bacteria (MTB), and cellular membrane, such as RBC, macrophage, or platelet [67]. Microorganisms often employ biological extensions such as cilia and flagella for movement even in complicated surroundings. In contrast to their movement on solid surfaces, their movement in an aquatic environment is well-understood since bacteria may push themselves with flagella or utilize magnetosomes to align themselves for directed movement (in the case of MTB). In contrast, they have developed to produce a greater number of flagella and the capacity to secrete surfactants that smooth the solid surface for their movement [68]. These inspirations from biological processes, biological micro/nanodevices, and biohybrids suggest the employment of various biological components to regulate propulsion. MTB are the most often utilized microorganisms, despite the fact that achieving their design while keeping their function is quite difficult. These bacteria possess a chain of magnetic nanoparticles that allow them to align in response to a magnetic field and cause self-motion.

Numerous species of animals, including birds, insects, and fish, have been observed swarming together. It is a catch-all word for things such as completing tasks, gaining what they desire, and avoiding predators. Inspired by this, researchers have created command-obeying nanobot swarms [69,70]. The swarming behavior of nanomotors can be triggered by optical or magnetic stimulation, or they can swarm when exposed to enzymes. Hortelao et al. have recently created a nano-motor utilizing porous silica and gold nanoparticles to power swarming enzymes [71]. The construct was radiolabeled with iodine-124 (I^{124}) for it to be tracked in real-time during positron emission tomography (PET) scans. Mice bladders exhibited swarming and collective movement of the constructs upon I^{124} activation. However, the use of radioactive elements presents ethical considerations and may disturb physiological systems in humans. Manamanchaiyaporn et al. created a magnetite nanoparticle-based swarm that leveraged the hydrodynamic effect to gather tissue plasminogen activator (t-PA) in a magnetic field, consequently resolving this issue [72]. By quickly spinning at the site of the clot, a swarm of nanobots carrying caged t-PA molecules promoted thrombolysis in this study. In thrombolytic *in-vitro* experiments, this swarm showed promise by reducing a 9.0 mm clot to 3 mm in less than two hours [72]. The nonviral delivery of Metallothionein to prostate cancer cells was also the subject of a separate study published; powered by a 0.025% fuel medium, the Au-Ag-based biocompatible nanobots were integrated into cancer cells and stored in endosomes within 30 minutes [73]. Chemically driven nanobots can resolve issues associated with traditional DNA transfection techniques and direct protein delivery in general. However, because of its possible cytotoxicity, H_2O_2 utilization is restricted.

These are some of the methods used for the propulsion of nanobots. The choice of propulsion method depends on the specific application and the desired performance of the nanobot. Researchers are continuously working on developing new and more efficient methods of propulsion to enable the widespread adoption of nanobots in a variety of fields.

11.5   REGULATIONS FOR NANOMEDICINES: THE CHALLENGES

Nano drugs, which are still relatively novel in the pharmaceutical sector, may require additional evaluation parameters in addition to those used to analyze more established drugs. The current challenges are as follows:

1. Lack of standardization: nanomedicines are a new and rapidly evolving field, and there is currently a lack of standardization in terms of their production, characterization, and testing.
2. Safety concerns: because nanomedicines are so small, they have the potential to interact with biological systems in unexpected ways, which raises safety concerns.
3. Testing requirements: testing the safety and efficacy of nanomedicines can be challenging due to their unique properties and the need for specialized techniques and equipment.
4. Approval process: the regulatory approval process for nanomedicines can be lengthy and complex, requiring extensive data on their safety, efficacy, and quality.
5. Preclinical and clinical data: the availability of high-quality preclinical and clinical data is essential for regulatory approval, but it can be difficult to obtain for nanomedicines due to the challenges in testing and characterizing them.

6. Lack of regulatory harmonization: different countries have different regulations for nanomedicines, which can lead to inconsistent standards and difficulties in bringing new products to market globally.

The FDA has taken a proactive approach to addressing the challenges posed by nanomedicine and ensuring that these products are safe and effective for patients. To this end, the FDA has released several guidance documents to address the specific challenges posed by nanomedicines, including guidance on their development, preclinical testing, clinical trials, and regulatory approval [74]. The FDA uses a science-based approach to the regulation of nanomedicines, taking into account the unique properties and potential risks posed by these products. In addition, the FDA has adopted a risk-based approach to evaluate the safety and efficacy of nanomedicines, taking into account the latest scientific knowledge and data. The FDA collaborates with stakeholders, including industry, academia, and patient groups, to ensure that the regulatory framework for nanomedicines is up-to-date and responsive to the latest scientific advances. The FDA recognizes the potential benefits of nanomedicines for patients and encourages innovation in this field while ensuring that new products are safe and effective. Finally, the FDA works with international regulatory agencies to promote regulatory harmonization and facilitate global development and approval of nanomedicines.

11.6 SUMMARY

Developing delivery vehicles capable of delivering the medicine across the blood–brain barrier with targeted imaging of the sick tissue constitutes an advanced method of drug delivery. Co-delivery of pharmaceuticals enables tailored patient therapy; hence, it is necessary that the delivery vehicle be able to transport drug mixtures. Active targeting of magnetic nanoparticles by external magnetic fields must also be investigated further, as animal and human parameters may vary. Brain cancer has remained the disease with the fewest or no viable treatments.

Nanotechnology, particularly magnetic nanoparticles, is in high demand due to their medicinal and diagnostic characteristics.

Magnetic nanoparticles can be utilized for drug delivery, hyperthermia, cell tracking, medication biodistribution, and accurate bioimaging. These polymeric MNPs have the potential to alter the worldwide outlook on cancer treatment/diagnosis and represent a viable tool for the future generation of medicine. Carbon nanomaterial is a potent drug delivery agent that can be utilized to diagnose and treat cancer. By using organic components in the production of CNMs, toxicity concerns have been resolved. Developing and identifying novel anticancer medications or agents will facilitate the creation of more efficient delivery methods.

Future research should investigate how nucleation/growth processes influence structure/properties, how to manage their morphology/size, and how to identify photoluminescence pathways. VLPs have evolved to transport and distribute cargo, making them ideal drug delivery specialists. Large dosages of VLPs are often well tolerated, but proteolytic breakdown ensures their quick and thorough elimination, resulting in fewer adverse effects. As the sector evolves and more items undergo clinical testing and development, efforts must be concentrated on enhancing process development and large-scale production processes. In medical research, artificial nanobots are developing as a demanding technology for dealing with nanoscale-tailored medication delivery and diagnostics.

Therapeutic techniques based on bacteriophages and plant viruses are on the verge of entering clinical development. This is an exciting period for the research, and we anticipate that developing viral nanotechnologies will soon move from the laboratory to the clinic. By eliminating hazardous fuels or fuels that generate harmful byproducts during propulsion and exploiting biological components, it is possible to create biocompatible nanomotors. Biohybrids consisting of non-pathogenic bacteria, viruses, blood cells, and DNA origami have also shown great potential. Despite this continual development, the following difficulties must be resolved before biological nanobots may be utilized in the real world.

Despite the substantial advances in nanobots creation over the past five years, the applications of these devices are not yet enough to satisfy unmet biological demands. Nanomotors are anticipated to be used in the future to deliver medications to specific areas, drill through biomaterials, remove blood clots, and perform surgery. Advanced nanomaterials or biological carriers should provide new prospects for achieving high levels of efficiency and propulsion speed with increased biocompatibility and control.

REFERENCES

[1] O. Sumant, Nanomedicine Market Global Opportunity Analysis and Industry Forecast, 2021–2030, Allied Market Research (2022). https://www.alliedmarketresearch.com/nanomedicine-market.

[2] A. Sultana, M. Zare, V. Thomas, T.S.S. Kumar, S. Ramakrishna, Nano-based drug delivery systems: Conventional drug delivery routes, recent developments and future prospects, Med. Drug Dis. 15 (2022) 100134. doi:10.1016/j.medidd.2022.100134.

[3] A. Al Ragib, R. Chakma, K. Dewan, T. Islam, T. Kormoker, A.M. Idris, Current advanced drug delivery systems: Challenges and potentialities, J Drug Deliv Sci Technol. 76 (2022) 103727. doi:10.1016/j.jddst.2022.103727.

[4] M.L. Etheridge, S.A. Campbell, A.G. Erdman, C.L. Haynes, S.M. Wolf, J. McCullough, The big picture on nanomedicine: The state of investigational and approved nanomedicine products, Nanomed. Nanotechnol. Biol. Med. 9 (2013) 1–14. doi:10.1016/j.nano.2012.05.013.

[5] K. Brindhadevi, H.A. Garalleh, A. Alalawi, E. Al-Sarayreh, A. Pugazhendhi, Carbon nanomaterials: Types, synthesis strategies and their application as drug delivery system for cancer therapy, Biochem. Eng. J. (2023) 108828. doi:10.1016/j.bej.2023.108828.

[6] M. Monthioux, Carbon Meta-Nanotubes: Synthesis, Properties and Applications, John Wiley & Sons, New York (2011).

[7] L. Liu, Q. Ma, J. Cao, Y. Gao, S. Han, Y. Liang, T. Zhang, Y. Song, Y. Sun, Recent progress of graphene oxide-based multifunctional nanomaterials for cancer treatment, Cancer Nano. 12 (2021) 18. doi:10.1186/s12645-021-00087-7.

[8] S. Joshi-Barr, C. de Gracia Lux, E. Mahmoud, A. Almutairi, Exploiting oxidative microenvironments in the body as triggers for drug delivery systems, Antioxid. Redox. Signal. 21 (2014) 730–754. doi:10.1089/ars.2013.5754.

[9] R. Majumder, T. Pal, A. Basumallick, C. Das Mukhopadhyay, Functionalized carbon nano onion as a novel drug delivery system for brain targeting, J. Drug Deliv. Sci. Technol. 63 (2021) 102414. doi:10.1016/j.jddst.2021.102414.

[10] X. Wei, X. Chen, M. Ying, W. Lu, Brain tumor-targeted drug delivery strategies, Acta Pharm. Sinica B. 4 (2014) 193–201. doi:10.1016/j.apsb.2014.03.001.

[11] F. Alexis, E. Pridgen, L.K. Molnar, O.C. Farokhzad, Factors affecting the clearance and biodistribution of polymeric nanoparticles, Mol. Pharm. 5 (2008) 505–515. doi:10.1021/mp800051m.

[12] A. Camisasca, S. Giordani, Carbon nano-onions in biomedical applications: Promising theranostic agents, Inorganica Chim. Acta. 468 (2017) 67–76. doi:10.1016/j.ica.2017.06.009.

[13] B. Pakhira, M. Ghosh, A. Allam, S. Sarkar, Carbon nano onions cross the blood brain barrier, RSC Adv. 6 (2016) 29779–29782. doi:10.1039/C5RA23534K.

[14] A. Bhowmik, R. Khan, M.K. Ghosh, Blood brain barrier: A challenge for effectual therapy of brain tumors, BioMed Res. Int. 2015 (2015) e320941. doi:10.1155/2015/320941.

[15] T.T. Nguyen, T.T.D. Nguyen, N.-M.-A. Tran, G. Van Vo, Lipid-based nanocarriers via nose-to-brain pathway for central nervous system disorders, Neurochem. Res. 47 (2022) 552–573. doi:10.1007/s11064-021-03488-7.

[16] B. Joshi, A. Joshi, Polymeric magnetic nanoparticles: A multitargeting approach for brain tumour therapy and imaging, Drug Deliv. Transl. Res. 12 (2022) 1588–1604. doi:10.1007/s13346-021-01063-9.

[17] A.K. Gupta, R.R. Naregalkar, V.D. Vaidya, M. Gupta, Recent advances on surface engineering of magnetic iron oxide nanoparticles and their biomedical applications, Nanomed. 2 (2007) 23–39. doi:10.2217/17435889.2.1.23.

[18] N. Andhariya, B. Chudasama, R.V. Mehta, R.V. Upadhyay, Biodegradable thermorespon-sive polymeric magnetic nanoparticles: A new drug delivery platform for doxorubicin, J. Nanopart Res. 13 (2011) 1677–1688. doi:10.1007/s11051-010-9921-6.

[19] B.D. Kels, A. Grzybowski, J.M. Grant-Kels, Human ocular anatomy, Clin. Dermatol. 33 (2015) 140–146. doi:10.1016/j.clindermatol.2014.10.006.

[20] T. Meng, V. Kulkarni, R. Simmers, V. Brar, Q. Xu, Therapeutic implications of nanomed-icine for ocular drug delivery, Drug Dis. Today. 24 (2019) 1524–1538. doi:10.1016/j.drudis.2019.05.006.

[21] A. Bochot, E. Fattal, Liposomes for intravitreal drug delivery: A state of the art, J. Con. Rel. 161 (2012) 628–634. doi:10.1016/j.jconrel.2012.01.019.

[22] B. Chiang, J.H. Jung, M.R. Prausnitz, The suprachoroidal space as a route of administration to the posterior segment of the eye, Adv. Drug Deliv. Rev. 126 (2018) 58–66. doi:10.1016/j.addr.2018.03.001.

[23] L. Lalu, V. Tambe, D. Pradhan, K. Nayak, S. Bagchi, R. Maheshwari, K. Kalia, R.K. Tekade, Novel nanosystems for the treatment of ocular inflammation: Current paradigms and future research directions, J. Con. Rel. 268 (2017) 19–39. doi:10.1016/j.jconrel.2017.07.035.

[24] J. Rodríguez Villanueva, M.G. Navarro, L. Rodríguez Villanueva, Dendrimers as a promising tool in ocular therapeutics: Latest advances and perspectives, Int. J. Pharm. 511 (2016) 359–366. doi:10.1016/j.ijpharm.2016.07.031.

[25] A. Mandal, R. Bisht, I.D. Rupenthal, A.K. Mitra, Polymeric micelles for ocular drug delivery: From structural frameworks to recent preclinical studies, J. Con. Rel. 248 (2017) 96–116. doi:10.1016/j.jconrel.2017.01.012.

[26] J.L. Perry, K.P. Herlihy, M.E. Napier, J.M. DeSimone, PRINT: A novel platform toward shape and size specific nanoparticle theranostics, Acc. Chem. Res. 44 (2011) 990–998. doi:10.1021/ar2000315.

[27] G. Acharya, C.S. Shin, M. McDermott, H. Mishra, H. Park, I.C. Kwon, K. Park, The hydrogel template method for fabrication of homogeneous nano/microparticles, J. Con. Rel. 141 (2010) 314–319. doi:10.1016/j.jconrel.2009.09.032.

[28] B. Hosnedlova, M. Kepinska, C. Fernandez, Q. Peng, B. Ruttkay-Nedecky, H. Milnerow-icz, R. Kizek, Carbon nanomaterials for targeted cancer therapy drugs: A critical review, Chem. Rec. 19 (2019) 502–522. doi:10.1002/tcr.201800038.

[29] Y.H. Chung, H. Cai, N.F. Steinmetz, Viral nanoparticles for drug delivery, imaging, immunotherapy, and theranostic applications, Adv. Drug Deliv. Rev. 156 (2020) 214–235. doi:10.1016/j.addr.2020.06.024.

[30] A. Puiggalí-Jou, L.J. del Valle, C. Alemán, Drug delivery systems based on intrinsically conducting polymers, J. Con. Rel. 309 (2019) 244–264. doi:10.1016/j.jconrel.2019.07.035.

[31] N.F. Steinmetz, Biological and evolutionary concepts for nanoscale engineering, EMBO Rep. 20 (2019) e48806. doi:10.15252/embr.201948806.

[32] C. Wang, V. Beiss, N.F. Steinmetz, Cowpea mosaic virus nanoparticles and empty virus-like particles show distinct but overlapping immunostimulatory properties, J. Virol. 93 (2019) e00129. doi:10.1128/JVI.00129-19.

[33] A.O. Elzoghby, W.M. Samy, N.A. Elgindy, Protein-based nanocarriers as promising drug and gene delivery systems, J. Con. Rel. 161 (2012) 38–49. doi:10.1016/j.jconrel.2012.04.036.

[34] N. Ferrer-Miralles, E. Rodríguez-Carmona, J.L. Corchero, E. García-Fruitós, E. Vázquez, A. Villaverde, Engineering protein self-assembling in protein-based nanomedicines for drug delivery and gene therapy, Crit. Rev. Biotechnol. 35 (2015) 209–221. doi:10.3109/07388551.2013.833163.

[35] U. Unzueta, M.V. Céspedes, E. Vázquez, N. Ferrer-Miralles, R. Mangues, A. Villaverde, Towards protein-based viral mimetics for cancer therapies, Tr. Biotech. 33 (2015) 253–258. doi:10.1016/j.tibtech.2015.02.007.

[36] C.E. Ashley, E.C. Carnes, G.K. Phillips, P.N. Durfee, M.D. Buley, C.A. Lino, D.P. Padilla, B. Phillips, M.B. Carter, C.L. Willman, C.J. Brinker, J. do C. Caldeira, B. Chackerian, W. Wharton, D.S. Peabody, Cell-specific delivery of diverse cargos by bacteriophage MS2 virus-like particles, ACS Nano. 5 (2011) 5729–5745. doi:10.1021/nn201397z.

[37] T.C. Johnstone, K. Suntharalingam, S.J. Lippard, The next generation of platinum drugs: Targeted pt(II) agents, nanoparticle delivery, and pt(IV) prodrugs, Chem. Rev. 116 (2016) 3436–3486. doi:10.1021/acs.chemrev.5b00597.

[38] C.E. Franke, A.E. Czapar, R.B. Patel, N.F. Steinmetz, Tobacco mosaic virus-delivered cisplatin restores efficacy in platinum-resistant ovarian cancer cells, Mol. Pharmaceut. 15 (2018) 2922–2931. doi:10.1021/acs.molpharmaceut.7b00466.

[39] R.D. Lin, N.F. Steinmetz, Tobacco mosaic virus delivery of mitoxantrone for cancer therapy, Nanoscale. 10 (2018) 16307–16313. doi:10.1039/C8NR04142C.

[40] P. Lam, R.D. Lin, N.F. Steinmetz, Delivery of mitoxantrone using a plant virus-based nanoparticle for the treatment of glioblastomas, J. Mater. Chem. B. 6 (2018) 5888–5895. doi:10.1039/C8TB01191E.

[41] M. Galetti, S. Rossi, C. Caffarra, A.G. Gerboles, M. Miragoli, Chapter 9 - Innovation in nanomedicine and engineered nanomaterials for therapeutic purposes, in: N. Marmiroli, J.C. White, J. Song (Eds.), Exposure to Engineered Nanomaterials in the Environment, Elsevier, Cambridge (2019): pp. 235–262. doi:10.1016/B978-0-12-814835-8.00009-1.

[42] A. Gupta, S. Soni, N. Chauhan, M. Khanuja, U. Jain, Nanobots-based advancement in targeted drug delivery and imaging: An update, J. Con. Rel. 349 (2022) 97–108. doi:10.1016/j.jconrel.2022.06.020.

[43] M. Luo, Y. Feng, T. Wang, J. Guan, Micro-/nanorobots at work in active drug delivery, Adv. Funct. Mater. 28 (2018) 1706100. doi:10.1002/adfm.201706100.

[44] J. Wang, Y. Dong, P. Ma, Y. Wang, F. Zhang, B. Cai, P. Chen, B.-F. Liu, Intelligent micro-/nanorobots for cancer theragnostic, Adv. Mater. 34 (2022) 2201051. doi:10.1002/adma.202201051.

[45] G. Giri, Y. Maddahi, K. Zareinia, A brief review on challenges in design and development of nanorobots for medical applications, Appl. Sci. 11 (2021) 10385. doi:10.3390/app112110385.

[46] J.C. Barnes, C.A. Mirkin, Profile of Jean-Pierre Sauvage, Sir J. Fraser Stoddart, and Bernard L. Feringa, 2016 Nobel Laureates in Chemistry, Proc. Natl. Acad. Sci. U.S.A. 114 (2017) 620–625. doi:10.1073/pnas.1619330114.

[47] V. Balzani, M. Clemente-León, A. Credi, B. Ferrer, M. Venturi, A.H. Flood, J.F. Stoddart, Autonomous artificial nanomotor powered by sunlight, Proc. Natl. Acad. Sci. U.S.A. 103 (2006) 1178–1183. doi:10.1073/pnas.0509011103.

[48] R. Tripathi, A. Kumar, A. Kumar, Chapter thirteen - architecture and application of nanorobots in medicine, in: A.T. Azar (Ed.), Control Systems Design of Bio-Robotics and Bio-Mechatronics with Advanced Applications, Academic Press, Cambridge (2020): pp. 445–464. doi:10.1016/B978-0-12-817463-0.00013-7.

[49] A. Nourhani, E. Karshalev, F. Soto, J. Wang, Multigear bubble propulsion of transient micromotors, Res. 2020 (2020). doi:10.34133/2020/7823615.

[50] Y. Wu, Z. Song, G. Deng, K. Jiang, H. Wang, X. Zhang, H. Han, Gastric acid powered nanomotors release antibiotics for in vivo treatment of helicobacter pylori infection, Small. 17 (2021) 2006877. doi:10.1002/smll.202006877.

[51] P. Díez, E. Lucena-Sánchez, A. Escudero, A. Llopis-Lorente, R. Villalonga, R. Martínez-Máñez, Ultrafast directional Janus Pt–mesoporous silica nanomotors for smart drug delivery, ACS Nano. 15 (2021) 4467–4480. doi:10.1021/acsnano.0c08404.

[52] M. Mathesh, E. Bhattarai, W. Yang, 2D Active nanobots based on soft nanoarchitectonics powered by an ultralow fuel concentration, Angew. Chem., Int. Ed. Engl. 61 (2022) e202113801. doi:10.1002/anie.202113801.

[53] H. Wang, G. Zhao, M. Pumera, Beyond platinum: Bubble-propelled micromotors based on Ag and MnO_2 catalysts, J. Am. Chem. Soc. 136 (2014) 2719–2722. doi:10.1021/ja411705d.

[54] Y. Yang, X. Arqué, T. Patiño, V. Guillerm, P.-R. Blersch, J. Pérez-Carvajal, I. Imaz, D. Maspoch, S. Sánchez, Enzyme-powered porous micromotors built from a hierarchical micro- and mesoporous UiO-type metal–organic framework, J. Am. Chem. Soc. 142 (2020) 20962–20967. doi:10.1021/jacs.0c11061.

[55] B. Khezri, M. Pumera, Metal–organic frameworks based nano/micro/millimeter-sized self-propelled autonomous machines, Adv. Mater. 31 (2019) 1806530. doi:10.1002/adma.201806530.

[56] N.V.S. Vallabani, S. Singh, A.S. Karakoti, Magnetic nanoparticles: Current trends and future aspects in diagnostics and nanomedicine, Curr. Drug Metabol. 20 (n.d.) 457–472.

[57] A.A. Harraq, B.D. Choudhury, B. Bharti, Field-induced assembly and propulsion of colloids, Langmuir. 38 (2022) 3001–3016. doi:10.1021/acs.langmuir.1c02581.

[58] G.Y. Karaca, F. Kuralay, E. Uygun, K. Ozaltin, S.E. Demirbuken, B. Garipcan, L. Oksuz, A.U. Oksuz, Gold–nickel nanowires as nanomotors for cancer marker biodetection and chemotherapeutic drug delivery, ACS Appl. Nano Mater. 4 (2021) 3377–3388. doi:10.1021/acsanm.0c03145.

[59] T. Xu, W. Gao, L.-P. Xu, X. Zhang, S. Wang, Fuel-free synthetic micro-/nanomachines, Adv. Mater. 29 (2017) 1603250. doi:10.1002/adma.201603250.

[60] X. He, H. Jiang, J. Li, Y. Ma, B. Fu, C. Hu, Dipole-moment induced phototaxis and fuel-free propulsion of ZnO/Pt Janus micromotors, Small. 17 (2021) 2101388. doi:10.1002/smll.202101388.

[61] Y. Xing, S. Tang, X. Du, T. Xu, X. Zhang, Near-infrared light-driven yolk@shell carbon@silica nanomotors for fuel-free triglyceride degradation, Nano Res. 14 (2021) 654–659. doi:10.1007/s12274-020-3092-2.

[62] D. Xu, J. Hu, X. Pan, S. Sánchez, X. Yan, X. Ma, Enzyme-powered liquid metal nanobots endowed with multiple biomedical functions, ACS Nano. 15 (2021) 11543–11554. doi:10.1021/acsnano.1c01573.

[63] H. Shahsavan, A. Aghakhani, H. Zeng, Y. Guo, Z.S. Davidson, A. Priimagi, M. Sitti, Bioinspired underwater locomotion of light-driven liquid crystal gels, Proc. Natl. Acad. Sci. U.S.A. 117 (2020) 5125–5133. doi:10.1073/pnas.1917952117.

[64] S. Zheng, Y. Wang, S. Pan, E. Ma, S. Jin, M. Jiao, W. Wang, J. Li, K. Xu, H. Wang, Biocompatible nanomotors as active diagnostic imaging agents for enhanced magnetic resonance imaging of tumor tissues in vivo, Adv. Funct. Mater. 31 (2021) 2100936. doi:10.1002/adfm.202100936.

[65] S.S. Andhari, R.D. Wavhale, K.D. Dhobale, B.V. Tawade, G.P. Chate, Y.N. Patil, J.J. Khandare, S.S. Banerjee, R.D. Wavhale, K.D. Dhobale, B.V. Tawade, G.P. Chate, Y.N. Patil, J.J. Khandare, S.S. Banerjee, Self-propelling targeted magneto-nanobots for deep tumor penetration and pH-responsive intracellular drug delivery, Sci. Rep. 10 (2020) 4703. doi:10.1038/s41598-020-61586-y.

[66] P.-P. Yang, Y.-G. Zhai, G.-B. Qi, Y.-X. Lin, Q. Luo, Y. Yang, A.-P. Xu, C. Yang, Y.-S. Li, L. Wang, H. Wang, NIR light propulsive Janus-like nanohybrids for enhanced photothermal tumor therapy, Small. 12 (2016) 5423–5430. doi:10.1002/smll.201601965.

[67] W. Xu, H. Qin, H. Tian, L. Liu, J. Gao, F. Peng, Y. Tu, Biohybrid micro/nanomotors for biomedical applications, Appl. Mater. Today. 27 (2022) 101482. doi:10.1016/j.apmt.2022.101482.

[68] S. Klumpp, D. Faivre, Magnetotactic bacteria, Eur. Phys. J. Spec. Top. 225 (2016) 2173–2188. doi:10.1140/epjst/e2016-60055-y.

[69] S.N.A. Yusof, N.A.C. Sidik, Y. Asako, W.M.A.A. Japar, S.B. Mohamed, N.M. Muhammad, A comprehensive review of the influences of nanoparticles as a fuel additive in an internal combustion engine (ICE), Nanotechnol. Rev. 9 (2020) 1326–1349. doi:10.1515/ntrev-2020-0104.

[70] J. Wang, Z. Xiong, J. Tang, The encoding of light-driven micro/nanorobots: From single to swarming systems, Adv. Intell. Syst. 3 (2021) 2000170. doi:10.1002/aisy.202000170.

[71] A.C. Hortelao, C. Simó, M. Guix, S. Guallar-Garrido, E. Julián, D. Vilela, L. Rejc, P. Ramos-Cabrer, U. Cossío, V. Gómez-Vallejo, J. Patiño, J. Llop, S. Sánchez, Swarming behavior and in vivo monitoring of enzymatic nanomotors within the bladder, Sci. Robot. 6 (2021). doi:10.1126/SCIROBOTICS.ABD2823.

[72] L. Manamanchaiyaporn, X. Tang, Y. Zheng, X. Yan, Molecular transport of a magnetic nanoparticle swarm towards thrombolytic therapy, IEEE Robot. Autom. Lett. 6 (2021) 5605–5612. doi:10.1109/LRA.2021.3068978.

[73] A. Ressnerova, F. Novotny, H. Michalkova, M. Pumera, V. Adam, Z. Heger, Efficient protein transfection by swarms of chemically powered plasmonic virus-sized nanorobots, ACS Nano. 15 (2021) 12899–12910. doi:10.1021/acsnano.1c01172.

[74] R. Nijhara, K. Balakrishnan, Bringing nanomedicines to market: Regulatory challenges, opportunities, and uncertainties, Nanomed. Nanotechnol. Biol. Med. 2 (2006) 127–136. doi:10.1016/j.nano.2006.04.005.

12 Journey of Nano-Drug Delivery Systems from Lab to Clinics
Case Studies

12.1 AN OVERVIEW OF THE DRUG DEVELOPMENT PROCESS

The process of turning a molecule from a drug candidate (the result of the discovery phase) into a product that has been given the green light for commercialization by the relevant regulatory bodies is known as drug development. For two key reasons, efficient drug development is essential to its economic success.

- Development expenditures make up around two-thirds of all R&D expenses. The investment per project rises significantly when the project enters the final stages of clinical assessment and is significantly higher during the development stage. The administration is very concerned about controlling these expenditures. Late-stage compound failure results in significant financial loss.
- Time devoted to development may reduce the length of patent exclusivity when the medicine enters the market, therefore development speed is a crucial element in defining sales income. When the patent runs out, generic competitive rivalry severely cuts down on sales income.

In spite of widespread recognition in the pharmaceutical sector of the need to cut costs and speed up research, both have significantly grown during the past two decades. This is mostly a result of external causes, notably the regulatory bodies' increasing vigilance in evaluating the efficacy and safety of emerging medications [1,2]. As a result, organizations increasingly need to enhance their effectiveness in this field to be profitable and competitive as the weight of development tends to rise.

There is a significant amount of "unplannability" in drug discovery, which means that it is inherently an investigation of the unexplored. Successful initiatives may produce molecules that are completely different from those sought-after compounds. In contrast, drug development does have a clearly defined objective: to develop the medicine in a commercial version and to get regulatory approval to commercialize it as soon as feasible for use in the intended indication(s) [3,4]. There are three primary categories of work involved in this: technical, investigative, and management.

DOI: 10.1201/9781003358114-12

- Technological development is the process of overcoming synthesis and formulation-related technical issues with the goal of primarily ensuring the standard of the finished product. The principal tasks of technical development involve chemical and pharmaceutical development.
- Investigational studies to determine the product's safety and effectiveness, including a determination of its pharmacokinetic (PK) suitability for clinical application in humans. Pharmacokinetics, toxicology, safety pharmacology, and clinical development are the primarily involved aspects of these studies.
- Coordination is a management task that involves controlling logistics, communications, and decision-making in a sizable interdisciplinary project to ensure high-quality information and prevent unwarranted delays. Project management, documentation, and regulatory affairs are the primary roles involved in this aspect.

An interesting difference between the technical and investigatory parts of the formulation is that when dealing with technical issues, it is presumed that a solution already exists, and the team's task is to find and optimize it as soon as possible. In contrast, when evaluating safety and efficacy, it could not be believed that the drug meets the necessary standards; instead, the component is to explore this as quickly and inexpensively as possible. In another sense, technical development is primarily a problem-solving practice, as opposed to clinical and toxicological research, which is a continuous examination of the compound's qualities. Technical issues, such as an unacceptably complicated and poor-yielding synthesizing route or difficulty in generating an acceptable formulation, can result in the termination of the endeavor, which is relatively rare. Nonetheless, failure due to the drug's biological characteristics, such as toxicity, ineffectiveness, or suboptimal pharmacokinetics, is highly frequent and primarily explains why only around 10% of compounds undergoing Phase I clinical studies were ultimately marketed. Establishing "no-go" guidelines and testing the drug against them as promptly as feasible thus becomes a crucial component of managing drug development initiatives [4,5].

Development is significantly more "plannable" than discovery since it follows much more well-defined paths, especially in nonclinical investigations where the majority of the necessary work may be done using established experimental techniques. This is true for Phase I clinical investigations as well. Nevertheless, unforeseen findings that need additional research prior to clinical trials would begin, such as poor oral absorption in humans or species-specific harmful effects, may cause delays. Since a drug's action mechanism is wholly new, the technical phase is frequently prolonged as off-target symptoms are investigated (occasionally at the regulating authority's demand) [1,6].

Following Phase I, the path to be taken is typically considerably less clearly mapped, and success rests largely on the project team's tactical planning regarding which clinical objectives must be explored. They must determine, for instance, whether it will be simple or difficult to enroll patients for the study, which selection criteria must be employed, what therapeutic result assessments must be utilized, and how extensive the therapy and evaluation phases should be.

To expedite registration, it may, for instance, be practical to choose a fairly low but rapid clinical objective for the early studies and to conduct those trials concurrently with longer trials in the principal target. The patient group chosen for the study needs to be carefully considered in order to increase the likelihood of success in reaching a definitive outcome. Experience has shown that bad choices of this nature frequently result in ambiguous clinical studies, which are a significant reason for rejection or lag in drug development. An adaptable trial strategy may provide a more accurate assessment of the drug when the indication permits it [2,3].

12.2 DOXIL®—THE FIRST NANOMEDICINE AUTHORIZED BY THE FDA

12.2.1 NEED AND DEVELOPMENT OF DOXIL®

An antibiotic called doxorubicin (DOX) is generated by the bacteria Streptomyces peucetius. Since the 1960s, it has been widely used as a chemotherapeutic drug. The chemotherapy drug class known as anthracyclines also includes DOX, epirubicin, idarubicin, and daunorubicin. DOX is frequently used as a medication to treat solid tumors in both children and adults. The most crucial clinical factor in choosing DOX as a chemotherapeutic agent is that it is among the most potent anticancer medications ever discovered, making it one of the principles of "first line" anticancer medications from nearly the time of its invention and continuing until today. Compared to other classes of chemotherapeutic medicines, it is efficacious for numerous cancer types, notably blood cancers, lymphomas, and breast, ovarian, uterine, and lung cancers [7,8].

DOX does have toxicity and adverse effects, nevertheless, just like the majority of other anticancer medications. The most hazardous effect of this medication is cumulative dosage-dependent cardiotoxicity, which severely reduces its effectiveness (the maximum cumulative dose permitted is 550 mg/m^2). The adverse effects of DOX include vomiting, nausea, extreme myelosuppression, and skin infections [9–11].

Doxil®, the first nano-drug to get FDA approval (1995), is a formulation made with doxorubicin liposome containing polyethylene-glycol. To minimize the cardiotoxicity of the medication, DOX has been recommended for delivery in the liposome-associated formulation, relying on pathological findings in preclinical models of animals employing various liposome compositions as well as the decreased cardiac absorption of DOX that has been liposome-encapsulated. The prospective advantages of such nanocarriers for anticancer drug delivery systems have recently expanded owing to the emergence of novel formulations of long-circulating liposomes exhibiting decreased absorption by the RES and improved retention in tumors [12]. Liposome-assisted DOX has been demonstrated to circulate with extremely extended half-lives in the 15 to 30 hours in investigations with dogs and mice using some novel formulations [12,13]. When DOX is transported by long-circulating lipid nanoparticles like liposomes, an enhanced drug accumulation is observed in transplantable mouse tumors and ascitic tumor exudates. As compared to unbound DOX in several animal models, DOX entrapped in long-circulating liposomes exhibits superior therapeutic anticancer efficacy and less toxicity [14,15]. As a result, long-circulating liposomes seem to have a dual benefit as a method of delivering anticancer drugs: toxicity neutralization, similar to other liposome formulations in the past, and selective tumor aggregation, which results in increased antitumor activity.

Moreover, the nano-drug system based on liposomes should demonstrate some common attributes for their approval by FDA or other regulatory bodies. Those characteristics are as follows:

- To avail of the advantages of an EPR effect and extravasate through the blood capillaries at the tumor within the tumor tissue, the liposomes employed need to be on the nanoscale (nano-liposomes). Such liposomes might be regarded as "nano-drugs." Unfortunately, getting a suitable amount and sustainability of drug loading is quite difficult when approaching nano-scales. The extremely small dimension of the nano-liposomes is the reason for this issue. Since DOX requires a large dosage to be therapeutically effective ($10–50$ mg/m^2 [9,10], this may be particularly challenging.
- These liposomes must reach the tumors supplied with a reasonable level of drug amount for better therapeutic efficiency.
- Nano-liposomes must regulate the pharmacokinetics (PK) and biodistribution (BD) of the drug molecules; specifically, the liposomal drug must exhibit a significantly longer plasma circulation interval, which is governed by the carrier's extended circulation time. This will permit the sustained concentration of the drug over the tumor.
- The drug must be accessible to tumor cells either through the release of the drug at the tumor site or through tumor cell internalization of drug-loaded nano-liposomes.

Doxil® did follow these characteristics and was approved by FDA in 1995. This nano-drug is centered around three independent principles: 1. RES minimization and extended drug circulation time as a result of PEGylated nano-liposome utilization; 2. A transdermal ammonium sulfate gradient drives consistent and elevated remote loading of DOX, facilitating sustained drug release to the tumor; and 3. possessing the elevated Tm (53 °C) phosphatidylcholine and cholesterol in a "liquid regulated" phase with the liposome lipid bilayer. The DOX in Doxil® is "passively targeted" to tumors as a result of the EPR effect, and it is released and made accessible to tumor cells by as-yet-unidentified mechanisms [16].

12.2.2 How and Where Doxil® Was Developed

To accomplish all the characteristics mentioned earlier and create a workable liposomal doxorubicin product, Liposome Technology Inc. (LTI) integrated and applied two distinct and original ideas that developed into two unique, innovative technologies and gave rise to two distinct and separate patent portfolios. The first one addresses how to load drugs into nano-liposomes in a manner that satisfies all the previously mentioned requirements, and the second one makes it possible to increase the duration that nano-liposomes spend in the plasma while preventing RES. Previously, neither technology had been tested. The major aspects such as extended circulation time, higher loading capacity, delivery of drug molecules to the targeted sites, and drug penetration through the EPR effect have been investigated in a parallel manner at four different sites as follows [16].

- LTI labs at Menlo Park, Calif., by LTI scientists.
- Papahadjopoulos's lab at UCSF by Gabizon (continued later at Gabizon's lab at Hadassah University Hospital in Jerusalem).
- Terry Allen's lab at the University of Alberta in Canada.
- Hebrew University-Hadassah Medical School in Jerusalem.

Working together, LTI, Terry Allen, and Alberto Gabizon/Dimitri Papahadjopoulos were able to produce liposomes with prolonged circulation and RES avoidance that, because of their nanoscale size, may benefit from the EPR effect. EPR was predicted to cause preferential extravasation of nanoparticles from the tumor vasculature to the tumor tissue. Dr. Frank Martin of LTI called the liposomes "Stealth®" liposomes, and this special characteristic of liposomes was referred to as "Stealthness," which signifies undetected or undiagnosed particulates by the RES. Simultaneously, Yechezkel Barenholz and his student Gilad Haran invented a unique remote and robust loading mechanism for weak amphipathic bases like DOX into nanoliposomes. The Doxil® nano-liposomes were able to enter the tumor site loaded with an adequate dosage and release that was required to achieve therapeutic effectiveness in individuals attributable to their techniques, which successfully satisfied all the major objectives [17,18]. Such loading allowed for the intra-tumoral release of the drug in contrast to "Stealth cisplatin," which prevented the drug from reaching the tumor cells and was a "dead end." [16,19–21].

12.2.3 Doxil® Performance in Humans

12.2.3.1 Pharmacokinetics

Yechezkel Barenholz conducted a "first-in-man Doxil® clinical trial" investigation between 1991 and 1994 to demonstrate the pharmacokinetics of Doxil®. They have concluded that the proposed nanoformulation of Doxil® has presented selective and higher localization of tumors [18]. The findings serve as the first demonstration of the EPR effect caused by human malignancies by targeted delivery **(Figure 12.1)** [16,18]. Gabizon and colleagues provided further evidence for the buildup of Doxil® in human cancers through direct fluorescence microscopy of patient samples [22].

Nearly 53 Doxil® courses are included in the Yechezkel Barenholz research that was previously stated. The objective was to compare free (non-liposomal) doxorubicin delivered in what was regarded as "standard treatment" with Doxil®'s I.V. plasma PK and buildup in tumor utterings in cancer patients. After Doxil® delivery compared to free doxorubicin, this research convincingly showed significantly increased amounts of the drug in both tumor cells and interstitial fluids. They have discovered that >98 % of the plasma DOX following Doxil® I.V. injection is liposome linked employing the cationic ion exchanger Dowex-50 [23,24]. At DOX concentrations of 25 and 50 mg/m^2, PK was evaluated. The half-lives for Doxil®'s plasma clearance

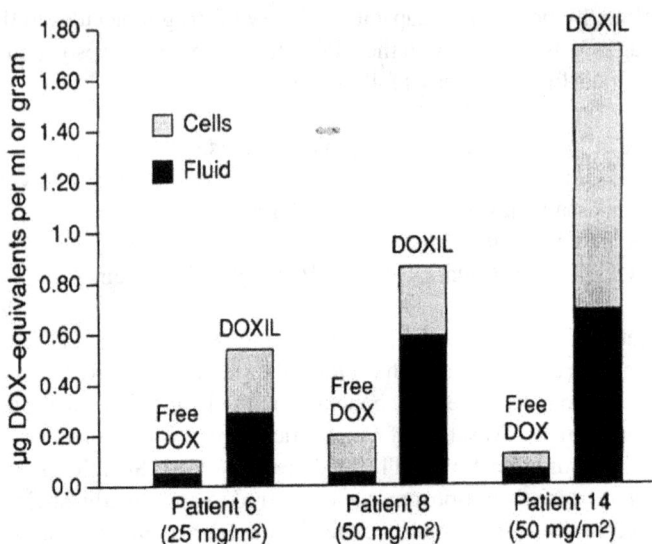

FIGURE 12.1 Doxorubicin Concentrations in Tumor Samples from Patients: A Comparison of Free DOX and Doxil. [Reprinted with permission from *Y. Barenholz (2012)*] [16].

period were 2 and 45 h, with the higher half-life clearing the majority of the dosage from plasma. There was also a significant disparity in the amount of distribution (4 L for Doxil® versus 254 L for free DOX). The rate of elimination for DOX extracted from Doxil® was also much lower (0.1 L/h for Doxil® vs. 45 L/h for free DOX).

The DOX metabolites produced by Doxil® doxorubicin in patients' urine remained the same as those produced in patients who received free DOX injections, but the Doxil® group's cumulative daily urinary output was much lower. The data on drug levels at cancerous outpourings were four to 16 times greater than following free DOX delivery, which is the most promising. Moreover, drug levels in tumors maximized around three and seven days following DOX injection, indicating that the tumor cell is exposed to the drug for a considerably longer period of time and at significantly greater concentrations than after free doxorubicin delivery [18,25]. Their results show that sustained remote loading of DOX into long-circulating nano-liposomes is a good strategy for passively targeting doxorubicin to tumors [25] and are in perfect accord with our preclinical experiments. Gabizon et al. (2003) have thoroughly demonstrated the improved PK effectiveness of Doxil®. A summary of the PK characteristics in humans at dosages between 10 and 80 mg/m^2 can be found in their study [19]. The PK has one or two stages of distribution: a first stage with a half-life of 1–3 h and a second stage, which is in charge of the majority of the elimination and has a half-life of 30–90 h.

As compared to free drugs, the AUC following a 50 mg/m^2 dosage is almost 300 times higher. There is a significant reduction in distribution volume and clearance. These results highlight the significance of dosage scheduling that takes into account the unique pharmacokinetic properties of PEGylated nano-liposomal DOX [16].

12.2.3.2 Toxicity

Doxil® significantly increases the daily adherence of patients, and of particular interest is the drastic decrease in cardiotoxicity (in comparison to regular care), which permits raising the cumulative dose and prolonging the length of therapy. Doxil® has recently been found to have a unique substantial immunological modulatory impact on patients. The first-line platinum-based chemotherapeutics, which is the recommended therapy for ovarian cancer therapy, has an exceptionally high success rate when used early in the course of the disease. Yet most patients with severe stages of the disease ultimately show signs of recurrent illness, and they are then given carboplatin doublets as a kind of treatment. More than 15% of individuals who get carboplatin again exhibit significant hypersensitivity reactions (HSRs). Such reactions, which have been deadly in a few cases, are caused by IgG to platinum, which also explains certain cross-reactivity with cisplatin and infrequently with oxaliplatin. Nevertheless, similar effects were not seen when Doxil® and carboplatin were administered concurrently [16,26].

Also, it is quite interesting to note that newly published crossover studies found that the conjunction of doublet carboplatin and taxol is substantially more frequently linked to carboplatin responses than the conjunction of doublet carboplatin and Doxil® (Caelyx) [27]. In particular, Doxil® appears to have immunosuppressive properties that inhibit or lessen the secondary (IgG-mediated) HRSs to carboplatin.

Despite Doxil®'s general tolerability advantage over DOX, there have been two adverse events that were not characteristic of the free drug standard of care therapy. The very first, more severe case, known as palmar plantar erythrodysthesia (PPE) or "foot and hand syndrome," causes underestimating dermatitis in grades 2 or 3. The PPE manifests as skin that is red, sensitive, and peeling, as was earlier shown in initial FIM research [18] and published by Solomon and Gabizon [25]. In comparison to DOX in the same treatment protocol, the Doxil® dose that may be administered is constrained by the frequency of this adverse effect. In addition to the aforementioned extension in treatment intervals, there is currently no comprehensive cure for this effect [25]. The second consequence is an unfavorable immunological phenomenon that Doxil®, along with numerous other nano-systems, can cause; it is an infusion-related response that manifests as flushing and breathlessness. It is, in fact, a complement activation-related pseudo-allergy (CARPA). CARPA is an abrupt hypersensitivity, or infusion response, and is so named due to the causative involvement of complement activation in its patho-mechanism in place of IgE binding [28]. Sluggish infusion rates and premedication can also help to lower CARPA. There is a strong likelihood that minimizing these two side effects and, in particular, minimizing or overcoming the negative PPE impact might enhance Doxil®'s overall efficacy and broaden its applicability.

12.2.4 NEXT-GENERATION DOXIL®-LIKE LIPOSOMES

In light of the efficacy of Doxil®, other innovative drug formulations, such as improved Doxil® or even other nano-drugs relying on Stealth liposomes loaded with other medications or medication combinations, are now being developed at distinctive phases. The adverse impacts of Doxil®, PPE, and acute infusion responses must have been minimized (or eliminated) by these innovative nano-drug compositions. One method to lessen them is to employ liposomal DOX with a relatively short half-life by using glucuronate instead of the sulfate counterion of the ammonium being used for remote loading. In tumor-bearing animals, the administration of glucuronate, which has a permeability coefficient equivalent to sulfate yet fails to cause intra-liposome drug deposition, causes DOX to circulate more quickly, albeit without sacrificing its therapeutic efficacy [16,29]. A very little but noticeable impact on the PK is anticipated to lessen the buildup of DOX in the skin, lessening the intensity of PPE. There are additional ways to enhance nano-liposome-based chemotherapy and have improved control over drug release, including 1. the use of external methods like intensive ultrasound or hyperthermia; 2. the use of drug combinations by remotely loading two medications that work synergistically inside one liposome; and 3. the pairing of two distinct therapeutic approaches, like Doxil® and interleukin-2 (IL-2) [30].

After chemotherapy, the idea of triggering the host immune system to eliminate any remaining tumor cells has long been advocated. Since DOX is significantly less harmful to innate immunity when given as Doxil® than when provided alone, it is used in conjunction with IL-2 considering IL-2 supplied in liposomes after Doxil® will be very much effective. The theory underlying this chemo-immunotherapy regimen is that Doxil® may keep a hold on the majority of the tumor volume. In contrast, the immunotherapy evoked by the IL-2 will boost the still-functioning immune response, permitting it to eliminate the remaining tumor cells [30]. When liposomal IL-2 is used, its toxicity is reduced, and its lifetime in circulation is prolonged without losing any of its effectiveness [31,32].

The strategy employed lately by Jain and colleagues is highly promising. As a result, losartan, which suppresses collagen I formation, was utilized to alter the extracellular tumor environment, boosting the accumulation of Doxil® (and other nanoparticles) in tumors and enhancing the therapeutic effectiveness of Doxil® [33].

12.3 DOCETAXEL-PNP FROM BASICS TO CLINICAL USE

Docetaxel (DTX) is frequently utilized as an anticancer agent used alone or in combination for non-small cell pulmonary, ovarian, breast, gastrointestinal, neck, prostate, and throat cancers. Its tumor-fighting system is the suppression of the mitotic spindle through binding to microtubules, causing the spindle and microtubules to stabilize [34,35]. While DTX is a powerful anticancer agent, a drug for the therapy of a variety of cancers in unique chemical entities at different phases, it also has a few unfavorable cytotoxic consequences [36]. In a clinical context, the most serious non-hematological side effects of any taxane cytotoxic drug are central neurotoxicity and hypersensitivity [37].

Polymeric nanoparticles (PNPs), being a difficult but also well-regulated drug delivery approach, take advantage of the water-insoluble medicines' enhanced permeability and retention (EPR) impact in malignancies [38]. PNP-assisted targeted drug delivery is anticipated by oncologists to enhance the chemotherapeutic benefits of drugs on tumor tissues and lessen any negative effects on healthy tissue. Yet since PNP also serves as an exogenous substance that possesses the potential to produce toxicity due to its chemical characteristics, its biodegradability is essential to the efficacy of this medication.

The effectiveness of the PNP encapsulated by docetaxel (PNP-DTX) was evaluated by Song et al. (2016) in preclinical animal models, and the maximum tolerated dosage (MTD) was established using clinical testing [36]. Specialized mice models, such as orthotopic and subcutaneous, were employed for conducting the investigation. Both the quantification of *in-vivo* imaging and the tumor development delay in the orthotopic model was assessed. Advanced tumors were the focus of a single-center, retrospective, open-label phase I clinical investigation. Starting at 20 mg/m², the intravenous injection of PNP-DTX was increased to 35 mg/m², 45 mg/m², 60 mg/m², and 75 mg/m². In their study, the toxicities, tumor responses, and pharmacokinetics were assessed effectively.

The preclinical findings demonstrated that PNP-DTX nanoformulation has a more effective antitumor activity compared to docetaxel (DTX). The subcutaneous model, meanwhile, did not show any distinction among PNP-DTX and DTX. A test for tubulin polymerization revealed that PNP-DTX maintained the original mechanism of action of DTX. The 18 participants in phase I clinical study were examined. The MTD was estimated to be 75 mg/m², and grade 4 neutropenia that did not last longer than seven days was the most prevalent adverse effect. According to observations, the C_{max} of 60 mg/m² PNP-DTX and AUC_{last} of 45 mg/m² PNP-DTX are equivalent to those of 75 mg/m² DTX (**Figure 12.2**) [36]. Four patients have experienced partial remission (PR), which was just about 22% of the total number of patients. The orthotopic animal model particularly demonstrated the effectiveness of PNP-DTX. Although the MTD of PNP-DTX would hardly be confirmed, it was tentatively estimated as 75 mg/m². The pharmacokinetic profile of the 45 mg/m² PNP-DTX was identical to that of the 75 mg/m² DTX.

During the clinical trials, although one trial patient died unexpectedly well before the second therapy session, the responses of 18 trial patients were evaluated. PR was present in two (11%) patients. Eight (44%) of the patients were determined to have SD (stable disease), whereas the remaining eight (44%) had progressing disease (PD). Those who demonstrated PR were assigned to Group 4 (60 mg/m²), where there was a 40% objective response rate (2/5 patients). PR was attained for the maximum response in four (22%) of the 18 patients. Six patients (33%) exhibited SD, whereas eight patients (44%) displayed PD. The clinical results over the tumors by PNP-DTX in each of the patients are provided in **Table 12.1** [36]. Through a preclinical investigation of an orthotopic mouse model, they have shown that PNP-DTX is much more effective against pancreatic cancer.

12.4 SUMMARY

In this chapter, we have highlighted the significance and steps involved in the drug development process. The technical, investigative, and managerial operations comprised in these processes were also addressed, which entails the guidelines required for a nano-drug to acquire approval from regulatory authorities like FDA. In line with this, the important aspects of Doxil® being the first nano-drug formulation approved by the FDA have been described with its importance, PK, and toxicological investigation. Doxil®, a chemotherapeutic nano-drug, performed better therapeutically than free DOX (standard of care) in a number of neoplastic disorders because

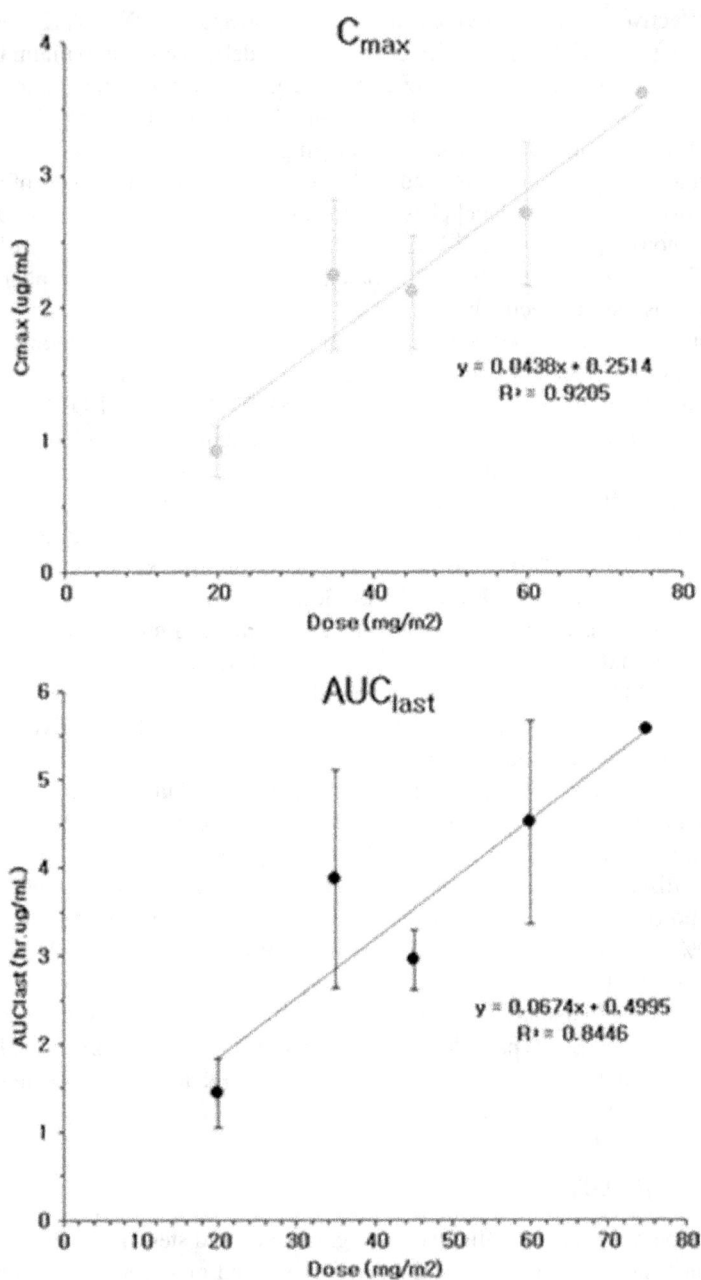

FIGURE 12.2 Pharmacokinetic (PK) Outcomes of PNP-DTX during Phase I Clinical Trials [36].

TABLE 12.1

Response of Tumors to PNP-DTX in Each Patient [36].

Group (Dose)	No	Primary Disease	Response after Second Cycle	Maximal Response
1 (20mg/m^2)	11	Colon	PD	PD
	12	Colon	PD	PD
	13	Rectum	SD	SD
	14	Colon	SD	SD
	15	Colon	SD	SD
	16	Colon	PD	PD
2 (35mg/m^2)	21	Colon	PD	PD
	22	Cervix	PD	PD
	23	Colon	PD	PD
3 (45mg/m^2)	31	Breast	SD	PR
	32	Bladder	SD	SD
	33	Colon	PD	PD
4 (60mg/m^2)	41	Breast	SD	SD
	42	Adrenal	PD	PD
	43	NSCLC	N/A*	N/A*
	44	Breast	PR	PR
	45	Bladder	PR	PR
	46	Kidney	SD	SD
5 (75mg/m^2)	51	Pancreas	SD	PR

of its distinct EPR-related PK and biodistribution, which lessen side effects (especially notable is the massive decline in cardiotoxicity) and increase patient adherence and life expectancy altogether. In combination with the remote loading of DOX into the long-circulating nano-liposomes, they have increased the anticancer therapeutic effectiveness of DOX as compared to conventional DOX (in specific cancers, like ovarian cancer). This illustrates why Doxil® enjoys the most widespread clinical usage out of the >12 liposomal medications authorized for clinical use. Furthermore, the preclinical assessments of potential PNP-based nano-drug delivery systems (PNP-DTX) were described, which suggest the suitable efficacy of these formulations. However, a comprehensive investigation of toxicological and biodistribution aspects is obligatory, along with the clinical trials, for their approval.

REFERENCES

[1] L. Mller, A. Lhe, Preclinical Safety Testing, in: The Textbook of Pharmaceutical Medicine, Wiley-Blackwell, Oxford (2009): pp. 101–136. doi:10.1002/9781444317800.ch3.

[2] P.N. Confalone, Principles of Process Research and Chemical Development in the Pharmaceutical Industry by Oljan Repic. John Wiley & Sons, New York (1998): pp. xvi, 213, 16 × 24 cm. ISBN 0-471-16516-6. $74.95. doi:10.1021/jm980248n.

[3] H.P. Rang, R.G. Hill, Drug Development, 2nd ed., Elsevier, Cambridge (2013): pp. 203–209. doi:10.1016/B978-0-7020-4299-7.00014-7.

[4] P.D. Stonier, Development of medicines: Full development, in: The Textbook of Pharmaceutical Medicine, Wiley-Blackwell, Oxford (2009): pp. 270–284. doi:10.1002/9781444317800. ch9.

[5] S. Warrington, Purpose and design of clinical trials, in: The Textbook of Pharmaceutical Medicine, Wiley-Blackwell, Oxford (2009): pp. 185–206. doi:10.1002/9781444317800. ch6.

[6] P. Rolan, V. Molnr, Clinical pharmacokinetics, in: The Textbook of Pharmaceutical Medicine, Wiley-Blackwell, Oxford (2009): pp. 167–184. doi:10.1002/9781444317800.ch5.

[7] R.B. Weiss, The anthracyclines: Will we ever find a better doxorubicin? Semin. Oncol. 19 (1992) 670–686. http://europepmc.org/abstract/MED/1462166.

[8] G. Minotti, P. Menna, E. Salvatorelli, G. Cairo, L. Gianni, Anthracyclines: Molecular advances and pharmacologic developments in antitumor activity and cardiotoxicity, Pharmacol. Rev. 56 (2004) 185–229. doi:10.1124/pr.56.2.6.

[9] X. Peng, The cardiotoxicology of anthracycline chemotherapeutics: Translating molecular mechanism into preventative medicine, Mol. Interv. 5 (2005) 163–171. doi:10.1124/ mi.5.3.6.

[10] C.H. Takimoto, E. Calvo, Principles of oncologic pharmacotherapy, Cancer Manag. Multidiscip. Approach. 11 (2008) 1–9.

[11] J. Kenyon, Chemotherapy and Cardiac Toxicity—the Lesser of Two Evils, Dr. Lounge Website (2010). https://www.ncbi.nlm.nih.gov/pmc/articles/PMC7736167/.

[12] A. Gabizon, R. Shiota, D. Papahadjopoulos, Pharmacokinetics and tissue distribution of doxorubicin encapsulated in stable liposomes with long circulation times, J. Natl. Cancer Inst. 81 (1989) 1484–1488. doi:10.1093/jnci/81.19.1484.

[13] A.A. Gabizon, Y. Barenholz, M. Bialer, Prolongation of the circulation time of doxorubicin encapsulated in liposomes containing a polyethylene glycol-derivatized phospholipid: Pharmacokinetic studies in rodents and dogs, Pharm. Res. 10 (1993) 703–708. doi:10.1023/A:1018907715905.

[14] D. Papahadjopoulos, T.M. Allen, A. Gabizon, E. Mayhew, K. Matthay, S.K. Huang, K.D. Lee, M.C. Woodle, D.D. Lasic, C. Redemann, Sterically stabilized liposomes: Improvements in pharmacokinetics and antitumor therapeutic efficacy, Proc. Natl. Acad. Sci. 88 (1991) 11460–11464. doi:10.1073/pnas.88.24.11460.

[15] A.A. Gabizon, Selective tumor localization and improved therapeutic index of anthracyclines encapsulated in long-circulating liposomes, Cancer Res. 52 (1992) 891–896. http://www.ncbi.nlm.nih.gov/pubmed/1737351.

[16] Y. (Chezy) Barenholz, Doxil®—the first FDA-approved nano-drug: Lessons learned, J. Control. Release. 160 (2012) 117–134. doi:10.1016/j.jconrel.2012.03.020.

[17] D. Peer (Ed.), Handbook of Harnessing Biomaterials in Nanomedicine, Jenny Stanford Publishing, Dubai (2021). doi:10.1201/9781003125259.

[18] A. Gabizon, R. Catane, B. Uziely, B. Kaufman, T. Safra, R. Cohen, F. Martin, A. Huang, Y. Barenholz, Prolonged circulation time and enhanced accumulation in malignant exudates of doxorubicin encapsulated in polyethylene-glycol coated liposomes, Cancer Res. 54 (1994) 987–92. http://www.ncbi.nlm.nih.gov/pubmed/8313389.

[19] A. Gabizon, H. Shmeeda, Y. Barenholz, Pharmacokinetics of pegylated liposomal doxorubicin, Clin. Pharmacokinet. 42 (2003) 419–436. doi:10.2165/00003088-200342050-00002.

[20] Y. Barenholz, Relevancy of drug loading to liposomal formulation therapeutic efficacy, J. Liposome Res. 13 (2003) 1–8. doi:10.1081/LPR-120017482.

[21] J. Szebeni, C.R. Alving, L. Rosivall, R. Bünger, L. Baranyi, P. Bedőcs, M. Tóth, Y. Barenholz, Animal models of complement-mediated hypersensitivity reactions to liposomes and other lipid-based nanoparticles, J. Liposome Res. 17 (2007) 107–117. doi:10.1080/08982100701375118.

[22] Z. Symon, A. Peyser, D. Tzemach, O. Lyass, E. Sucher, E. Shezen, A. Gabizon, Selective delivery of doxorubicin to patients with breast carcinoma metastases by stealth liposomes, Cancer. 86 (1999) 72–78. doi:10.1002/(SICI)1097-0142(19990701) 86:1<72::AID-CNCR12>3.0.CO;2-1.

[23] S. Druckmann, A. Gabizon, Y. Barenholz, Separation of liposome-associated doxorubicin from non-liposome-associated doxorubicin in human plasma: Implications for pharmacokinetic studies, Biochim. Biophys. Acta-Biomembr. 980 (1989) 381–384. doi:10.1016/0005-2736(89)90329-5.

[24] S. Amselem, Y. Barenholz, A. Gabizon, Optimization and upscaling of doxorubicin-containing liposomes for clinical use, J. Pharm. Sci. 79 (1990) 1045–1052. doi:10.1002/ jps.2600791202.

[25] R. Solomon, A.A. Gabizon, Clinical pharmacology of liposomal anthracyclines: Focus on pegylated liposomal doxorubicin, Clin. Lymphoma Myeloma. 8 (2008) 21–32. doi:10.3816/CLM.2008.n.001.

[26] D.S. Alberts, P.Y. Liu, S.P. Wilczynski, M.C. Clouser, A.M. Lopez, D.P. Michelin, V.J. Lanzotti, M. Markman, Randomized trial of pegylated liposomal doxorubicin (PLD) plus carboplatin versus carboplatin in platinum-sensitive (PS) patients with recurrent epithelial ovarian or peritoneal carcinoma after failure of initial platinum-based chemotherapy. Southwest Onc. Gynecol. Oncol. 108 (2008) 90–94. doi:10.1016/j.ygyno.2007.08.075.

[27] F. Joly, I. Ray-Coquard, M. Fabbro, M. Donoghoe, K. Boman, A. Sugimoto, M. Vaughan, A. Reinthaller, I. Vergote, G. Ferrandina, T. Dell'Anna, J. Huober, E. Pujade-Lauraine, Decreased hypersensitivity reactions with carboplatin-pegylated liposomal doxorubicin compared to carboplatin-paclitaxel combination: Analysis from the GCIG CALYPSO relapsing ovarian cancer trial, Gynecol. Oncol. 122 (2011) 226–232. doi:10.1016/j. ygyno.2011.04.019.

[28] J. Szebeni, Y.C. Barenholz, Complement activation, immunogenicity, and immune suppression as potential side effects of liposomes, in: Advances in Clinical Immunology, Medical Microbiology, COVID-19, Big Data, Jenny Stanford Publishing, Dubai (2021): pp. 55–75.

[29] A. Gabizon, Y. Barenholz, Method for Drug Loading in Liposomes, US 2005/0129753 A1 (2005).

[30] A. Cabanes, S. Even-Chen, J. Zimberoff, Y. Barenholz, E. Kedar, A. Gabizon, Enhancement of antitumor activity of polyethylene glycol-coated liposomal doxorubicin with soluble and liposomal interleukin 21, Clin. Cancer Res. 5 (1999) 687–693.

[31] E. Kedar, Y. Rutkowski, E. Braun, N. Emanuel, Y. Barenholz, Delivery of cytokines by liposomes. I: Preparation and characterization of interleukin-2 encapsulated in long-circulating sterically stabilized liposomes, J. Immunother. 16 (1994). https://journals. lww.com/immunotherapy-journal/Fulltext/1994/07000/Delivery_of_Cytokines_by_ Liposomes__I__Preparation.5.aspx.

[32] E. Kedar, E. Braun, Y. Rutkowski, N. Emanuel, Y. Barenholz, Delivery of cytokines by liposomes. II: Interleukin-2 encapsulated in long-circulating sterically stabilized liposomes: Immunomodulatory and anti-tumor activity in mice, J. Immunother. 16 (1994). https://journals.lww.com/immunotherapy-journal/Fulltext/1994/08000/Delivery_ of_Cytokines_by_Liposomes__II_.5.aspx.

[33] B. Diop-Frimpong, V.P. Chauhan, S. Krane, Y. Boucher, R.K. Jain, Losartan inhibits collagen I synthesis and improves the distribution and efficacy of nanotherapeutics in tumors, Proc. Natl. Acad. Sci. 108 (2011) 2909–2914. doi:10.1073/pnas.1018892108.

[34] A.-M.C. Yvon, P. Wadsworth, M.A. Jordan, Taxol suppresses dynamics of individual microtubules in living human tumor cells, Mol. Biol. Cell. 10 (1999) 947–959. doi:10.1091/mbc.10.4.947.

[35] R. Pazdur, A.P. Kudelka, J.J. Kavanagh, P.R. Cohen, M.N. Raber, The taxoids: Paclitaxel (Taxol®) and docetaxel (Taxotere®), Cancer Treat. Rev. 19 (1993) 351–386. doi:10.1016/0305-7372(93)90010-O.

[36] S.Y. Song, K. Kim, S.-Y. Jeong, J. Park, J. Park, J. Jung, H.K. Chung, S.-W. Lee, M.H. Seo, J. Lee, K.H. Jung, E.K. Choi, Polymeric nanoparticle-docetaxel for the treatment of advanced solid tumors: Phase I clinical trial and preclinical data from an orthotopic pancreatic cancer model, Oncotarget. 7 (2016) 77348–77357. doi:10.18632/oncotarget.12668.

[37] B. van Oijen, M. Pleunis, F. Erdkamp, R. Prevoo, H. van der Kuy, Toxic dermatitis in patients treated with Taxotere® (docetaxel): Three case reports, Int. J. Clin. Pharmacol. Ther. 49 (2011) 46–48. doi:10.5414/CPP49046.

[38] J.M. Chan, P.M. Valencia, L. Zhang, R. Langer, O.C. Farokhzad, Polymeric nanoparticles for drug delivery, in: S.R. Grobmyer, B.M. Moudgil (Eds.), Cancer Nanotechnology Methods Protocols, Humana Press, Totowa, NJ (2010): pp. 163–175. doi:10.1007/978-1-60761-609-2_11.

Index

For Product Safety Concerns and Information please contact our EU
representative GPSR@taylorandfrancis.com
Taylor & Francis Verlag GmbH, Kaufingerstraße 24, 80331 München, Germany

www.ingramcontent.com/pod-product-compliance
Lightning Source LLC
Chambersburg PA
CBHW052118230326
41598CB00080B/3849

9 781032 414478